Mental Health and Psychopathology

This volume is a compilation of articles that shed light on psychopathology, how the one struggling with it experiences its implications, and how it affects everyday life.

For one to be categorized as exhibiting positive mental health, an individual should not experience psychopathology, and additionally exhibit high levels of emotional well-being as well as high levels of psychological and social functioning. The dual-factor model of mental health suggests that enhancing positive mental health and alleviating psychopathology do not automatically go together and are not opposite of one another. There is accumulating evidence that psychopathology and positive mental health function along two different continua that are only moderately interrelated. However, to know what wellbeing is, understand good mental health, and enhance adaptive functioning, we need to explore and understand psychopathology, and how it affects us. The volume is divided into three conceptual sections: *The Experience of Psychopathology*, which is devoted to describing what it is and how it is experienced; *The Effect of Psychopathology on Everyday Life*, describes various effects that psychopathology has on the daily life of the sufferer; *Coherence, Resilience and Recovery*, which focuses on dealing with it, coping with the symptoms, and developing resilience.

The chapters in this book were originally published in *The Journal of Psychology*.

Ami Rokach is a clinical psychologist who has been researching and teaching about loneliness, human sexuality, and psychotherapy for the past 40 years. Ami is Executive Editor of *The Journal of Psychology: Interdisciplinary and Applied*, and a clinical psychologist who combines offering individual, couple and sex therapy with teaching and research. He is member of the psychology departments at York University in Canada, and Walden University in the USA.

Mental Health and Psychopathology

Edited by
Ami Rokach

Routledge
Taylor & Francis Group

LONDON AND NEW YORK

First published 2022
by Routledge
2 Park Square, Milton Park, Abingdon, Oxon OX14 4RN

and by Routledge
605 Third Avenue, New York, NY 10158

Routledge is an imprint of the Taylor & Francis Group, an informa business

British Library Cataloguing in Publication Data
A catalogue record for this book is available from the British Library

ISBN: 978-1-032-15313-1 (hbk)
ISBN: 978-1-032-15318-6 (pbk)
ISBN: 978-1-003-24360-1 (ebk)

DOI: 10.4324/9781003243601

Typeset in Minion Pro
by Newgen Publishing UK

Publisher's Note
The publisher accepts responsibility for any inconsistencies that may have arisen during the conversion of this book from journal articles to book chapters, namely the inclusion of journal terminology.

Disclaimer
Every effort has been made to contact copyright holders for their permission to reprint material in this book. The publishers would be grateful to hear from any copyright holder who is not here acknowledged and will undertake to rectify any errors or omissions in future editions of this book.

Contents

Citation Information

The following chapters were originally published in various issues of *The Journal of Psychology*. When citing this material, please use the original citations and page numbering for each article, as follows:

Chapter 1

Fifty Shades of Darkness: A Socio-Cognitive Information-Processing Framework Applied to Narcissism and Psychopathy
B. Lopes, H. Yu, C. Bortolon, and R. Jaspal
The Journal of Psychology, volume 155, issue 3 (2021), pp. 309–333

Chapter 2

Self-Stigma Is Associated with Depression and Anxiety in a Collectivistic Context: The Adaptive Cultural Function of Self-Criticism
John Jamir Benzon R. Aruta, Benedict G. Antazo, and Judith L. Paceño
The Journal of Psychology, volume 155, issue 2 (2021), pp. 238–256

Chapter 3

Language and the Symptoms of Mental Illness Connection via Abstract Representations of the Self and the World
Yaşar Kuzucu, Ömer Faruk Şimşek, and Çiğdem Koşe-Demiray
The Journal of Psychology, volume 154, issue 3 (2020), pp. 214–232

Chapter 4

Personality Trait Interactions in Risk for and Protection against Social Anxiety Symptoms
Patryk Łakuta
The Journal of Psychology, volume 153, issue 6 (2019), pp. 599–614

Chapter 5

Insecure Attachment and Subclinical Depression, Anxiety, and Stress: A Three-Dimensional Model of Personality Self-Regulation as a Mediator
Ahmad Valikhani, Zahra Abbasi, Elham Radman, Mohammad Ali Goodarzi, and Ahmed A. Moustafa
The Journal of Psychology, volume 152, issue 7–8 (2018), pp. 548–572

For any permission-related enquiries please visit:
www.tandfonline.com/page/help/permissions

Notes on Contributors

Zahra Abbasi has a master's degree in Clinical Psychology from Islamic Azad University, Science and Research Branch. Her research interests concern clinical and health psychology, in particular, mindfulness and self-regulation.

Benedict G. Antazo received his MA in Counseling from De La Salle University, and is currently pursuing his PhD in Educational Psychology at the same institution. At present, he is a part-time professor at the department of psychology of Jose Rizal University. His research interests include general mental health, mental health stigma and attitudes, and psychometrics.

Kimberly A. Arditte Hall (PhD) obtained her doctorate at Clinical Psychology from University of Miami, and is currently a post-doctoral fellow at the National Center for Posttraumatic Stress Disorder within the VA Boston Healthcare System.

John Jamir Benzon R. Aruta is an assistant professorial lecturer at De La Salle University, Manila, Philippines. He also has a private practice in counseling and psychotherapy. His research interests include the role of culture on mental health, and application of psychological principles towards environmental sustainability.

Cristina Baleizão has a master's degree in Clinical Psychology, Department of Psychology, School of Social Sciences, University of Evora.

Casey N.-H. Batterbee is a student of psychology at the University of Michigan, USA.

Elisardo Becoña, PhD, is Professor in Clinical Psychology, and Director of the Smoking Cessation and Addictive Disorders Unit, University of Santiago de Compostela (Spain). His research interest areas are psychological treatment of smoking, cannabis, cocaine, gambling and new technologies.

C. Bortolon is Maitre de Conferences en Psicologie Clinique at the University of Grenoble in France. She is an international expert on cognitive and behavioral theory and treatments with a particular focus on psychosis. She is also an expert on neuroscience and mental health disorders.

Federica Bottazzi, MSc, recently received her master's degree in Psychology from the University of Genoa, Italy. She plans to pursue a PsyD in clinical psychology, with research interests in aggression and emotion.

Berta Caçador has a master's degree in Clinical Psychology, Department of Psychology, School of Social Sciences, University of Evora.

Rui C. Campos is a professor in the Department of Psychology, School of Social Sciences, University of Evora, Portugal. He is also a clinical psychologist by the Portuguese Psychologists Board and a researcher in the Research Centre for Education and Psychology (CIEP-UE).

Julia Y. Carbonella (MS) is a doctoral student in Clinical Psychology at University of Miami, and is currently completing her clinical internship.

Vincenzo Caretti, PhD, is Full Professor at the Department of Human Sciences of LUMSA University in Rome, Italy. His research interests currently focus on psychopathy and addictive behaviors. He has been scientific advisor to several academic and inter-institutional programs aimed at understanding, preventing, and treating violent behaviors.

Edward C. Chang is Professor of Psychology and Social Work in the Department of Psychology and the School of Social Work at the University of Michigan. His interests involve optimism/pessimism, perfectionism, coping and cultural influences on behavior.

Olivia D. Chang is a student at the Research in Action AcademyTM, USA.

Rie Chiba is Professor in the Department of Nursing, Graduate School of Health Sciences, Kobe University, Japan. Areas of interest are positive psychology, psychiatric nursing, and personal recovery among people with mental illness.

Elena Fernández del Río, PhD, is Assistant Professor in the Department of Psychology and Sociology in the University of Zaragoza (Spain). Her research interests are health psychology, personality, and addictive behaviors.

Liesbeth H.M. Eurelings-Bontekoe is Emeritus Professor at Leiden University. She is a clinical psychologist, psychotherapist, and researcher. Her main research interests are the assessment and treatment of personality pathology, and the role of personality attributes as a risk factor for the development of psychopathology.

Lisa Fiksenbaum is a part-time lecturer of psychology at the University of Toronto, Scarborough, and York University. Her areas of research include stress, coping, burnout, and work-family conflict.

Ana Sofia Fragata has a master's degree in Clinical Psychology, Department of Psychology, School of Social Sciences, University of Evora.

Akiko Funakoshi is Professor at the Kobe City College of Nursing, Japan. Areas of interest are psychiatric nursing, and personal recovery among people with mental illness.

Francisco Garcia-Santos is a member of NECO - Center for Behavioral Economics Lisboa. His research interests include attitudes to liquidity, money and assets traded in financial markets.

Carlo Garofalo, PhD, is Assistant Professor at the Department of Developmental Psychology of Tilburg University, The Netherlands. His main research interests concern the role of emotion regulation in the development and manifestation of personality pathology and antisociality, with a specific focus on psychopathic traits.

Simon Ghinassi completed his degree in Psychology at the University of Florence. His main research interests concern the study of relationships between personality characteristics and psychosocial well-being across life span.

Mohammad Ali Goodarzi is a professor of Clinical Psychology at Shiraz University. His research interests include cognitive and clinical psychology and cognitive psychotherapy.

Esther Greenglass is a professor of psychology at York University. She is Fellow of the Canadian Psychological Association (CPA), American Psychological Association (APA), and International Association of Applied Psychology (IAAP), and is widely cited for her work on stress and coping.

Yu Gu is a student of psychology at The University of British Columbia, Canada.

Yuncheng Guo is a student of psychology at Gettysburg College, USA.

Jiaying He is a student of psychology at the University of International Business and Economics, China.

Jameson K. Hirsch is Associate Professor in the Department of Psychology at East Tennessee State University. His interests involve personality, culture and health, psychopathology, coping and suicide prevention.

Ronald R. Holden is a registered clinical psychologist in Ontario, Canada and a professor of Psychology at Queen's University, Kingston, Ontario, Canada. His research interests are in suicide, scale construction, and test dissimulation.

R. Jaspal is Professor of Psychology at Nottingham Trent University, UK, and Fellow of the British Psychological Society. He developed Identity Process Theory in liaison with Dame Glynis Breakwell and is an international expert on identity and mental and sexual health.

Zunaira Jilani is a graduate student in the Department of Psychology at the University of Michigan. Her interests involve the study of mindfulness, domestic violence, sexual assault and mental health, and the psychology of South Asians.

Tetsuya Kawamoto is a project assistant professor at the Center for Advanced School Education and Evidence-based Research (CASEER) in the University of Tokyo, Japan. He received his Ph.D. from the University of Tokyo. His research interests include personality development and the evolution of personality traits.

Stefan Kempke is a postdoctoral researcher at the University of Leuven. His research interests include the role of maladaptive perfectionism in functional somatic disorders, such as chronic fatigue and fibromyalgia. His postdoctoral research focuses on the role of epigenetics in chronic fatigue syndrome, with a special emphasis on DNA methylation of genes involved in the HPA axis.

Jurrijn A. Koelen is a psychologist and researcher, currently working with the outpatient clinic for mood and anxiety disorders at Dimence, Deventer. His current research interests are attachment and emotional awareness, their manifestation as transdiagnostic risk and resilience factors, and their impact on the process of psychotherapy.

Çiğdem Koşe-Demiray is a clinical psychologist and she works with children and adolescents. Her main areas of research interest are cognitive behavioral therapy, child and adolescent psychopathology.

Yaşar Kuzucu is an associate professor in the Department of Counseling and Guidance at the Adnan Menderes University. His research focuses on mental health of adolescents and using advanced statistical analyses such as growth curve modeling.

Patryk Łakuta is now a PhD candidate. His main research interests are within the broad field of adult mental health, especially adults with chronic conditions. Many of his current projects focus explicitly on affective disorders, with a primary focus on improving the understanding of risk and protective factors, and their use in selecting potential targets and promising strategies for interventions.

Pengzi Li is a student of psychology at the University of Toronto, Canada.

Xiaoqing Li is a student of psychology at Boston University, USA.

Jiachen Lin is a student in the Department of Psychology at the University of Michigan. Her interests involve dental care seeking behaviors, sexual assault victimization, loneliness, and psychological adjustment.

B. Lopes is Clinical Psychologist and Senior Researcher at the Center for Research in Neuropsychology and Cognitive and Behavioral Intervention (CINEICC), University of Coimbra, Portugal. She is an expert on cognitive and behavioral theory and treatments, with particular focus on psychosis.

Ana López-Durán, PhD, is Associated Professor in University of Santiago de Compostela, and coordinator of the Smoking Cessation and Adictive Disorders Unit (University of Santiago de Compostela, Spain). Her research interests are related to addictive behaviors, and psychological treatment of smoking, cannabis and cocaine.

Abigael G. Lucas is a student of psychology at the University of Michigan, USA.

Zdravko Marjanovic is an assistant professor of psychology at Concordia University of Edmonton. He studies various topics that span across personality, social, and health psychology.

Carmela Martínez-Vispo is a PhD student in Neuroscience and Clinical Psychology, University of Santiago de Compostela, and therapist of the Smoking Cessation and Adictive Disorders Unit (University of Santiago de Compostela, Spain). Her research interests are related to smoking cessation treatment, health psychology, depression and smoking comorbidity.

Teresa Mayordomo, PhD, is a professor in the Catholic University of Valencia. She focuses her investigation on coping, well-being, and resilience in aging and dementia, method, and analysis of results.

Juan C. Meléndez, PhD, is a professor in the Faculty of Psychology, University of Valencia. His main field of study focuses on coping, well-being, and resilience in aging and dementia; nonpharmacological treatments in aging and dementia; and the method and analysis of results.

Yuki Miyamoto is Associate Professor, Department of Psychiatric Nursing, Graduate School of Medicine, The University of Tokyo, Japan. Areas of interest are psychiatric nursing, and personal recovery among people with mental illness.

Ahmed A. Moustafa is a senior lecturer in Cognitive and Behavioural Neuroscience at Western Sydney University and Qatar University. His research interests lie at the intersection of computational modeling, cognitive neuroscience, and clinical neuropsychology. He is interested in understanding learning and cognitive function in various psychiatric and neurological disorders.

Mine Muyan is a graduate student in the Department of Educational Sciences at Middle East Technical University. Her interests involve international psychology and the study of hope, loneliness, perfectionism, intimate partner violence, and coping as predictors of adjustment in adults.

Judith L. Paceño is affiliated with the University of Santo Tomas Counseling and Career Center. Her ten years of professional experience in the school setting include psychological assessment, counseling, and management for special cases. Her research interests are LGBT special population group, suicidal and self-harming behaviors, help-seeking behavior, and psychological distress. Currently, she is pursuing her Doctoral Degree in Counseling Psychology at De La Salle University, Manila, Philippines.

Lucia Ponti, PhD in Psychology, is a psychologist and psychotherapist with a research position at the School of Psychology at the University of Florence. She's a member of Italian Society of Behavioral and Cognitive Therapy. Her main research interests concern the study of risk and protective factors on the psychological and relational well-being across life span.

Elham Radman has a master's degree in Clinical Psychology from Islamic Azad University of Arak. Her research interests include personality and mental disorders.

Keith D. Renshaw is an associate professor in the Department of Psychology at George Mason University. His current research interests include anxiety, stress and trauma, and romantic relationships.

Rubén Rodríguez-Cano, PhD, is a therapist of the Smoking Cessation and Adictive Disorders Unit (University of Santiago de Compostela, Spain). His research interest areas are addictive behaviors, cancer prevention, health psychology and transdiagnostic processes underlying emotional disorder, and substance use disorder comorbidity.

Alicia Sales, PhD, is a professor in the Faculty of Psychology, University of Valencia. Her main field of study focuses on neuropsychological aspects in healthy older people and dementia patients, and nonpharmacological treatments in aging for improving successful and well-being aging.

Encarnación Satorres, PhD, is a research technician in the Faculty of Psychology, University of Valencia. Her research focuses on aging and dementia, neuropsychological assessment, and coping and well-being in aging.

Carmen Senra, PhD, is a titular professor in Psychopathology in University of Santiago de Compostela (Spain). Her research interests are related to clinical psychology, psychopathology and development of depressive disorders and eating disorders.

Ashley M. Shaw (PhD) obtained her doctorate in Clinical Psychology from University of Miami, and is currently a post-doctoral fellow at University of Miami.

Ömer Faruk Şimşek is a professor at Istanbul Rumeli University, Department of Psychology. His main areas of research interest are subjective well-being and its relation to narrative processes, language use and mental health, personal sense of uniqueness, and self-consciousness. He is also interested in using advanced statistical analyses such as multitrait-multimethod analyses and growth curve modeling.

Yingrui Sun is a student of psychology at Boston College, USA.

Franca Tani, psychologist and psychoanalyst, member of the International Psychoanalytical Association (IPA), is Full Professor of Developmental Psychology at the Department of Health Sciences and dean of the School of Psychology in the University of Florence, Italy. Her main research interests concern the analysis of the relationships among intrapsychic dynamics and the development of social and relational competence across lifespan, with particular reference to networks of close relationships (parent-child relationship, friendship, romantic relationship), and risk and protection factors in the intergenerational transmission.

Kiara R. Timpano (PhD) is an associate professor of Psychology in the Adult Division at the University of Miami.

Ahmad Valikhani is a researcher at Shiraz University. His research interests include personality, clinical, health, and positive psychology. His research interests are mainly focused on mindfulness, patience, personality disorders, attachment, and self-regulation.

Patrizia Velotti, PhD, PsyD, is Associate Professor at the Department of Educational Sciences of the University of Genoa, Italy. She studies the role of emotion regulation and other intersecting mechanisms linked with mental health and psychopathology. She is the head of the Emotion Regulation Interpersonal and Intergroup Relations Lab where she conducts research projects addressing these issues in laboratory, field, and clinical settings.

Paz Viguer, PhD, is a professor in the Faculty of Psychology, University of Valencia. Her research focuses on developmental psychology and aging. She has examined the psychological influences on well-being and how to promote successful aging.

Liangqiu Wan is a student of psychology at the University of Michigan, USA.

Yingjie Wang is a student of psychology at Coventry University, UK.

Hilary Weingarden is a doctoral candidate at George Mason University. Her current research interests include the role of emotions and cognitions in anxiety disorders and obsessive compulsive related disorders.

Yoshihiko Yamazaki is Professor in the Faculty of Social Welfare, Nihon Fukushi University, Japan. Areas of interest are Health Sociology and Sense of Coherence.

H. Yu is Senior Lecturer in Psychology at De Montfort University in the UK. She has expertise in data mining and in cross-cultural research with a particular focus on emotional regulation strategies and mental health accross cultures.

Tina Yu is a student in the Department of Psychology at the University of Michigan. Her interests involve ethnic/racial psychology, sexual assault and trauma, eating disturbances, chronic illness, and cultural variations in adjustment.

Zhan Zhang is a student of psychology at Mount Holyoke College, USA.

Introduction: How is it to experience psychopathology, and how it affects everyday life

Ami Rokach

"Mental illness, mental health, psychological sanity, psychological pathology, state of mind (French état d'âme, literally "state of soul") are terms by which we refer and understand ourselves as possessing mental and emotional, that is, psychological condition. As such, they have been at the center of philosophical discussions, especially in philosophical currents that focus on inner wellbeing … Looking for ways to link between a psychological and a historical perspective in regards to the subject of psychological wellbeing, or mental health, requires the examination of … the relation between mental health and the state of illness"

(Rotman, 2021; p. 22–23)

For one to be categorized as exhibiting positive mental health, an individual should not experience psychopathology, and additionally exhibit high levels of emotional well-being as well as high levels of psychological and social functioning (Trompetter, 2017). The dual-factor model of mental health suggests that enhancing positive mental health and alleviating psychopathology do not automatically go hand-in-hand, and are not opposite of one another (Keyes, 2005). There is accumulating evidence that psychopathology and positive mental health function along two different continua that are only moderately interrelated (Keyes 2005; Lamers et al. 2015). However, in order to know what wellbeing is, understand good mental health, and enhance adaptive functioning, we need to explore and understand psychopathology, and how it affects us. This volume is a compilation of articles that shed light on psychopathology, how the one struggling with it experiences its implications, and how it affects everyday life. The volume was divided into three conceptual sections: *The experience of psychopathology*, which is devoted to describing what it is and how it is experienced; *The effect of psychopathology on everyday life* describes various effects that psychopathology has on the daily life of the sufferer; *Coherence, resilience & recovery*, which focuses on dealing with it, coping with the symptoms, and developing resilience.

The experience of psychopathology

Lopes, Yu, Bortolon & Jaspal (2021) explored a socio-cognitive information-processing framework for narcissism and psychopathy in order to explain how psychopathic and narcissistic schemata influence the activation of psychological processes that interact with social and cultural contexts to display those personalities at a sub-clinical level. Their model enabled them to predict maladaptive behavior and to explain how personality disorders are developed in sub-clinical narcissists and psychopaths. The SCIPNP emphasizes the role of culture in shaping motives, appraisals, behavior and affect. Recommendations for future research are provided.

Aruta, Antazo & Paceno (2021) aimed to understand what are the mechanisms underlying the effect of self-stigma on depression and anxiety in a collectivistic culture such as the Philippines, since all previous research on psychological aspects of mental health were carried out in individualistic societies. They measured self-stigma, self-criticism, interdependent self-construal, depression, and anxiety symptoms on 312 adolescents in rural communities in the Philippines, which was utilized as an example of a collectivistic society. The authors found indirect effects of self-stigma on both depression and anxiety via self-criticism. Their findings confirmed that interdependent self-definition attenuate the detrimental impact of self-criticism on depression and anxiety in collectivistic contexts.

Kuzucu, Simsek & Kose-Demiray (2020) explored the mediatory processes through which language contributes to the symptoms of mental illness. Their investigation tested a structural equation model in which the need for the absolute truth about self and worry mediated the relationship of the gap between inner psychological experience and language with anxiety and depression. The results supported the model and indicated that the gap, indeed, predicts both the need for absolute truth and the tendency to worry which, in turn, predict the levels of anxiety and depression.

Lakuta (2019) was interested in personality traits that enhance a tendency towards social anxiety (SA). Lakuta, utilizing 135 participants aged 18–50 years, explored how interactions between the Big Five personality factors predict SA symptoms. Results revealed that low emotional stability was an independent predictor of higher levels of SA. They also discovered two significant interactions: the interactions between extraversion and openness, where high openness was correlated with agreeableness and predicted SA symptoms. At high openness, higher extraversion was associated with significantly lower levels of SA. It was therefore suggested that extraverts are likely to be protected against SA symptoms, but more so the more open they are. Additionally, at high levels of agreeableness, low openness has been shown to be uniquely predictive for higher levels of SA symptoms, indicating that the combined effect of openness with agreeableness may be more important to SA than either trait separately. Thus, extraverts are likely to be protected against SA symptoms, but more so the more open they are.

Valikhani, Abbasi, Radman, Goodarzi & Moustafa (2018) aimed to investigate the mediating and moderating role of the three-dimensional model of personality self-regulation in the relationship between insecure attachment and subclinical depression, anxiety, and stress. The study involved four hundred Iranian students. Their results indicated that there was a moderate correlation among all the variables under study, namely adult attachment, depression, anxiety, stress, integrative self-knowledge, mindful attention awareness, self-control, and self-compassion, in the expected directions. Analyses indicated that regarding the relationship between insecure attachment and depression, the components of integrative self-knowledge, self-control, and self-compassion functioned as mediators. As far as the relationship between insecure attachment and anxiety and stress, it was shown that integrative self-knowledge, mindfulness, and self-compassion relatively functioned as mediators. Their results pointed out that only mindfulness and self-compassion were identified as moderators in the relationship between insecure attachment and depression. The researchers concluded that insecure attachment may cause psychological damage due to deficiency in the components of the three-dimensional model of personality self-regulation.

Campos, Holden,Balezao, Cacador & Fragata (2018) set out to investigate whether the self-criticism and neediness predict suicide ideation when controlling for general distress. They studied two non-clinical samples. One of 202 community adults and the second, of 207 college students. Study 1 yielded that self-criticism, but not neediness, together with suicide ideation interacted with distress. Neediness also tended to interact with self-criticism in the prediction of suicide ideation. Results from Study 2 were similar and confirmed results which the authors found in Study 1. Changes in self-criticism, but not changes in neediness, predicted changes in suicide ideation. Changes in the interaction between self-criticism and distress, predicted changes in suicide ideation and changes in the interaction between self-criticism and neediness tended to predict changes in suicide ideation.

Shaw, Carbonella, Arditte Hall & Timpano (2017) were interested in investigating obsessive-compulsive disorder (OCD), since not much is known about which factors explain the overlap between obsessive-compulsive symptoms (OCS) and depressive symptoms. It was hypothesized that OCS and depressive symptoms may be related via depressive cognitive styles, such as rumination or dampening. This study, which involved 250 participants, evaluated the associations of OCS dimensions with depressive symptoms and cognitive styles, as well as the associations of OCS dimensions with depressive symptoms and cognitive styles, and the indirect effects of rumination and dampening in the relationship between OCS and depressive symptoms. Results indicated greater depressive symptoms, rumination, and dampening were associated with greater levels of all OCS dimensions. They also found a significant indirect effect of depressive cognitive styles on the relationship between OCS and depressive symptoms, through rumination and dampening. The authors recommended that their study be replicated on clinical populations, which stands to reason.

Velotti, Garofalo, Bottazzi & Caretti (2017) explored shame experiences and their associations with other aspects of psychological functioning and well-being. Their sample was composed of 308 people from the community of which 66% were women. Their female participants reported higher levels of shame (in particular, bodily and behavioral shame), guilt, psychological distress, emotional reappraisal, and hostility. Males on the other hand, showed higher levels of self-esteem, emotional suppression, and physical aggression. Shame feelings, across genders, were associated with low self-esteem, hostility, and psychological distress. Only women showed associations between characterological shame and emotional suppression, as well as between bodily shame and anger. Moreover, they found that characterological and bodily shame enhanced the prediction of low self-esteem, hostility, and psychological distress above and beyond the influence of trait shame. Lastly, and only among females, emotional suppression mediated the influence of characterological shame on hostility and psychological distress.

Koelen, Eurelings-Bontekoe & Kempe (2016) looked at the picture of a clinical sample made of 120 patients with somatoform disorder (SFD) which complained of the presence of chronic physical complaints that are not fully explained by a general medical condition or another mental disorder. The authors noted that insecure attachment patterns are common in this patient group, which are often associated with interpersonal difficulties.

In the present study, the mediational role of two types of alexithymia and negative affectivity (NA) was examined in the association between attachment styles and interpersonal problems in a group of 120 patients with SFD. Patients were requested to fill out several self-report questionnaires for the assessment of attachment strategies, alexithymia, NA, and interpersonal problems. The inability to identify and verbalize emotions, termed cognitive alexithymia mediated the relationship between avoidant attachment patterns and interpersonal problems.

Fiksenbaum, Marjanovic, Greenglass & Garcia-Santos (2017) tested the extent to which perceived economic hardship is associated with psychological distress, exemplified by suicide ideation and confusion, after controlling for personal characteristics. The authors also explored whether perceived financial threat (being unsure about the stability and security of one's personal financial situation) mediates the relationship between economic hardship and psychological distress outcomes. Their research involved 211 Canadian students and compared them to 161 community people. Their findings indicated that in both samples, greater experience of economic hardship increased with financial threat, which in turn increased with levels of suicide ideation and confusion.

The effect of psychopathology on everyday life

Ponti, Ghinassi & Tani (2020) aimed to analyze the direct and indirect relationships between the two phenotypes of narcissism, vulnerable and grandiose, and whether it enhances the tendency to perpetrate psychological abuse, and exploring the mediating role of romantic jealousy. They studied 473 participants, males and females, aged 18–30 years which were involved in a stable romantic relationship. Results show that the two forms of narcissism are both linked to psychological perpetrated abuse, but in different ways. Vulnerable narcissism was only indirectly linked to psychological abuse, through romantic jealousy; while grandiose narcissism was positively and directly associated with psychological abuse within the romantic relationship. Results applied to both genders.

Kawamoto (2019) focused on the differential susceptibility model in relation to middle adulthood regarding personality stability and change. The study was done on 1051, 534 of them females, Japanese middle adults [mean age= 41]. Model analyses revealed substantial mean-level declines in Agreeableness and Honesty–Humility. Of interest were the results which pointed to the influences of some life events on personality change and which are moderated by individual susceptibility to one's environment. Based on these findings the authors suggested that the trends of personality development may differ between Western and non-Western countries and that differential susceptibility model may play an important role in deriving individual differences in personality stability and change.

Martinez-Vispo, Lopez-Duran, Rodriguez-Cano, Fernandez del Rio, Senra & Becona (2019) studied loneliness and its association with depression, cigarette dependence, and the role of sex in this relationship. Their sample was composed of 275 adult treatment-seeking daily smokers, aged on average 45 years. Results showed a significant correlation between higher scores of loneliness, depressive symptoms, and cigarette dependence. In addition, there was a significant indirect effect of loneliness on cigarette dependence, via depressive symptoms. Sex was shown to significantly moderate the relationship between depressive symptoms and cigarette dependence. Results echo previous research that indicated that, in treatment seeking smokers, loneliness is a significant predictor of depressive symptoms, and through this relation, it predicts cigarette dependence.

Weingarden & Renshaw (2016) examined body dysmorphic disorder, and how appearance-based teasing affects the person, as well as functional impairment (i.e., social, occupational, family impairment), and depression in a nonclinical sample of undergraduates. Findings indicated that appearance-based teasing was positively correlated with body dysmorphic symptoms, and that correlation stronger than that between teasing and obsessive-compulsive symptom severity, which was also examined. Additionally, body dysmorphic symptom severity and appearance-based teasing interacted in predicting functional impairment and depression, in that appearance-based teasing was positively associated with depression and functional impairment only in those with elevated body dysmorphic symptoms. The interaction was nonsignificant for those with obsessive-compulsive symptoms.

Coherence, resilience & recovery

Mayordomo, Viguer, Sales, Satorres & Melendez (2016) examined well being and what may affect it. Based on the idea that development involves changes in individuals' adaptive capacity to meet their needs over time, the changes that occur in the second half of life require effort to adapt to the new reality. This study used a structural model to test the effects of coping strategies and resilience on well-being in a sample of 305 mid-life adults. Several constructs were measured: coping strategies, resilience, and well-being. A final model was obtained with good fit indices; psychological well-being was positively predicted by resilience and negatively by emotional coping. Moreover, positive reappraisal and avoidance form part of both coping strategies (problem-focused and emotion-focused).

Chang, Wan, Li, Guo, He, Gu et al. (2017) examined loneliness and future orientation as predictors of suicidal risk, namely, due to depression and suicide ideation, in a sample of 228 college students. Future orientation was found to significantly augment the prediction model of both depressive symptoms and suicide ideation. Beyond loneliness and future orientation, the Loneliness × Future Orientation interaction term was found to further augment both prediction models of suicidal risk. Future orientation is, indeed, an important buffer of suicidal risk, among lonely students. The researchers found that those with high future orientation, compared to low future orientation, reported significantly lower levels of depressive symptoms and suicide ideation.

Muyan, Chang, Jilani, Yu, Lin & Hirsch (2016) examined the role of hope in understanding the link between loneliness and anxiety and depressive symptoms. Their sample was composed of 318 adults. As expected, loneliness was found to be a significant predictor of both anxiety and depressive symptoms. Hope was found to significantly augment the prediction of depressive symptoms. They also found evidence for a significant Loneliness × Hope interaction effect in predicting anxiety, noting that the association between loneliness and anxiety was weaker among high, compared to low, hope adults.

Chiba, Yamazaki, Miyamoto & Funakoshi (2021) looked at the process of recovery. Their sample included 195 respondents aged 20 or older that were tested in time 1 and time 2. Their study aimed to examine the relationships among the initial levels and longitudinal changes in personal recovery, benefit finding [BF], and sense of coherence [SOC] among people with chronic mental illness in Japan. Their conclusion indicated that the initial levels and changes in personal recovery, BF, and SOC were significantly and positively related to each other.

To conclude, this volume may serve as an indication to researchers and clinicians regarding what and how psychopathology is expressed, addressed and needs to be addressed in therapy. I hope that you will find the articles in this volume illuminating and enhancing your thinking regarding helping those who are diagnosed as suffering form psychopathology.

References

Keyes, C. L. M. (2005). Mental illness and/or mental health? Investigating axioms of the complete state model of health. *Journal of Consulting and Clinical Psychology*, 73(3), 539e548. http://doi.org/10.1037/0022-006X.73.3.539.

Lamers, S. M. A., Westerhof, G. J., Glas, C. A. W., & Bohlmeijer, E., T. (2015). The bidirectional relation between positive mental health and psychopathology in a longitudinal representative panel study. *Journal of Positive Psychology*. doi:10.1080/17439760.2015.1015156.

Rotman, Y. (2021). Moral psychopathology and mental health: Modern and ancient. *History of Psychology*, 24(1), 22–33.

Trompeter, H.R., Lamers, S.M.A., Westerhof, G.J. Fledderus, M. & Bohlmeijer, E.T. (2017). Both positive mental health and psychopathology should be monitored in psychotherapy: Confirmation for the dual-factor model in acceptance and commitment therapy. *Behaviour Research and Therapy*, 91, 58–63. http://dx.doi.org/10.1016/j.brat.2017.01.008

Part I

The Experience of Psychopathology

Fifty Shades of Darkness: A Socio-Cognitive Information-Processing Framework Applied to Narcissism and Psychopathy

B. Lopes (iD), H. Yu, C. Bortolon, and R. Jaspal

ABSTRACT

Existing trait-based and cognitive models of psychopathy and narcissism fail to provide a comprehensive framework that explains the continuum between sub-clinical and clinical presentations of those personalities and to predict associated maladaptive behavior in different social and cultural contexts. In this article, a socio-cognitive information-processing framework for narcissism and psychopathy (SCIPNP) is proposed to explain how psychopathic and narcissistic schemata influence the activation of psychological processes that interact with social and cultural contexts to display those personalities at a sub-clinical level. The proposed framework enables us to predict maladaptive behavior and to explain how sub-clinical narcissists and psychopaths develop personality disorders. The SCIPNP emphasizes the role of culture in shaping motives, appraisals, behavior and affect. Recommendations for future research are provided.

Introduction

Narcissism is characterized by ideas of self-grandiosity and a personal sense of self-entitlement and psychopathy by callousness, viciousness and antisocial behavior, and both traits share a lack of empathy, disagreeableness, exploitative and manipulative characteristics (see Paulhus & Williams, 2002). The traits of psychopathy and narcissism are increasingly categorized under the broader construct of "dark personalities" (see Furnham et al., 2013 for a review). The prevalence of psychopathy and narcissism has been increasing (e.g., Babiak et al., 2010; Stewart & Bernhardt, 2010), especially in specific social, cultural and occupational contexts (e.g., Coid et al., 2009; Stinson et al., 2008).

There are two major paradigms in current research into clinical and sub-clinical presentations of narcissism and psychopathy: trait theories and cognitive theories. Trait theories, such as the trait circumplex model for the dark triad (Jones & Paulhus, 2011) tend to describe these personalities as a list of traits, while cognitive approaches such as that of Beck et al. (2015a) often focus on the general information-processing model. These paradigms are characterized by limitations which are addressed in the framework proposed in this article.

In this article, the Socio-Cognitive Information-Processing Framework for Narcissism and Psychopathy (SCIPNP) is outlined to explain the social, cognitive and affective dimensions of sub-clinical narcissism and psychopathy. In the SCIPNP, affective and behavioral responses to internal or external stimuli are viewed as resulting from a dynamic interaction between bottom-up and top-down processes, which incorporate information from one's cultural background and personal experiences, as well as situational cues. Moreover, the SCIPNP explains how the cognitive schemata and specific appraisal processes underpin the observed similarities and differences between psychopathy and narcissism.

Current Personality Theories

The Trait Theory

The Dark Personality Triad (Jones & Paulhus, 2011) is comprised of three distinctive but related socially aversive sub-clinical personality traits: narcissism, psychopathy and machiavellianism (Paulhus & Williams, 2002). All three dark triad personalities score low on agreeableness (Egan, 2009; Jakobwitz & Egan, 2006; Paulhus, 2001; Paulhus & Williams, 2002; Vernon et al., 2008; Widiger & Lynam, 1998). However, of the three dark personalities, psychopathy is associated with the least remorse and is most associated with callousness, impulsivity, thrill-seeking and criminal behavior, while narcissism is characterized by grandiosity, egocentrism and a sense of personal entitlement, and machiavellianism through strategic manipulation of others (Jones & Paulhus, 2011).

The Dark Triad is considered to be a descriptive, rather than functional and process-based personality model (Collins et al., 2017; Mischel & Shoda, 1995). It does not explain the mental processes that underpin the personalities or the causal factors underlying sub-clinical manifestations of psychopathy or narcissism; the role of social context in fluctuations in behavior and emotions (Mischel & Shoda, 1995); or how mental processes and the social context interact to affect the display of behavior and emotion (i.e., individual processes-based constructs) and their variability over time (Collins et al., 2017).

The notion of a unified and trait-based dark triad personality can also be challenged. For instance, psychopathy and machiavellianism have been found to be negatively related to openness and conscientiousness whereas narcissism is not (Jakobwitz & Egan, 2006; Paulhus & Williams, 2002). Moreover, psychopathy is much more associated with deviant behavior and predicts delinquency and criminality, while machiavellianism and narcissism do not (e.g., Buckels et al., 2014; Williams & Paulhus, 2004). Therefore, the three dark personalities may actually be less unified than previously thought.

In light of studies that suggest that machiavellianism is conceptually separate from narcissism and is a sub-dimension of psychopathy (Giammarco & Vernon, 2014; LeBreton et al., 2006; Persson et al., 2019) and in contrast to trait perspectives, we argue that machiavellianism is best conceptualized not as a distinct personality but as a selfish and manipulative strategy employed mainly by psychopaths to manipulate others (see

Clempner, 2017) but that it can also be used to a lesser degree by narcissists (Malesza, 2020).

Furthermore, trait-based personality theories often postulate that personality is fixed and immutable. However, some research suggests that there are culturally specific aspects of these traits, and that they may vary across time, context and culture (e.g., Youli & Chang, 2015).

The Cognitive Model of Personality Disorders

In their cognitive model of personality, Beck et al. (2015a) suggest that personality traits can be conceptualized as an overt expression of the schemata that organize, select and synthesize incoming information. Thus, the activation of a specific schema will impact on the evaluation of the stimulus, the affective and motivation arousal, and on the selection and implementation of specific strategies. The authors suggest that the dysfunctional schemata found in personality disorders are the product of an interaction between the individual's genetic predisposition and exposure to (adverse) life events. Accordingly, they argue that "personality disorders represent an exaggeration of adaptive personality strategies" (p. 19) which become inflexible and overgeneralized as a consequence of challenging experiences. Although these strategies may be considered adaptive in evolutionary terms, their rigid nature renders them maladaptive in most contexts. The model suggests that personality disorders can also be understood as cognitive profiles—each personality disorder is characterized by a composite of beliefs, attitudes, affect, and behavior. Nevertheless, this model does not describe the general narcissistic and psychopathic underlying personal needs/motives, cognitive appraisals and processes, or their behavioral and affective manifestations in sub-clinical populations. Moreover, it does not address how different processes are shaped and how they interact with social and cultural contexts, or their relationship with distinct personalities.

Fifty Shades of Darkness: The Sub-Clinical and Clinical Presentations

The SCIPNP is a framework oriented toward explaining sub-clinical presentations of narcissism and psychopathy while explaining why individuals with sub-clinical narcissism and psychopathy may gradually develop clinical presentations of narcissism and psychopathy.

Research has examined both quantitative (e.g., degree of severity) and qualitative (e.g., type of features, e.g., self-confidence for non-clinical vs. exhibitionism for clinical narcissism) continuum between sub-clinical and clinical presentations of narcissism and psychopathy (Aslinger et al., 2018; Edens et al., 2006; Vyas, 2015; Woodmass & O'Connor, 2018). For example, individuals with both sub-clinical and clinical presentations of narcissism and psychopathy have been found to be egocentric, exploitative and to harm others, which can impede feelings of intimacy and relationship quality (Ali & Chamorro-Premuzic, 2010; Campbell & Foster, 2002). They tend to behave in this way in order to obtain personal gratification (psychopathy) (Hare, 1999, 2003) or to safeguard self-esteem (narcissism) (Campbell, 1999).

Also, both sub-clinical and clinical presentations of narcissism and psychopathy have more or less adaptive facets and sub-types. For example, research has found four distinct facets of leadership/authority (more adaptive) vs. exhibitionism/exploitativeness (less adaptive) for narcissism (see Grijalva et al., 2015) and four distinct facets for psychopathy: affective/interpersonal (more adaptive) vs. lifestyle/antisocial (less adaptive) (Hare, 2003). A distinction has been made between two different types of narcissism: grandiose (high self-esteem, interpersonal dominance, tendency to over-estimate one's capabilities) vs. vulnerable narcissism (low self-esteem, insecure, hypervigilant of criticism) (Malesza & Kaczmarek, 2018). Similarly, a distinction has been made between two types of psychopathy: primary (selfish, manipulative) vs. secondary psychopathy (antisocial, impulsive) (Skeem et al., 2003) that have distinct behavioral and affective outcomes (see Gray et al., 2019 – primary psychopathy is considered to be more adaptive whereas secondary psychopathy is considered to be less adaptive and to be related to impulsive and antisocial behavior).

Generally, it appears that sub-clinical psychopaths and narcissists present mostly adaptive, less severe and flexible features (in comparison to clinical psychopaths and narcissists who mostly exhibit rigid, severe, maladaptive and dysfunctional features) (Curry et al., 2011; Johnston et al., 2014; Persson, 2013). However, this means that such individuals are less likely to achieve communal success and, as such, may experience difficulties in maintaining strong friendships, family bonds and romantic attachments (Campbell, 1999; Gervais et al., 2013). Nevertheless, it is likely that sub-clinical psychopaths and narcissists tend to exploit only their subordinates, while attempting to preserve their relationships with their close family and friends and with people in power for personal gain (Babiak et al., 2010; Braun, 2017). Conversely, clinical psychopathy and narcissism feature mostly severe, maladaptive and rigid features (e.g., persistent antisocial and criminal behavior; interpersonally harmful behaviors) (see Persson, 2013).

Not all individuals who exhibit sub-clinical narcissism and or psychopathy develop clinical narcissism and psychopathy [see Diagnostic Statistic Manual (DSM)-5 criteria, 2013]. Based on the proposed framework, we argue that (1) the readiness and inflexibility/rigidity of schemata availability and use; (2) the inability to adopt different schemata; (3) the activation and lack of self-regulation of malfunctioning "normal" processes e.g., biased cost-benefit analysis; (4) the lack of self-regulation in relation to the activation of narcissistic and psychopathic schemata and of consequent behavior and affect; and (5) specific brain changes/abnormalities that might sustain dysfunctional behavior, collectively, underpin the onset of clinical narcissism and psychopathy.

First, it is argued that some individuals develop narcissistic and or psychopathic schemata early on due to the influences of their culture, personal history and needs. These types of schema were once adaptive because they served a function and helped fulfill underlying motives/needs (e.g., need for power and success) but become maladaptive and dysfunctional due to their *rigidity and inflexibility* (see Beck et al., 2015a), thereby leading to clinical presentations of narcissism and psychopathy.

Second, while clinical psychopaths and narcissists persistently activate their psychopathic and narcissistic schemata in any kind of situation, thus leading to an over-generalization and lack of self-regulation in relation to psychopathic and narcissistic behavior, the sub-clinical individual will use the narcissistic and or psychopathic schemata only in specific social contexts in which they benefit from activating these schemata to pursue self-serving motives and needs.

Third, the maintenance of maladaptive appraisals in clinical narcissism and psychopathy is thought to be supported by an extremely distorted, rigid and consistent *biased cost-benefit analysis* and associated *externalizing blame and empathy biases,* which may prompt clinical psychopaths' transgressive and antisocial behavior, irrespective of the potential costs that this type of behavior entails for them and in particular for others (DeLisi et al., 2014).

Finally, it is proposed that the *empathy deficits* that are observed in clinical presentations of narcissism and psychopathy may be maintained by brain changes and abnormalities that are not generally observable in sub-clinical presentations, thus helping to sustain the dysfunctional behavior in clinical presentations (Hare, 1999; Hoppenbrouwers et al., 2016; Ronningstam, 2017).

The Socio-Cognitive Information-Processing Framework for Narcissism and Psychopathy (SCIPNP)

The SCIPNP proposes that personality consists not only of individual traits but also of cognitive patterns, that is, overarching schemata and styles of appraisal. Consistent with a functionalist contextual approach (Biglan & Hayes, 1996; Gifford & Hayes, 1999), we argue that, in order to explain narcissistic and psychopathic personalities, it is necessary first to understand the inherent motivations underpinning affect and behavior in response to particular social and cultural cues (Gifford & Hayes, 1999). From an evolutionary perspective, motives are conceptualized as drives that enable human beings to survive and to leave their genes behind (Gilbert, 2001) and are usually associated with personal needs (basic e.g., physiological needs and socially driven e.g., need for power success and control) which must be satisfied (Dweck, 2017; Gilbert, 2001). They are also psychological drives that are culturally tailored and enable action in pursuit of a goal (Dweck, 2017). Hence, personalities can be thought of as the individual's drive to satisfy culturally specific needs and motives through personal interactions, which subsequently become part of the individual's personality schemata (see Dweck, 2017).

The SCIPNP also takes an information-processing approach, by drawing on cognitive theories of human behavior, evolutionary theories of psychopathology that focus on representations of social mentalities (see Gilbert, 2001), and social learning theory (Bandura, 1977), and proposes a stage-based framework (Beck et al., 2015a, 2015b) to understand narcissistic and psychopathic personalities' cognitive, affective and behavioral presentations. In contrast to Beck et al.'s (2015a) model, the SCIPNP emphasizes the role of culture in shaping narcissistic and psychopathic mental representations of needs/motivations and their context-dependent and schemata-driven appraisals at a sub-clinical level.

The following cognitive stages are proposed: Appraisal of the Antecedent, Organization of Response (Affect and Behavior domains), and the Appraisal of the Consequences (see Figure 1). These cognitive stages are sequential, with each stage influencing the next during decision-making and action-taking. Moreover, there are appraisal processes (and affective, behavioral and socio-cultural processes, such as

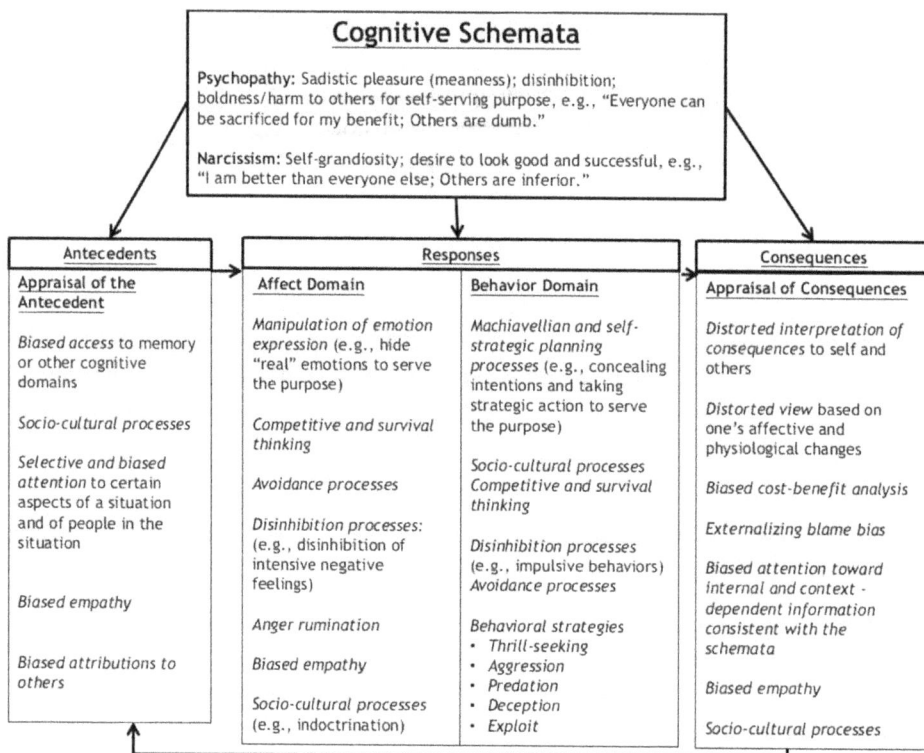

Figure 1. SCIPNP: Cognitive Schemata and Appraisal and Socio-Cultural Processes associated with each Cognitive Stage of Information-Processing of an Event.

ideological indoctrination, enculturation and cultural assimilation) in each cognitive stage that operationalize the display of both narcissistic and psychopathic behavior and affect (see Figure 1).

Cognitive Schemata

A cognitive schema is conceptualized as a pattern of thought that organizes and categorizes information and the relationships between them (see for example, Young, 1999). It is composed of beliefs or cognitions, values, and appraisals related to oneself, others and the social environment. The beliefs or cognitions and appraisals that form part of a particular schema are thought to be socially constructed and, as such, have moral and emotional meanings attached to them which vary cross-culturally.

According to the SCIPNP, cognitive schemata are at the heart of information-processing, decision-making, behavior and subjective feelings. Most schemata have evolutionary and social roots and self-serving and self-protecting functions. For example, when competing for self-survival, maintaining self-superiority and taking revenge against others may be adaptive and are common patterns observed in both narcissists and psychopaths (Campbell & Miller, 2012; Nathanson, 2008). Consequently, narcissists' and psychopaths' ways of thinking are not fundamentally different from those of the

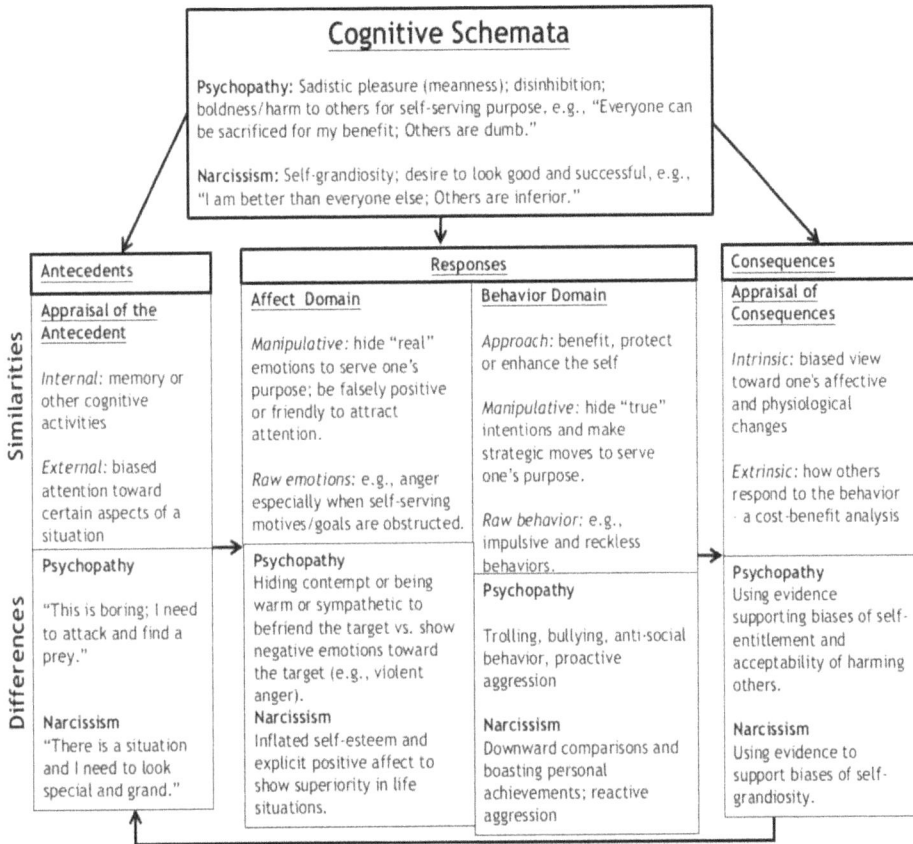

Figure 2. SCIPNP: Narcissistic and Psychopathic Cognitive Schemata and their similarities and differences in appraisals, affect and behavior.

general population. Psychopathic and narcissistic schemata are thought to be adaptive in some situations because they help fulfill underlying needs and the pursuit of personal motives and goals according to specific cultural norms and values and the social context (McCain & Campbell, 2018). However, they become maladaptive when the person is unable to deactivate those types of schema and associated malfunctioning processes. Depending on the type of schema that is activated, some appraisal processes may be absent at a given time and thus the behavior, cognitions and affect that are displayed may be a different subset of the common patterns. Appraisals, behavior and affect commonly observed in psychopathy and narcissism are summarized in Figure 2.

The most common schemata of psychopathic thinking include beliefs of the acceptability and entitlement to harm others for self-benefit; beliefs about the positivity of bold behavior (e.g., "Fortune favors the bold"); of the superiority of the individual's needs over morals and rules (e.g., "I am entitled to have fun even if it is illegal and breaks the rules"); non-remorseful beliefs (e.g., "I have no remorse after hurting others"); defiant beliefs against the authority ("The police does not deter me from doing what I want") and impulsivity/disinhibition ("I can do whatever I want how I want") (Hare, 1999, 2003).

These social predatory strategies must have been successfully implemented by our ancestors in the long evolutionary path to ensure our existence in the absence of cooperation (Dawkins & Krebs, 1978). Therefore, self-serving at others' expense and prioritizing individual needs are long-standing. Even some of the perpetrators of the most horrific crimes (such as the Holocaust) have not been considered to be clinical psychopaths (Greiner & Nunno, 1994). Psychopathic behavior may be enacted so that the individual can fulfill particular goals and associated underlying motives/needs that are ideologically indoctrinated (e.g., Nazi ideology) and under specific conditions, such as moving up the ranks or being commended by others. Hence, it seems that psychopathic mindsets still serve an adaptive role in some contexts, such as the workplace. For example, a high prevalence of psychopathic tendencies has been observed in senior management and among company chief executive officers (CEOs) (e.g., Babiak et al., 2010; Body, 2017; see also Landay et al., 2019 for a meta-analysis). This research suggests that psychopathy is associated with power, high social rank and "success"—in Western cultures at least.

Although psychopathy may be characteristic of powerful individuals and serves the purpose of obtaining success and power by favoring selfish interests at the expense of others, this behavior is likely to vary in accordance with social context. For instance, a CEO may exhibit psychopathic behaviors in the workplace but not when interacting with his children in the family home. Thus, the deactivation of the psychopathic schemata is likely to occur in domains in which they do not serve an adaptive function. Therefore, there may be a degree of flexibility and of self-regulation of psychopathic schemata and behavior at the sub-clinical level (see Vyas, 2015).

Narcissism, on the other hand, is characterized by self-grandiose views and the distorted belief that one is essentially superior to others, which can provide feelings of self-satisfaction (Campbell & Miller, 2012). This personality too has evolutionary and social roots. Human societies have long evolved into intricate hierarchies that determine the individual's worth, rank, status and role he/she plays and, as such, individuals have to compete with each other for resources and status, and defeat in social situations leads to shame and low social status and rank (see Gilbert, 2001). Hence, narcissism may be an evolutionary strategy that serves the purpose of adapting to challenging and competitive social contexts, promoting self-survival and personal success in hierarchical and status-based relationships.

In modern Western, industrialized societies, in which individualism is the dominant cultural orientation and interpersonal competitiveness is a key tenet of this cultural orientation, it is easy to see why narcissism might still perform an adaptive function. In particular, there is also an observed correlation between narcissism and success in leadership roles (Braun, 2017; Grijalva & Newman, 2015).

Although some narcissists never develop psychopathic features, some do (Miller et al., 2010). This may occur when individuals with narcissistic tendencies also possess psychopathic schemata, such as impulsive, antisocial and violent traits. The psychopathic schemata are sometimes also present in a narcissistic individual (see Kernberg & Caligor, 2005; Ronningstam, 2005). Thus, there are clinical cases of narcissists and psychopaths who simultaneously exhibit characteristics of both narcissism and psychopathy, illustrating the continuum between the two (see Ronningstam, 2005).

How Are Narcissistic and Psychopathic Schemata Developed?

It is likely that cognitive schemata are long-standing and developed on the basis of early childhood experiences, including parent-child interactions, which contribute to mental representations of the self and others and the relationships between them.

Clinical psychologists emphasize the importance of childhood experiences in prompting the development of psychological disorders, including the development of personality disorders (see Beck et al., 2015a, 2015b). For example, severe childhood traumatic experiences of abuse and neglect have been associated with the more severe facets of adult psychopathy (antisocial behavior, criminality) (Craparo et al., 2013; Piquero et al., 2012). It is argued that the antisocial/impulsive facet of psychopathy that is characteristic of secondary psychopathy (see Skeem et al., 2003) reflects a detachment of emotions which can result from negative childhood experiences where the child learns to desensitize pain. The child thus develops working mental models of relationships based on their negative interactions with a caregiver (e.g., mother) that persist into adulthood and that focus on potential threat from others and insecure attachments. These mental models in adult psychopaths lead to ineffective and dysfunctional behavioral strategies (e.g., displaying excessive anger to elicit response from others) and to frustration to reward and non-response to punishment (Benning et al., 2003).

Consistent with attachment theory (see Bowlby, 1944), several studies have found positive associations between psychopathic traits and attachment insecurity in adults (Blanchard & Lyons, 2016; Christian et al., 2017; Craig et al., 2013). In particular, most studies reveal an association between the impulsive/irresponsible component of psychopathy and attachment avoidance (dismissive attachment style) and attachment anxiety (preoccupied attachment style) (Christian et al., 2017; Craig et al., 2013).

Concerning narcissism, clinical theorists have often argued that adult narcissism can result from extreme forms of dysfunctional parenting. On the one hand, both Kernberg (1975) and Kohut (1977) have argued that narcissism is the product of cold, indifferent, rejecting or harsh parenting (e.g., authoritarian) that is inadequate in meeting the needs of the child, which in turn leads the child to fulfill those needs (e.g., need for recognition) in adulthood. The inadequate and insensitive parenting that some narcissists receive during childhood is thought to be associated with the development of the vulnerable type of adult narcissism that is characterized by low self-esteem and feelings of inferiority that are then "disguised" by attempts to show a grandiose "façade" (Kohut, 1977). Conversely, Millon (1981) proposed that parenting that is over-indulgent and characterized by parents putting their children on a pedestal can lead them to develop a grandiose type of narcissism.

It is argued that parents that over-indulge their children are then contributing to the formation of self-schemata in children which reflect their internalization of their parents' views of them being "special" (Millon, 1981). To maintain these grandiose schemata, strategies are developed that include exhibitionism and the pursuit of activities that have the sole purpose of inflating the self in the social environment (see McCain & Campbell, 2018).

Empirical studies have examined the impact of childhood experiences and insecure attachment styles in developing adult narcissism. For example, some studies have found that overindulgent parenting (e.g., warmth and admiration) was linked especially to the grandiose type of narcissism in adults (e.g., Brummelman et al., 2015; Horton et al., 2006). Other studies have found that cold and rejecting parenting (e.g., lack of warmth) is linked especially to the vulnerable type of narcissism (Otway & Vignoles, 2006; Smolewska & Dion, 2005). Moreover, parenting characterized by lack of supervision, psychological control and other types of inadequate parenting (i.e., more permissive and or more authoritarian, harsh discipline) are also related to adult narcissism (Cater et al., 2011; Horton et al., 2006; Wink, 1991).

Children learn through interactions with parents and peers, internalizing views of themselves and others that subsequently guide their behavior in later life. Moreover, insecure attachment styles developed in childhood influence and confirm adult narcissistic and psychopathic patterns of thought and action. For example, disorganized and preoccupied attachment styles due to childhood experiences of parental rejection and/or abuse are commonly associated with adult narcissistic/psychopathic aggression and heightened displays of negative affect (Craparo et al., 2013). Therefore, aggressive behavior serves to confirm one's views of others as threatening and indicates difficulties in self-regulation that are present in both adult narcissism and psychopathy (Ronningstam, 2017; Schimmenti et al., 2014). Conversely, avoidant/dismissive attachments developed in childhood serve to confirm grandiose views of oneself in adulthood since one develops an over-reliance on oneself, which confirms the view that one is special (Brennan & Shaver, 1998; Craig et al., 2013). Experiences of abuse are particularly problematic, since both adult psychopaths and narcissists who suffer abuse during childhood and consequently have insecure attachment styles, experience difficulties in emotional, behavioral and cognitive self-regulation (see Schimmenti et al., 2014).

The Influence of Culture in Shaping Adult Narcissism and Psychopathy

Culture plays an important role in determining how an individual functions in a particular society by introducing values, norms and rules that guide cognition, affect and behavior. Cultural indoctrination uses *socialization and enculturation and assimilation processes* that teach culturally specific values/beliefs and needs and impose rules and behaviors that are socially expected within a particular culture. Hence, socialization of cultural values occurs early on, beginning within the family environment and in parental rearing practices and then later on are reinforced in the external environment (e.g., at school). According to social learning theory (see Bandura, 1977) children learn from very early on through observation and interaction with significant others the specific cultural values and norms to be followed. These values, beliefs and norms are internalized and, as such, define the child's needs/motives/goals and associated beliefs about themselves, others and the social world, guiding both their behavior and display of affect. For example, Chinese culture is based on Confucian values, and children are socialized and indoctrinated early on by their parents and in schools to respect elders, be obedient and obey authority. Confucian values also tend to celebrate group-orientation and assimilation within the group and co-operation. Therefore, children are encouraged to pursue collectivistic goals and to elaborate on their own inadequacies relative to other children in an effort to "blend in" or assimilate with others (Yu, 1996). Those beliefs also persist well into adulthood and shape adult life decisions and underlying motives and needs, such as marriage (Chen, 2006).

As a result of these socialization processes, people in Western and Eastern cultures tend to differ in the level of importance that they append to distinctiveness, with Westerners generally valuing individual distinctiveness vis-à-vis conformity which conversely is more valued by those in Eastern cultures (Triandis, 1989; Vignoles et al., 2000). In support of culturally specific socialization processes, several studies have examined parenting styles in Eastern and Western cultures, as well as cultural differences within some ethnic groups (see Markus & Kitayama, 1991). It is generally argued that Chinese parents are more authoritarian, perceive their children as being dependent on the family, and as having group responsibilities, thus promoting assimilation and interdependence (Peterson et al., 2003). In contrast, North American parents are reportedly less authoritarian and tend to praise children more often, focusing on attributes and behavior that differentiate their children from others, thereby promoting individual distinctiveness (Peterson et al., 2003).

There are thus likely to be cultural differences in the motives/needs and appraisals of both narcissistic and psychopathic individuals. For example, in Chinese culture filial piety is important, so the need of recognition from significant others may be displayed in a collective sense by Chinese narcissists (Gries et al., 2015), whereas individualistic cultures that over-praise children and over-indulge them in schools and within families may later lead to a more agentic type of narcissism characterized by grandiose self-displays of superiority to satisfy distinctiveness (McCain & Campbell, 2018).

In addition, studies show that, in collectivistic cultures, violence and anti-social behavior, which are characteristic of antisocial personality disorder (ASPD), are less observable and the prevalence of ASPD is lower than in individualistic cultures (see Compton et al., 2005- rates of ASPD between 0.10-0.20% in Taiwan vs. 1.49% to 5.66% in United States of America). Furthermore, Cooke (1996) and Gilbert (2005) argue that culturally specific socialization processes are important in explaining those differences. Individualistic cultures tend to allow displays of aggression more than collectivistic cultures (see Ekblad, 1990). Also, in contrast to collectivistic cultures, individualistic cultures seem to propagate the idea that compassion in certain contexts (e.g., the workplace) is a sign of weakness and thus is not conducive to individual gain and success in highly competitive environments (Gilbert, 2005). Therefore, individuals are socialized from early on to think that being compassionate is a weakness and that showing aggression and cruelty may be morally acceptable, especially if this leads to personal gain and success in competition, which are then characteristic of psychopathic leaders in the Western workplace (see Body, 2017).

In sum, it is argued that Western societies and/or any other societies that assimilate the individualistic neo-liberal cultural ideology of the *survival of the fittest* and *self-made man* will indoctrinate their citizens into the idea that using cut-throat and cruel tactics may be morally acceptable in certain contexts (e.g., competitive workplaces) and should be used to attain success and power and to move up in the social hierarchy (Gilbert, 2005; Pendergast, 2000). Moreover, Western societies also tend to promote narcissistic tendencies and to over-praise individuals indiscriminately e.g., Western celebrity adulation and mimicry display of narcissism and the Western parental over-praise and gratification of children (Gray, 2014). Therefore, those cultural tenets of individualistic Western societies might promote and shape the formation of sub-clinical psychopathic and narcissistic schemata in particular individuals. Thus, it is likely that, once activated, these schemata will help individuals achieve specific goals, e.g., being successful in the workplace, in the short term in specific contexts. Also, because individualistic Western cultures tend to accept and promote displays of egocentrism, manipulation, deceit and exploitation of others for self-benefit (see Gilbert, 2005; McCain & Campbell, 2018), one might assume that it is adaptive to develop sub-clinical narcissism and psychopathy to survive and cope with challenges that occur in specific contexts within individualistic Western cultures. However, this does not mean that those individuals will develop clinical narcissism or psychopathy. Instead, this only means that "non-clinical" individuals can develop sub-clinical narcissism and psychopathy because both serve a purpose (e.g., being useful in competitive contexts) and are thus promoted in certain cultures and contexts.

Appraisal of the Antecedent

Activation of schemata in this stage can be rather automatic, particularly if the set of schemata is the most readily available one, irrespective of the social context, or it can be a conscious activation (Beck et al., 2015a, 2015b). In this early stage of information-processing, the individual retrieves relevant past information from his/her database of past memories of similar events and of semantic knowledge and then applies them to the current situation.

The active schema may lead to *biased and/or selective attention to particular aspects of the situation* which are consistent with the schema's representation of the self, others and the world and the relationships between them. For example, if an individual has activated narcissistic and or psychopathic schemata, which include the belief "Other people can be exploited," then the individual may *pay selective attention* to people who appear to be easy to exploit and to manipulate (Book et al., 2013). The active schemata may also lead people to make *biased attributions* to others which guide his/her behavior (e.g., "He/she looks old, so he/she must be weak"). Conversely, the individual will downplay or ignore other information which is inconsistent with these schemata. Furthermore, the activated schemata are likely to influence the ways in which the individual evaluates whether a situation is agreeable or threatening. This perception depends on the underlying motive that is guiding the individual's behavior toward a specific person in any given situation (e.g., to befriend the person to appear more popular by association vs. to compete with the person for high status).

The individual's activated narcissistic and/ or psychopathic schemata may also lead to *biased empathy*, that is, the tendency to ignore or downplay the pain of others while paying biased attention to his/her own feelings (see Farah et al., 2009; Hepper et al., 2014). Moreover, a narcissistic or psychopathic individual may recall *biased memories*. For example, he/she may recall specifically his/her past successes in exploiting others without thinking about the pain he/she provoked in others (see Ritchie et al., 2015).

Socio-cultural processes may be activated in this stage thus influencing the biased recollection of memories that are culturally relevant and leading to biased attention processes in the situation (Aaker & Schmitt, 2001). For example, when exposed to individualistic cultures that value particular exterior signs of status (e.g., a specific luxurious brand) and when appraising the situation in individualistic cultures, individuals from collectivistic cultures may assimilate this specific value and themselves seek signs of status in others with the intent to culturally blend in (Aaker & Schmitt, 2001).

There is broad empirical support for the appraisal processes associated with psychopathic and narcissistic schemata outlined in Figure 1. For example, the Response Modulation Hypothesis for psychopathy (Newman & Baskin-Sommers, 2011) postulates that abnormalities in both fear and inhibition in psychopathy are due to the presence of an "attention bottleneck" in this personality profile which "interferes with the processing of information that is congruent with a current goal rather than limitations in later stages of selection" (p. 427). Similarly, in the SCIPNP, *biased attention processes* in psychopathy are said to lead to rigid behaviors in pursuit of a specific goal.

Organization of Responses (Affect and Behavior Domains)

Having appraised the social context, the individual will append affective meaning to it. The activated schemata play the most important role in determining the individual's affective and behavioral responses to a situation. Schemata and the consequent display of affect and behavior are heavily influenced by *socio-cultural processes*. For example, a study has found that Chinese and other collectivistic cultures value low arousal emotions in contrast to Western cultures that value high arousal emotions, such as anger, and thus they avoid displaying high arousal emotions whereas in Western cultures, the display of those emotions is more common (Nangyeon, 2016). Moreover, collectivistic cultures, such as, the Korean culture tend to show less self-expression in public compared to North Americans (Park, 1998). This may be tied to the need/motivation in North American culture relative to East Asian cultures to express themselves as a way to differentiate themselves from others and also to maintain self-esteem and self-regard (Aaker & Schmitt, 2001). Therefore, it is likely that behavioral and affective expressions of sub-clinical narcissists and psychopaths in Western cultures differ from those from Eastern cultures.

Individuals who activate narcissistic/psychopathic schemata in socially threatening situations (e.g., when publicly criticized by others) will most likely display *intensified negative affect* because they feel personally threatened (e.g., Durand, 2016; Falkenbach et al., 2013; Geukes et al., 2017; Hare, 2003). This perception of threat may be attributed to the individual's persistent *competitive and survival thinking* that may be more prominent in Western individualistic cultures (Gebauer et al., 2012). For instance, when an individual has to compete with someone else for a job but fails, instead of accepting that only one out of a number people can actually get the post, he/she may feel personally threatened and, thus, intensely angry and ashamed.

The narcissistic and psychopathic schemata may also lead to *difficulties in regulating negative affect* and to *disinhibition* in behavior (Gray et al., 2019). For example, it has been reported that offenders with high levels of psychopathy exhibited a higher cardiovascular response when they processed negative, rather than positive, information in comparison to those with low levels of psychopathy (Casey et al., 2013).

Psychopaths and narcissists may also use maladaptive emotional regulation strategies, such as excessive *anger rumination* (i.e., focusing on anger-related episodes and thoughts, see Sukhodolsky et al., 2001), which in turn can aggravate feelings of anger in the long term given its association with aggressive behaviors as coping responses (Bushman, 2002, Bushman et al., 2001). Indeed, anger rumination mediates the effect of narcissism on relational aggression, suggesting that narcissism leads to relational aggression only when anger rumination is also present (Ghim et al., 2015).

Psychopathic and narcissistic people also exhibit *biased empathy* (see Farah et al., 2009; Ronningstam, 2017), that is, they tend to ignore or downplay the emotions that others feel (especially negative emotions, e.g., pain) and instead only pay attention to their own emotions. For example, narcissists experience difficulty in recognizing the emotions of others, exhibit low distress tolerance (Baskin-Sommers et al., 2014; Farah et al., 2009) and experience difficulties in emotional regulation (Schulze et al., 2013).

Avoidance of negative affect such as shame might be also utilized by people with narcissistic and psychopathic tendencies. For example, if the individual has activated narcissistic schemata including the belief "I am superior to others, so other people should treat me in a special way," he/she might avoid situations in which other people do not treat him/her in a special way or make him/her feel inferior to others. This strategy is intended to downplay negative affect. Indeed, narcissists avoid situations that contradict their sense of self-worth in order to protect their own implicit self-esteem (e.g., Oltmanns & Balsis, 2011). Similarly, if the individual has activated narcissistic and/or psychopathic schemata that include beliefs such as "I don't have any weaknesses," he/she might exhibit *avoidant behaviors*, e.g., alcohol and drug overuse in order to escape from intolerable affects and a threatened self-image (Beck et al., 2015a; Kealy et al., 2017).

Moreover, people with narcissistic or psychopathic tendencies may feel entitled to display negative emotions, such as anger, and refuse to down regulate those negative emotions because they feel that other people in the situation are responsible for their own negative emotions (Ellis et al., 2017; Morrison & Gilbert, 2001). Consequently, they may exhibit *disinhibited* and or *non-regulated affect* in a situation of social threat, resulting in the display of immense anger toward other people (Durand, 2016). Moreover, reduced feelings of guilt make individuals with narcissistic and psychopathic tendencies less likely to make amends for their negative actions but more likely to engage in transgressive and vengeful behavior (Poless et al., 2018; Prado et al., 2016).

In contrast to this, narcissistic and psychopathic individuals with stable and consistent identities (characterized by self-esteem and devoid of insecurity) are less susceptible to such reactivity (e.g., Bateman, 1998) and, as such, are better adapted to challenging, socially threatening and competitive contexts. In this case, psychopaths, in particular, might be able to *manipulate their explicit affect* to achieve a specific motive. Thus, a psychopath might behave in a charming manner in order to win the trust of someone he/she actually intends to harm (see Hare, 1999).

Crucially, psychopathic and narcissistic individuals may also engage in calculated *manipulative* behavior, that is, *machiavellianism.* They may hide their "true" intentions and take strategic action to manipulate other people in line with their active schemata and underlying motives and associated goals. For example, under activated narcissistic schemata that include the belief that "Status is everything," narcissistic individuals may befriend popular people that they actually dislike with the underlying motive of boosting his/her self-superiority in relation to others (see Rose, 2007). In short, when narcissistic and psychopathic schemata are activated, individuals may feign (either successfully or not) calmness, agreeableness and positivity, in order to lure their target and manipulate them while retaining a positive public identity to display to others (see Porter et al., 2011). This strategy is designed for self-benefit and can be adaptive in certain contexts (White, 2014).

Other *behavioral strategies* that are selfish and self-protective, e.g., avoiding negative states like feeling inferior to others; self-enhancing behaviors and exploiting; thrill-seeking and bold behaviors; deceiving; attacking others to protect and benefit the self; as well as taking revenge against others are thought to be present in non-clinical presentations of narcissism and psychopathy (see Beck et al., 2015a, 2015b). While narcissists show *reactive aggression*, i.e., show aggression whenever they are provoked and particularly when their ego is being threatened, psychopaths do so not only when their ego is threatened but also when they are provoked physically (e.g., physical injury) (see Jones & Paulhus, 2010). Moreover, in contrast to narcissists, psychopaths tend to exhibit also *pro-active aggression*, that is, unprovoked aggression, which is associated with the poor impulse control in psychopathy (Perenc & Radochonski, 2014).

Appraisal of the Consequences

According to the SCIPNP, while pursuing a particular action, the individual will evaluate the consequences of his/her action. The individual with activated schemata will assess whether the behavior has either enabled him/her to react successfully to threat (which can be attributed to automatic/reactive self-protection) or has enabled him/her to meet his/her underlying motives/needs and conscious goals. The activated schemata will always lead to a schemata-driven and *biased cost-benefit analysis* of the consequences of one's behavior (see Clempner, 2017). For example, an individual may pay *biased attention to* and *distort* the meanings of his/her affective and physiological responses, i.e., a psychopathic individual may label sympathetic activation stimulated by the sight of discomfort in people being hurt (e.g., faster heartbeat) as pleasurable and exciting (Harenski et al., 2012), also exhibiting *biased empathy* (e.g., Baskin-Sommers et al., 2014; Farah et al., 2009).

The individual may also *pay biased attention* to aspects of the current situation, which lead to a *distorted interpretation of the consequences* of his/her behavior in general. Moreover, this can further lead to *distorted interpretations of the consequences of his/her behavior to the self and others* (e.g., "Others submitted to my showcase of power and of superiority, and I felt good"—*narcissism* and "I felt good putting down and harming other people and they seemed to fear me"—*psychopathy*), thereby reinforcing his/her original psychopathic and narcissistic logic and beliefs (e.g., "I am superior and others are inferior"—*narcissism* and "I am entitled to harm others to feel good about myself"—*psychopathy*).

The *biased cost-benefit analysis* is also linked to an *externalizing blame bias*, which is associated with psychopathic and narcissistic schemata (Bentall et al., 1994; Morrison & Gilbert, 2001). An externalizing blame bias is a type of bias that is observed when people blame others for negative outcomes and consequences of their behavior instead of blaming themselves (Morrison & Gilbert, 2001). Psychopathic and narcissistic individuals exhibit an externalizing blame bias because they are shame- and guilt-intolerant and have difficulties in regulating their emotions in socially threatening situations (Morrison & Gilbert, 2001). This is observable in both clinical and non-clinical populations (Campbell & Elison, 2005; Campbell & Miller, 2012; Morrison & Gilbert, 2001; Schalkwijk et al., 2016). Primary and secondary psychopathy (see Skeem et al., 2003) have a negative relationship with adaptive shame coping (e.g., submissive displays in a confrontation) and a positive relationship with externalizing blame (see Campbell & Elison, 2005). Moreover, in their study of delinquent and non-delinquent adolescents, Schalkwijk et al. (2016) found a strong positive relationship between narcissism and externalizing blame for negative and shaming outcomes.

In short, it is argued that people with sub-clinical psychopathic and narcissistic tendencies generally conduct a *biased cost-benefit analysis of the consequences of their behavior* in the appraisal of consequences stage and exhibit an *externalizing blame bias*. The objective is to distance the cause of the negative consequences of their behavior from themselves onto others. As such, they will pay attention only to the benefits of their behavior to themselves and to their own emotions in response to the situation (i.e., *biased empathy*), as well as to stimuli supporting their self-serving narcissistic and psychopathic underlying motivations, needs and schemata.

The Cognitive Loop: Reinforcement of the Schemata and Appraisals

The loop of cognitive stages may unfold several times during information-processing and action-taking in the current situation and may also unfold in another similar social situation in dynamic and flexible ways. Moreover, context-dependent appraisals are consistent with the activated schemata and reinforce the particular dominant narcissistic and or psychopathic belief. For example, the individual who possesses the belief "I am entitled to exploit others for my self-benefit" in response to an opportunity to exploit others may: (1) reevaluate the antecedent (e.g., "Is it a good opportunity to exploit?"); (2) evaluate his/her responses (e.g., predate, exploit, apologize, do nothing, e.g., "I am so brilliant and others are inferior and stupid" when using exploitative strategies) and (3) evaluate the consequences of his/her responses (e.g., "Is my endeavor successful? Shall I follow up?"). When the consequences of the behavior fulfill the underlying needs and motives and associated goals in response to a specific situation (e.g., the psychopathic need to obtain pleasure and the associated motive of obtaining self-benefits through harming others), they will reinforce the underlying psychopathic cognitions and schemata, which may become dominant in the long term. As such, the loop of cognitive stages that an individual experiences in a particular situation can be maintained in other analogous situations. Nevertheless, drawing from systems modeling (see Bramson, 2009), it is also argued that a dynamic system is not rigid. Hence, it is argued that, at a sub-clinical level, the SCIPNP system has a tipping point that occurs when it achieves a non-equilibrium state. For example, when costs severely outweigh the benefits, the system then shifts to a new state that is more adaptive, i.e., narcissistic and psychopathic schemata are de-activated and substituted by the activation of other schemata in response to a particular situation and as such, new behaviors are manifested. In conclusion, sub-clinical narcissistic and psychopathic behavior occurs in particular situations because it is adaptive in the short term and in specific contexts, thereby enabling the individual to achieve specific goals and to satisfy his/her motives/needs.

Future Research

Future research should examine whether the appraisal processes described in the SCIPNP are present in sub-clinical presentations of psychopathy and narcissism and whether they underpin the continuum between sub-clinical and clinical presentations. A longitudinal research design would be advantageous. Research should also examine which social contexts are more likely to activate narcissistic and psychopathic schemata and how the appraisal processes described in this framework influence the display of both narcissistic and psychopathic adaptive and maladaptive behaviors. It is important to explore how the SCIPNP can be applied to understand diverse adaptive and maladaptive behaviors (e.g., trolling, Lopes & Yu, 2017; and sexual risk-taking, Jaspal et al., 2021) in different social contexts and especially in under-researched cultural contexts, while testing SCIPNP-based practical interventions to reduce the incidence of maladaptive and antisocial behavior.

Conclusion

The proposed SCIPNP framework strives to provide a more comprehensive explanation of the continuum between clinical and sub-clinical presentations of psychopathy and narcissism than trait theory which has long dominated the field of personality research. In contrast to trait theories which do not generally explain the processing of information, the SCIPNP treats personality as a combination of cognition, affect and behavior which results from the dynamic interaction between the context (e.g., a situation in the workplace), culture and the cognitive schemata and appraisal processes that are activated at the present moment. The personalities' schemata serve as lenses through which one evaluates the situation, influencing affective and behavioral responses. In addition, the schemata also influence how one interprets the consequences of one's behavior and those consequences further reinforce the activation of the schemata under the next round of action in a perceived similar situation. The SCIPNP challenges the notion of fixed, consistent, universal traits by showing how human beings construct schemata or patterns of thinking that are situationally and culturally adaptive, flexible and advantageous.

Acknowledgements

We would like to thank Professor Shira Elqayam for her insightful ideas.

Declaration of Interest

The authors have no interests to declare.

ORCID

B. Lopes (iD) http://orcid.org/0000-0002-1400-020X

References

Aaker, J., & Schmitt, B. (2001). Culture-dependent assimilation and differentiation of the Self: Preferences for consumption symbols in the United States and China. *Journal of Cross-Cultural Psychology*, *32*(5), 561–576. https://doi.org/10.1177/0022022101032005003

Ali, F., & Chamorro-Premuzic, T. (2010). The dark side of love and life satisfaction: Associations with intimate relationships, psychopathy and Machiavellianism. *Personality and Individual Differences*, *48*(2), 228–233. https://doi.org/10.1016/j.paid.2009.10.016

American Psychiatric Association (APA). (2013). *Diagnostic and statistical manual of mental disorders* (5th ed.). American Psychiatric Association Publications. https://doi.org/10.1176/appi.books.9780890425596

Aslinger, E., Manuck, S., Pilkonis, P., Simms, L., & Wright, A. (2018). Narcissist or narcissistic? Evaluation of the latent structure of narcissistic personality disorder. *Journal of Abnormal Psychology*, *127*(5), 496–502. https://doi.org/10.1037/abn0000363

Babiak, P., Neumann, S. C., & Hare, D. R. (2010). Corporate psychopathy: Talking the walk. *Behavioral Sciences & Law*, *28*(2), 174–193. https://doi.org/10.1002/bsl.925

Bandura, A. (1977). Self-efficacy: Toward a unifying theory of behavioral change. *Psychological Review*, *84*(2), 191–215. https://doi.org/10.1037/0033-295X.84.2.191

Baskin-Sommers, A., Krusemark, E., & Ronningstam, E. (2014). Empathy in narcissistic personality disorder: From clinical and empirical perspectives. *Personality Disorders*, *5*(3), 323–333. https://doi.org/10.1037/per0000061

Bateman, A. W. (1998). Thick- and thin-skinned organisations and enactment in borderline and narcissistic disorders. *International Journal of Psychoanalysis*, *79*(1), 13–25.

Blanchard, A., & Lyons, M. (2016). Sex differences between primary and secondary psychopathy, parental bonding, and attachment style. *Evolutionary Behavioral Sciences*, *10*(1), 56–63. https://doi.org/10.1037/ebs0000065

Beck, A. T., Davis, D., & Freeman, D. (2015a). *Theory of personality disorders* (3rd ed.). Guilford Press.

Beck, A. T., Davis, D. D., & Freeman, A. (Eds.). (2015b). *Cognitive therapy of personality disorders*. Guilford Publications.

Benning, S. D., Patrick, C. J., Hicks, B. M., Blonigen, D. M., & Krueger, R. F. (2003). Factor structure of the Psychopathic Personality Inventory: Validity and implications for clinical assessment. *Psychological Assessment, 15*(3), 340–350. https://doi.org/10.1037/1040-3590.15.3. 340

Bentall, R., Kinderman, P., & Kaney, S. (1994). The self, attributional processes and abnormal beliefs: Towards a model of persecutory delusions. *Behaviour Research and Therapy, 32*(3), 331–341. https://doi.org/10.1016/0005-7967(94)90131-7

Biglan, A., & Hayes, S. C. (1996). Should the behavioral sciences become more pragmatic? The case for functional contextualism in research on human behavior. *Applied and Preventive Psychology, 5*(1), 47–57. https://doi.org/10.1016/S0962-1849(96)80026-6

Body, R. C. (2017). Psychopathic leadership: A case study of a corporate psychopath CEO. *Journal of Business Ethics, 145*, 141–156. https://doi.org/10.1007/s10551-015-2908-6

Book, A., Costello, K., & Camilleri, J. (2013). Psychopathy and victim selection: The use of gait as a cue to vulnerability. *Journal of Interpersonal Violence, 28*(11), 2368–2383. https://doi.org/ 10.1177/0886260512475315

Bowlby, J. (1944). Forty-four juvenile thieves: Their character and home-life. *International Journal of Psychoanalysis, 25*, 19–52.

Bramson, A. (2009). Formal measures of dynamical properties: Tipping, robustness and path dependence. *AAAI Fall Symposium: Complex Adaptive Systems and the Threshold Effect.*

Braun, S. (2017). Leader narcissism and outcomes in organizations: A review at multiple levels of analysis and implications for future research. *Frontiers in Psychology, 8*(773), 773. https://doi. org/10.3389/fpsyg.2017.00773

Brennan, K. A., & Shaver, P. R. (1998). Attachment styles and personality disorders: Their connections to each other and to parental divorce, parental death, and perceptions of parental caregiving. *Journal of Personality, 66*(5), 835–878. https://doi.org/10.1111/1467-6494.00034

Brummelman, E., Thomaes, S., Nelemans, S. A., Orobio de Castro, B., & Bushman, B. J. (2015). My child is God's gift to humanity: Development and validation of the Parental Overvaluation Scale (POS). *Journal of Personality and Social Psychology, 108*(4), 665–679. https://doi.org/10. 1037/pspp0000012

Buckels, E., Trapnell, P., & Paulhus, D. (2014). Trolls just want to have fun. *Personality and Individual Differences, 67*, 97–102. https://doi.org/10.1016/j.paid.2014.01.016

Bushman, B. J. (2002). Does venting anger feed or extinguish the flame? Catharsis, rumination, distraction, anger, and aggressive responding. *Personality and Social Psychology Bulletin, 28*(6), 724–731. https://doi.org/10.1177/0146167202289002

Bushman, B. J., Baumeister, R., & Phillips, M. C. (2001). Do people aggress to improve their mood? Catharsis beliefs, affect regulation, opportunity, and aggressive responding. *Journal of Personality and Social Psychology, 81*(1), 17–32. https://doi.org/10.1037/0022-3514.81.1.17

Campbell, S. J., & Elison, J. (2005). Shame coping styles and psychopathic personality traits. *Journal of Personality Assessment, 84*(1), 96–104. https://doi.org/10.1207/s15327752jpa8401_16

Campbell, W. K. (1999). Narcissism and romantic attraction. *Journal of Personality and Social Psychology, 77*(6), 1254–1270. https://doi.org/10.1037/0022-3514.77.6.1254

Campbell, W. K., & Foster, C. A. (2002). Narcissism and commitment in romantic relationships: An investment model analysis. *Personality and Social Psychology Bulletin, 28*(4), 484–495. https://doi.org/10.1177/0146167202287006

Campbell, W. K., & Miller, J. D. (2012). *The handbook of narcissism and narcissistic personality disorder: Theoretical approaches, empirical findings, and treatments.* John Wiley & Sons. https://doi.org/10.1002/9781118093108

Casey, H., Rogers, R. D., Burns, T., & Yiend, J. (2013). Emotion regulation in psychopathy. *Biological Psychology, 92*(3), 541–548. https://doi.org/10.1016/j.biopsycho.2012.06.011

Cater, T. E., Zeigler-Hill, V., & Vonk, J. (2011). Narcissism and recollections of early life experiences. *Personality and Individual Differences, 51*(8), 935–939. https://doi.org/10.1016/j.paid. 2011.07.023

Chen, C. (2006). From filial piety to religious piety: Evangelical Christianity reconstructing Taiwanese immigrant families in the United States. *International Migration Review, 40*(3), 573–602. https://doi.org/10.1111/j.1747-7379.2006.00032.x

Christian, E., Sellbom, M., & Wilkinson, R. B. (2017). Clarifying the associations between individual differences in general attachment styles and psychopathy. *Personality Disorders, 8*(4), 329–339. https://doi.org/10.1037/per0000206

Clempner, B. J. (2017). A game theory model for manipulation-based Machiavellianism: Moral and ethical behaviour. *Journal of Artificial Societies and Social Simulation, 20*(2), 1–16. https://doi.org/10.18564/jasss.3301

Coid, J., Yang, M., Ullrich, S., Roberts, A., & Hare, R. D. (2009). Prevalence and correlates of psychopathic traits in the household population of Great Britain. *International Journal of Law and Psychiatry, 32*(2), 65–73. https://doi.org/10.1016/j.ijlp.2009.01.002

Collins, D. M., Jackson, J. C., Walker, R. B., O'Connor, P. J., & Gardiner, E. (2017). Integrating the context-appropriate balanced attention model and reinforcement sensitivity theory: Towards a domain-general personality process model. *Psychological Bulletin, 143*(1), 91–106. https://doi.org/10.1037/bul0000082

Compton, W. M., Conway, K. P., Stinson, F. S., Colliver, J. D., & Grant, B. F. (2005). Prevalence, correlates, and comorbidity of DSM-IV antisocial personality syndromes and alcohol and specific drug use disorders in the United States: Results from the national epidemiologic survey on alcohol and related conditions. *The Journal of Clinical Psychiatry, 66*(06), 677–685. https://doi.org/10.4088/JCP.v66n0602

Cooke, D. (1996). Psychopathic personality in different cultures: What do we know? What do we need to find out? *Journal of Personality Disorders, 10*(1), 23–40. https://doi.org/10.1521/pedi.1996.10.1.23

Craig, R. L., Gray, N. S., & Snowden, R. J. (2013). Recalled parental bonding, current attachment, and the triarchic conceptualisation of psychopathy. *Personality and Individual Differences, 55*(4), 345–350. https://doi.org/10.1016/j.paid.2013.03.012

Craparo, G., Schimmenti, A., & Caretti, V. (2013). Traumatic experiences in childhood and psychopathy: A study on a sample of violent offenders from Italy. *European Journal of Psychotraumatology, 4*(1), 21471–21471. https://doi.org/10.3402/ejpt.v4i0.21471

Curry, O., Chesters, M. J., & Viding, E. (2011). The psychopath's dilemma: The effects of psychopathic personality traits in one-shot games. *Personality and Individual Differences, 50*(6), 804–809. https://doi.org/10.1016/j.paid.2010.12.036

Dawkins, R., & Krebs, J. R. (1978). Animal signals: Information or manipulation. In J. R. Krebs & N. B. Davies (Eds.), *Behavioral ecology: An evolutionary approach* (pp. 282–309). Blackwell.

DeLisi, M., Angton, A., Vaughn, V. M., Trulson, R. C., Caudill, W. J., & Beaver, K. (2014). Not my fault: Blame externalization is the psychopathic feature most associated with pathological delinquency among confined delinquents. *International Journal of Offender Therapy and Comparative Criminology, 58*(12), 1415–1430. https://doi.org/10.1177/0306624X13496543

Durand, G. (2016). A replication of "Using self-esteem to disaggregate psychopathy, narcissism, and aggression (2013)". *The Quantitative Methods for Psychology, 12*(2), r1–r5. https://doi.org/10.20982/tqmp.12.2.r001

Dweck, C. S. (2017). From needs to goals and representations: Foundations for a unified theory of motivation, personality, and development. *Psychological Review, 124*(6), 689–719. https://doi.org/10.1037/rev0000082

Edens, J. F., Marcus, D. K., Lilienfeld, S. O., & Poythress, N. G., Jr. (2006). Psychopathic, not psychopath: Taxometric evidence for the dimensional structure of psychopathy. *Journal of Abnormal Psychology, 115*(1), 131–144. https://doi.org/10.1037/0021-843X.115.1.131

Egan, V. (2009, July). The main predictors of aggression: Low A, low A, and low A? *Paper presented at meeting of the International Society for the Study of Individual Differences*. Iillinois.

Ekblad, S. (1990). The children's behaviour questionnaire for completion by parents and teachers in a Chinese sample. *Journal of Child Psychology and Psychiatry, and Allied Disciplines, 31*(5), 775–791. https://doi.org/10.1111/j.1469-7610.1990.tb00817.x

Ellis, J. D., Schroder, H. S., Patrick, C. J., & Moser, J. S. (2017). Emotional Reactivity and regulation in individuals with psychopathic traits: Evidence for a disconnect between neurophysiology and self-report. *Psychophysiology*, *54*(10), 1574–1585. https://doi.org/10.1111/psyp.12903

Falkenbach, D. M., Howe, J. R., & Falki, M. (2013). Using self-esteem to disaggregate psychopathy, narcissism, and aggression. *Personality and Individual Differences*, *54*(7), 815–820. https://doi.org/10.1016/j.paid.2012.12.017

Farah, A., Amorim, I. & Chamorro-Prezumic, T. (2009). Empathy deficits and trait emotional intelligence in psychopathy. *Personality and Individual Differences*, *47*(7), 758–762. https://doi.org/10.1016/j.paid.2009.06.016

Furnham, A., Richards, S., & Paulhus, D. (2013). The Dark Triad of personality: A 10 year review. *Social and Personality Psychology Compass*, *7*(3), 199–216. https://doi.org/10.1111/spc3.12018

Gebauer, J. E., Sedikides, C., Verplanken, B., & Maio, G. R. (2012). Communal narcissism. *Journal of Personality and Social Psychology*, *103*(5), 854–878. https://doi.org/10.1037/a0029629

Gervais, M. M., Kline, M., Ludmer, M., George, R., & Manson, J. H. (2013). The strategy of psychopathy: Primary psychopathic traits predict defection on low-value relationships. *Proceedings of the Royal Society B Biological Sciences*, *280*(1757), 20122773. https://doi.org/10.1098/rspb.2012.2773

Geukes, K., Nestler, S., Hutteman, R., Dufner, M., Küfner, A. C. P., Egloff, B., Denissen, J. J. A., & Back, M. D. (2017). Puffed-up but shaky selves: State self-esteem level and variability in narcissists. *Journal of Personality and Social Psychology*, *112*(5), 769–786. https://doi.org/10.1037/pspp0000093

Giammarco, A. E., & Vernon, A. P. (2014). Vengeance and the Dark Triad: The role of empathy and perspective taking in trait forgivingness. *Personality and Individual Differences*, *67*, 23–27. https://doi.org/10.1016/j.paid.2014.02.010

Gifford, E. V., & Hayes, S. C. (1999). Functional contextualism: A pragmatic philosophy for behavioral science. In W. O'Donohue & R. Kitchener (Eds.), *Handbook of behaviorism* (pp. 285–327). Academic Press. https://doi.org/10.1016/B978-012524190-8/50012-7

Gilbert, P. (2001). Evolutionary approaches to psychopathology: The role of natural defences. *The Australian and New Zealand Journal of Psychiatry*, *35*(1), 17–27. https://doi.org/10.1046/j.1440-1614.2001.00856.x

Gilbert, P. (2005). Compassion and cruelty: A biopsychosocial approach. In P. Gilbert (Ed.), *Compassion: Conceptualisations, research and use in psychotherapy* (pp. 9–74). Routledge. https://doi.org/10.4324/9780203003459

Ghim, S. C., Choi, D. H., Lim, J. J., & Lim, S. M. (2015). The relationship between covert narcissism and relational aggression in adolescents: Mediating effects of internalized shame and anger rumination. *International Journal of Information and Education Technology*, *5*(1), 21–26. https://doi.org/10.7763/IJIET.2015.V5.469

Gray, N. S., Weidacker, K., & Snowden, R. J. (2019). Psychopathy and impulsivity: The relationship of psychopathy to different aspects of UPPS-P impulsivity. *Psychiatry Research*, *272*, 474–482. https://doi.org/10.1016/j.psychres.2018.12.155

Gray, P. (2014). *Why is narcissism increasing among young Americans? Psychology Today*. Retrieved from https://www.psychologytoday.com/us/blog/freedom-learn/201401/why-is-narcissism-increasing-among-young-americans

Greiner, N., & Nunno, V. J. (1994). Psychopaths at Nuremberg? A Rorschach analysis of the records of Nazi criminals. *Journal of Clinical Psychology*, *50*(3), 415–429. https://doi.org/10.1002/1097-4679(199405)50:3<415::AID-JCLP2270500313>3.0.CO;2-M

Gries, P., Sanders, M., Stroup, D., & Cai, H. (2015). Hollywood in China: How American popular culture shapes Chinese views of the 'Beautiful Imperialist,' an experimental analysis. *The China Quarterly*, *224*, 1070–1082. https://doi.org/10.1017/S0305741015000831

Grijalva, E., Harms, P.D., Newman, D.A., Gaddis,B.H. & Fraley, R.C. (2015). Narcissism and leadership: A meta-analytic review of linear and nonlinear relationships. *Personnel Psychology*, *68*(1), 1–47. https://doi.org/10.1111/peps.12072

Grijalva, E., & Newman, D. A. (2015). Narcissism and counterproductive work behavior (CWB): Meta-analysis and consideration of collectivist culture, Big Five personality, and narcissism's facet structure. *Applied Psychology*, *64*(1), 93–126. https://doi.org/10.1111/apps.12025

Hare, R. D. (1999). *Without conscience: The disturbing world of the psychopaths among us.* Guilford.

Hare, R. D. (2003). *The Hare Psychopathy Checklist – revised* (2nd ed.). Multi-Health Systems.

Harenski, C. L., Thornton, D. M., Harenski, K. A., Decety, J., & Kiehl, K. A. (2012). Increased frontotemporal activation during pain observation in sexual sadism: Preliminary findings. *Archives of General Psychiatry*, *69*(3), 283–299. https://doi.org/10.1001/archgenpsychiatry.2011.1566

Hepper, E. G., Hart, C. M., & Sedikides, C. (2014). Moving Narcissus: Can narcissists be empathic? *Personality & Social Psychology Bulletin*, *40*(9), 1079–1091. https://doi.org/10.1177/0146167214535812

Hoppenbrouwers, S. S., Bulten, B. H., & Brazil, I. A. (2016). Parsing fear: A reassessment of the evidence for fear deficits in psychopathy. *Psychological Bulletin*, *142*(6), 573–600. https://doi.org/10.1037/bul0000040

Horton, R. S., Bleau, G., & Drwecki, B. (2006). Parenting Narcissus: What are the links between parenting and narcissism? *Journal of Personality*, *74*(2), 345–376. https://doi.org/10.1111/j.1467-6494.2005.00378.x

Jakobwitz, S., & Egan, V. (2006). The dark triad and normal personality traits. *Personality and Individual Differences*, *40*(2), 331–339. https://doi.org/10.1016/j.paid.2005.07.006

Jaspal, R., Lopes, B., Wignall, L., & Bloxsom, C. (2021). Predicting sexual risk behavior in British and European Union university students in the United Kingdom. *American Journal of Sexuality Education.* https://doi.org/10.1080/15546128.2020.1869129

Jones, D. N., & Paulhus, D. L. (2010). Different provocations trigger aggression in narcissists and psychopaths. *Social Psychological and Personality Science*, *1*(1), 12–18. https://doi.org/10.1177/1948550609347591

Jones, D. N., & Paulhus, D. L. (2011). Differentiating the Dark Triad within the interpersonal circumplex. In L. M. Horowitz & S. Strack (eds.), *Handbook of interpersonal psychology: Theory, research, assessment, and therapeutic interventions* (pp. 249–269). Wiley & Sons. https://doi.org/10.1002/9781118001868.ch15

Kealy, D., Ogrodniczuk, J. S., Rice, S. M., & Oliffe, J. L. (2017). Pathological narcissism and maladaptive self-regulatory behaviours in a nationally representative sample of Canadian men. *Psychiatry Research*, *256*, 156–161. https://doi.org/10.1016/j.psychres.2017.06.009

Kernberg, O. (1975). *Borderline conditions and pathological narcissism.* Jason Aronson.

Kernberg, O. F., & Caligor, E. (2005). A psychoanalytic theory of personality disorders. In M. F. Lenzenweger & J. Clarkin (Eds.), *Major theories of personality disorder* (pp. 114–156). Guilford Press.

Kohut, H. (1977). *The restoration of the self.* International Universities Press.

Landay, K., Harms, P. D., & Credé, M. (2019). Shall we serve the dark lords? A meta-analytic review of psychopathy and leadership . *The Journal of Applied Psychology*, *104*(1), 183–196. https://doi.org/10.1037/apl0000357

LeBreton, J., Binning, J., & Adorno, A. (2006). Subclinical psychopaths. In J. C. Thomas & D. Segal (Eds.), *Comprehensive handbook of personality and psychopathology. Vol. 1: Personality and everyday functioning* (pp. 388–411). Wiley.

Lopes, B., & Yu, H. (2017). Who do you troll and why? An investigation into the relationship between the Dark Triad Personalities and online trolling behaviours towards popular and less popular Facebook profiles. *Computers in Human Behavior*, *77*, 69–76. https://doi.org/10.1016/j.chb.2017.08.036

Malesza, M. (2020). The effects of the Dark Triad traits in prisoner's dilemma game. *Current Psychology*, *39*(3), 1055–1062. https://doi.org/10.1007/s12144-018-9823-9

Malesza, M., & Kaczmarek, C. M. (2018). Grandiose narcissism versus vulnerable narcissism and impulsivity. *Personality and Individual Differences*, *126*, 61–65. https://doi.org/10.1016/j.paid.2018.01.021

Markus, H., & Kitayama, S. (1991). Culture and self: Implications for cognition, emotion & motivation. *Psychological Review, 98*(2), 224–253. https://doi.org/10.1037/0033-295X.98.2.224

McCain, J. L., & Campbell, W. K. (2018). Narcissism and social media use: A meta-analytical review. *Psychology of Popular Media Culture, 7*(3), 308–317. https://doi.org/10.1037/ppm0000137

Miller, J. D., Dir, A., Gentile, B., Wilson, L., Pryor, R., & Campbell, L. W. (2010). Searching for a vulnerable dark triad: Comparing factor 2 psychopathy, vulnerable narcissism, and borderline personality disorder. *Journal of Personality, 78*(5), 1529–1564. https://doi.org/10.1111/j.1467-6494.2010.00660.x

Millon, T. (1981). *Disorders of personality: DSM III: Axis II*. John Wiley.

Mischel, W., & Shoda, Y. (1995). A cognitive-affective system theory of personality: Reconceptualizing situations, dispositions, dynamics, and invariance in personality structure. *Psychological Review, 102*(2), 246–268. https://doi.org/10.1037/0033-295x.102.2.246

Morrison, D., & Gilbert, P. (2001). Social rank, shame and anger in primary and secondary psychopaths. *The Journal of Forensic Psychiatry, 12*(2), 330–356. https://doi.org/10.1080/09585180110056867

Nangyeon, L. (2016). Cultural differences in emotion: Differences in emotional arousal level between East and West. *Integrative Medicine Research, 5*(2), 105–109. https://doi.org/10.1016/j.imr.2016.03.004

Nathanson, C. (2008). *Exploring the dynamics of revenge* [Unpublished PhD dissertation. University of British Colombia]. Canada. https://open.library.ubc.ca/cIRcle/collections/ubctheses/24/items/1.0066779

Newman, J. P., & Baskin-Sommers, A. (2011). Early selective attention abnormalities in psychopathy: Implications for self-regulation. In M. Posner (Ed.), *Cognitive neuroscience of attention* (pp. 421–440). Guilford Press.

Oltmanns, T. F., & Balsis, S. (2011). Personality disorders in later life: Questions about the measurement, course, and impact of disorders. *Annual Review of Clinical Psychology, 7*, 321–349. https://doi.org/10.1146/annurev-clinpsy-090310-120435

Otway, L. J., & Vignoles, V. L. (2006). Narcissism and childhood recollections: A quantitative test of psychoanalytic predictions. *Personality & Social Psychology Bulletin, 32*(1), 104–116. https://doi.org/10.1177/0146167205279907

Park, E. (1998). *Individualism/collectivism, self-concept, and social behavior: False-uniqueness and the spiral of silence hypothesis* [Unpublished PhD dissertation, Stanford University].

Paulhus, D. L. (2001). Normal narcissism: Two minimalist accounts. *Psychological Inquiry, 12*(4), 228–230.

Paulhus, D. L., & Williams, K. M. (2002). The dark triad of personality: Narcissism, Machiavellianism, and Psychopathy. *Journal of Research in Personality, 36*(6), 556–563. https://doi.org/10.1016/S0092-6566(02)00505-6

Pendergast, T. (2000). *Creating the modern man: American magazines and consumer culture: 1900–1950*. University of Missouri Press.

Perenc, L., & Radochonski, M. (2014). Psychopathic traits and reactive-proactive aggression in a large community sample of Polish adolescents. *Child Psychiatry & Human Development, 45*(4), 464–471. https://doi.org/10.1007/s10578-013-0432-4

Persson, B. (2013). *Sub-clinical psychopathy and empathy* [Unpublished Thesis submitted to achieve the Bachelor Degree in Cognitive Neuroscience, University of Skövde], pp. 1–53. https://www.diva-portal.org/smash/record.jsf?pid=diva2%3A646254&dswid=8129

Persson, B., Kajonius, J. P., & Garcia, D. (2019). Revisiting the structure of the Short Dark Triad. *Assessment, 26*(1), 3–14. https://doi.org/10.1177/1073191117701192

Peterson, G. W., Steinmetz, S. K., & Wilson, S. M. (2003). Cultural and cross-cultural perspectives on parent-youth relations. *Marriage & Family Review, 35*(3-4), 5–19. https://doi.org/10.1300/J002v35n03_02

Piquero, A. R., Farrington, D. P., Fontaine, N. M. G., Vincent, G., Coid, J., & Ullrich, S. (2012). Childhood risk, offending trajectories, and psychopathy at age 48 years in the Cambridge

Study in Delinquent Development. *Psychology, Public Policy, and Law, 18*(4), 577–598. https://doi.org/10.1037/a0027061

Poless, P. G., Torstveit, L., Lugo, R. G., Andreassen, M., & Sütterlin, S. (2018). Guilt and proneness to shame: Unethical behaviour in Vulnerable and Grandiose Narcissism. *Europe's Journal of Psychology, 14*(1), 28–43. https://doi.org/10.5964/ejop.v14i1.1355

Porter, S., ten Brinke, L., Baker, A., & Wallace, B. (2011). Would I lie to you? "Leakage" in deceptive facial expressions relates to psychopathy and emotional intelligence. *Personality and Individual Differences, 51*(2), 133–137. https://doi.org/10.1016/j.paid.2011.03.031

Prado, E. C., Treeby, M., & Crowe, S. (2016). Examining the relationships between sub-clinical psychopathic traits with shame, guilt, and externalising response tendencies to everyday transgressions. *The Journal of Forensic Psychiatry & Psychology, 27*(4), 569–585. https://doi.org/10.1080/14789949.2016.1167933

Ritchie, T. D., Walker, W. R., Marsh, S., Hart, C., & Skowronski, J. J. (2015). Narcissism distorts the fading affect bias in autobiographical memory. *Applied Cognitive Psychology, 29*(1), 104–114. https://doi.org/10.1002/acp.3082

Ronningstam, E. (2005). *Identifying and understanding narcissistic personality*. Oxford University Press.

Ronningstam, E. (2017). Intersect between self-esteem and regulation in narcissistic personality disorder- implications for alliance building and treatment. *Borderline Personality Disorders and Emotion Dysregulation, 4*(3), 2–13. https://doi.org/10.1186/s40479-017-0054-8

Rose, P. (2007). Mediators of the association between narcissism and compulsive buying: The roles of materialism and impulse control. *Psychology of Addictive Behaviors, 21*(4), 576–581. https://doi.org/10.1037/0893-164X.21.4.576

Schalkwijk, F. W., Dekker, J., Peen, J., & Stams, J. (2016). Narcissism, self-esteem, shame regulation and juvenile delinquency. *Forensic Science & Criminology, 1*(1), 1–5. https://doi.org/10.15761/FSC.1000105

Schimmenti, A., Passanisi, A., Pace, U., Manzella, S., Di Carlo, G., & Caretti, V. (2014). The relationship between attachment and psychopathy: A study with a sample of violent offenders. *Current Psychology, 33*(3), 256–270. https://doi.org/10.1007/s12144-014-9211-z

Schulze, L., Dziobek, I., Vater, A., Heekeren, H. R., Bajbouj, M., Renneberg, B., Heuser, I., & Roepke, S. (2013). Gray matter abnormalities in patients with narcissistic personality disorder. *Journal of Psychiatric Research, 47*(10), 1363–1369. https://doi.org/10.1016/j.jpsychires.2013.05.017

Skeem, J. L., Poythress, N., Edens, J. F., Lilienfeld, S. O., & Cale, E. M. (2003). Psychopathic personality or personalities? Exploring potential variants of psychopathy and their implications for risk assessment. *Aggression and Violent Behavior, 8*(5), 513–546. https://doi.org/10.1016/S1359-1789(02)00098-8

Smolewska, K., & Dion, L. K. (2005). Narcissism and adult attachment: A multivariate approach. *Self and Identity, 4*(1), 59–68. https://doi.org/10.1080/13576500444000218

Stewart, K. D., & Bernhardt, P. C. (2010). Comparing millennials to pre-1987 students and with one another. *North American Journal of Psychology, 12*(3), 579–602.

Stinson, F. S., Dawson, D. A., Goldstein, R. B., Chou, S. P., Huang, B., Smith, S. M., Ruan, W. J., Pulay, A. J., Saha, T. D., Pickering, R. P., & Grant, B. F. (2008). Prevalence, correlates, disability, and comorbidity of DSM-IV narcissistic personality disorder: Results from the wave 2 national epidemiologic survey on alcohol and related conditions . *The Journal of Clinical Psychiatry, 69*(7), 1033–1045. https://doi.org/10.4088/jcp.v69n0701

Sukhodolsky, D. G., Golub, A., & Cromwell, E. N. (2001). Development and validation of the Anger Rumination Scale. *Personality and Individual Differences, 31*(5), 689–700. https://doi.org/10.1016/S0191-8869(00)00171-9

Triandis, H. C. (1989). The self and social behavior in different cultural contexts. *Psychological Review, 96*(3), 289–506. https://doi.org/10.1037/0033-295X.96.3.506

Vernon, P. A., Villani, V. C., Vickers, L. C., & Harris, J. A. (2008). A behavioral genetic investigation of the Dark Triad and the Big 5. *Personality and Individual Differences, 44*(2), 445–452. https://doi.org/10.1016/j.paid.2007.09.007

Vignoles, V. L., Chryssochoou, X., & Breakwell, G. M. (2000). The distinctiveness principle: Identity, meaning, and the bounds of cultural relativity. *Personality and Social Psychology Review*, 4(4), 337–354. https://doi.org/10.1207/S15327957PSPR0404_4

Vyas, K. (2015). *Psychopathic traits and everyday social behaviour* [Unpublished PhD dissertation, University College London].

White, A. B. (2014). Who cares when nobody is watching? Psychopathic traits and empathy in prosocial behaviors. *Personality and Individual Differences*, 56, 116–121. https://doi.org/10.1016/j.paid.2013.08.033

Widiger, T. A., & Lynam, D. R. (1998). Psychopathy as a variant of common personality traits: Implications for diagnosis, etiology, and pathology. In T. Millon (Ed.), *Psychopathy: Antisocial, criminal, and violent behavior* (pp. 171–187). Guilford Press.

Williams, K. M., & Paulhus, D. L. (2004). Factor structure of the Self-Report Psychopathy scale (SRP II) in nonforensic samples. *Personality and Individual Differences*, 37(4), 765–778. https://doi.org/10.1016/j.paid.2003.11.004

Wink, P. M. (1991). Two faces of narcissism. *Journal of Personality and Social Psychology*, 61(4), 590–597. https://doi.org/10.1037/0022-3514.61.4.590

Woodmass, K., & O'Connor, B. P. (2018). What is the opposite of psychopathy? A statistical and graphical exploration of the psychopathy continuum. *Personality and Individual Differences*, 131, 254–260. https://doi.org/10.1016/j.paid.2018.05.004

Youli, H., & Chang, L. (2015). A comparative study between the dark personality and the Big Five. *Canadian Social Science*, 11(1), 93–98. https://doi.org/10.3968/5715

Young, J. E. (1999). *Practitioner's resource series. Cognitive therapy for personality disorders: A schema-focused approach* (3rd ed.). Professional Resource Press/Professional Resource Exchange.

Yu, A. (1996). Ultimate life concerns, self and Chinese achievement motivation. In M. Bond (Ed.), *The handbook of Chinese psychology* (pp. 227–246). Oxford Press.

Self-Stigma Is Associated with Depression and Anxiety in a Collectivistic Context: The Adaptive Cultural Function of Self-Criticism

John Jamir Benzon R. Aruta (iD), Benedict G. Antazo, and Judith L. Paceño

ABSTRACT

Literature on the cultural psychological aspect of mental health suggests that antecedents of mental health in individualistic cultures, or societies that prioritize independence, autonomy, and personal uniqueness do not always apply in collectivistic cultures, or societies that prioritize interdependence, social connection, interpersonal harmony, and norms. The aim of the present study was to determine the mechanisms underlying the impact of self-stigma on depression and anxiety in a collectivistic culture such as the Philippines. Specifically, this study sought to examine: (1) the mediating role of self-criticism on the impact of self-stigma on depression and anxiety, and (2) the moderating role of interdependent self-construal on the impact of self-criticism on depression and anxiety in Filipinos. Surveys measuring self-stigma, self-criticism, interdependent self-construal, depression, and anxiety symptoms were administered to 312 adolescents in rural communities in the Philippines. Using structural equation modeling, findings revealed indirect effects of self-stigma on both depression and anxiety *via* self-criticism. Findings confirmed that interdependent self-construal attenuate the detrimental impact of self-criticism on depression and anxiety in collectivistic contexts. This study offers novel insights about the underlying mechanisms that operate in the impact of self-stigma on depression and anxiety symptoms among individuals in collectivist contexts. We highlight that self-criticism may have both adaptive and maladaptive functions in collectivist cultures. The study provides implications on the importance of culturally sensitive clinical interventions in preventing depression and anxiety by combating self-stigma and the negative aspect of self-criticism in collectivist cultures. Limitations and future directions are discussed.

Introduction

Global Rate of Depression and Anxiety

Mental health has emerged as a paramount public health concern in recent years. Recent research estimated that 792 million people lived with a mental health disorder, representing more than 10% of the global population (Ritchie & Roser, 2018). For example, 45 million people were diagnosed with bipolar disorder, 50 million individuals with Alzheimer's disease and other dementias, and Schizophrenia and other psychoses have been affecting approximately 20 million people across the globe (World Health Organization [WHO], 2019). With the prevalence of mental problems, anxiety and depression are considered as the most common. WHO's International Classification of Diseases (ICD-10) identifies anxiety with frequent symptoms of apprehension (worries, misfortune, lack of concentration), motor tension (restless fidgeting, tension, trembling), and autonomic overactivity (lightheadedness, sweating, epigastric discomfort). WHO (2019) described depressive symptoms as characterized by sadness, loss of interest or pleasure, feelings of guilt, low self-worth, disturbed sleep or appetite, tiredness, and low concentration. The long-lasting or recurrent effect of depression can substantially impair a person's daily functioning either at work or school and impede coping (WHO, 2019). Statistics show that around 2% to 6% or an estimated 264 million people worldwide experience depression and there could be much more who experience its milder forms. Moreover, the largest number of people experience anxiety disorders varying from 2.5% to 7% globally, with an estimated 286 million people making it the most prevalent mental health disorder (Ritchie & Roser, 2018). Despite the global rate of mental health problems, there is a paucity of studies that examines mental health problems in a wider sociocultural context. The present study aims to investigate the role of internal self-criticism on the impact of self-stigma on depression and anxiety within the cultural context in the Philippines.

Mental Health Condition in the Philippines

In the Philippines, 10% to 15% of Filipino children, aged 5 to 15, experience mental health problems, while between 17% and 20% of Filipino adults disclosed psychiatric disorders (Magtubo, 2016). The National Statistics Office revealed that mental health illnesses are the third most common form of morbidity for Filipinos reporting 88 cases of mental health problems for every 100,000 Filipinos. Despite these statistics, the figures may still be underreported due to stigma and taboo related to the country's mental health problems (Dalida et al., 2018; Rivera & Antonio, 2017). In a country where both natural and manmade disasters are common, psychological problems are probable, yet mental health has not been a top priority (Tolentino, 2004). In 2019, the Philippine Mental Health Act (RA NO. 11036) came into force to establish access to comprehensive and integrated mental health services for all Filipinos facing mental health concerns. Despite this significant progress, the country's mental health system needs to be strengthened and developed (Lally et al., 2019). There are only two mental hospitals available with an occupancy rate of about 92%, five government hospitals with psychiatric facilities intended for children, 46 outpatient facilities, and only an average of two mental health professionals per 100,000 people (WHO, 2007). Access to mental health facilities is uneven across the country, putting those in the rural areas in a more disadvantaged position. The National Center for Mental Health (NCMH), which is located in the National Capital Region (NCR), houses 77% (4200) beds for mental disorders, and the rest (22%) are distributed across the remaining regions. Similarly, 58% of the psychiatrists in the country, together with 44% board-certified specialists (Tolentino, 2004) practice in the capital region of Metro Manila (Samaniego, 2017). The lack of access to mental health services and information in the country contributes to the stigma and taboo associated with mental health (Rivera & Antonio, 2017). The present study attempts to address this limitation by focusing on individuals from rural communities in the Philippines.

Impact of Stigma on Depression and Anxiety

Stigmatized identities have been linked to engender psychological distress, predisposing people from developing mental health problems (e.g. Yen et al., 2005; Zahn et al., 2015). Stigma is defined as a form of deviance that leads others to judge an individual as illegitimate for social interaction (Brohan et al., 2010). Social cognitive models of stigma argue that stigma develops when a person holds negative mental illness stereotypes. While many researches explored prejudice and discrimination relating to mental illness (Kenny et al., 2018), interpretation of stigma has evolved and can now be categorized as public, personal, and self-stigma (Curcio & Corboy, 2020). The current study focuses on self-stigma, which is defined as the acceptance of the negative attitudes of others, which involves internalization and application of stigmatized beliefs toward the self (Corrigan & Watson, 2002). One model that offers a theoretical foundation for self-stigma research is Corrigan's Progressive Model of Self-Stigma. The model proposed that people who internalize mental health illness stigma go through four stages of internalization: stereotype awareness, personal agreement, self-concurrence, harm to self (i.e. self-esteem) (Corrigan et al., 2011), resulting in detrimental mental health consequences (Göpfert et al., 2019). Recent research (Garg & Raj, 2019) estimated that a third to half of the patients with mental disorders experience high levels of internalized stigma indicating the role of self-stigma in aggravating mental health illnesses. Past research shows that self-stigma is strongly associated with both depression (Yen et al., 2005; Zahn et al., 2015) and anxiety (Busby Grant et al., 2016). Consequently, individuals with mental health concerns avoid seeking treatment and social support (Corrigan & Matthews, 2003; Corrigan & Wassel, 2008; Vogel et al., 2007). Given that people with depression and anxiety tend to be more sensitive and vulnerable to negative stereotypes, it reflects that they tend to suffer from numerous negative mental health consequences (Ociskova et al., 2013).

Despite the ubiquitous evidence on the predictors of mental health problems such as depression and anxiety (e.g. Gao et al., 2020; Park & Kim, 2020), little progress has been made in understanding the cultural mechanisms that promote and protect people from the impact of stigma on depression and anxiety symptoms. The limited systematic research on the role of culture on developing depression and anxiety symptoms (e.g. Chen et al., 2020; Rawlings & Bains, 2020; Wong & Fisher, 2009) is a critical limitation given the global nature of these mental health concerns. The present study attempts to address this gap by examining the cultural function of self-criticism on the impact of self-stigma on depression and anxiety in a collectivistic context such as the Philippines.

Self-Criticism and Culture as Underlying Mechanisms

Self-criticism is a construct related to a negative cognitive style representing a negative evaluation of self, believing that others share one's pernicious view (Blatt, 1974). It involves constant, harsh self-evaluation, as well as a chronic fear of others' criticism, disapproval, and rejection (Blatt & Homann, 1992). Thompson and Zuroff (2004) explored the two variations of self-criticism based on Blatt's theory (1974). One form is comparative self-criticism, which involves externalized criteria operating under the belief that oneself lacks compared to others (Thompson & Zuroff, 2004). In this study, the second variation, which is the internalized self-criticism, was employed. Thompson and Zuroff (2004) described internal self-criticism as the negative view of the self that operates by a chronic sense of inferiority on one's impossibly high standards. Thus, there is no satisfaction in achieving one's personal standards.

Western theory and evidence demonstrated that people who unfairly criticize themselves for the adverse outcomes that they encounter are highly vulnerable to developing mental health problems including depression and anxiety (Abela et al., 2006; Bagby et al., 1992; Beck, 1964, 1983; Kessler et al., 1998). Internally self-critical people fit the negative outcomes to their problematic view of themselves, worsening their irrational core beliefs and increasing one's tendency to manifest depression and anxiety symptoms (Abela et al., 2006; Beck, 1964, 1983). Evidence from cultural psychology points out that findings from WEIRD (Western, Educated, Industrialized, Rich, and Democratic) countries cannot always be generalized to non-WEIRD populations due to the strong influence of sociocultural factors on several psychological constructs and processes (Heine, 2003; Markus & Kitayama, 1991). Self-construal theory (Markus & Kitayama, 1991) proposed that people from WEIRD cultures or individualistic societies, usually European countries and the US, tend to have higher independent self-construal leading them to view the self as unique and distinct from others and the social world, and place high importance on self-expression. On the other hand, people from non-WEIRD cultures or collectivistic societies, usually East Asian countries, tend to endorse an interdependent self-construal leading them to view the self as fundamentally interconnected with other people and value relationships over self-expression. We reason that self-criticism may operate differently in an interdependent culture like the Philippines due to its role in facilitating culturally-valued outcomes such as maintaining social harmony and preserving relationships (Markus & Kitayama, 1991; Yamaguchi et al., 2014). Cultural psychology proposed that self-criticism may serve an adaptive function in interdependent cultures because it allows people to reflect on their shortcomings and adjust themselves in accordance with the unwritten social rules and expectations (Heine, 2003; Heine et al., 1999; Markus & Kitayama, 1991). Taken together, we propose that in a predominantly interdependent culture like the Philippines, the detrimental influence of internal self-criticism on depression and anxiety may be weaker among those with greater levels of interdependent self-construal because of the positive social consequences that self-criticism could provide in such cultures.

The Philippine Culture

The Philippines, as an interdependent culture (Aruta, 2016, 2020; Aruta et al., 2020; Datu, 2017), places a high premium on adjusting to social norms, maintaining social face, and preserving social harmony (Aruta et al., 2019). To observe social norms, Filipinos tend to reflect on the appropriateness of their behaviors with the social environment, which requires a certain degree of self-criticism (Aruta et al., 2020). For instance, many Filipinos practice *pagninilay-nilay,* or a process of introspection and self-reflection, for the purpose of reflecting on personal mistakes and further improvement as a person (Pe-Pua & Protacio-Marcelino, 2000). To maintain social face or personal and family reputation, Filipinos are conscious about *kahihiyan,* or one's sense of propriety or embarrassment. To avoid *hiya* (embarrassment), Filipinos constantly observe whether their actions are in accordance with unwritten social expectations (Enriquez, 1994; Pe-Pua & Protacio-Marcelino, 2000). To preserve social harmony, Filipinos place great value on relationship-oriented cultural virtues such as *pakikibagay* (in conformity with others), *pakikipagkapwa-tao* (together with the person), and *pakikiramdam* (sensitivity to others' feelings and situations) to avoid interpersonal conflict and to preserve harmony in the social environment (Enriquez, 1986, 1994; Reyes, 2015). Recent research pointed out that these cultural virtues motivate Filipinos to engage in a certain degree of internal self-criticism, which provides an adaptive function to better mental health (Aruta et al., 2020). Putting together, the above-mentioned Filipino virtues may explain the importance of a certain degree of adaptive self-criticism in reaping several personal and social benefits, potentially protecting Filipinos from the negative consequences of the maladaptive manner of self-criticism on mental health.

The Present Study

Guided by the above-mentioned arguments, the present study examined the impact of self-stigma on both depression and anxiety symptoms using Filipino samples. We hypothesized that people who internalize greater levels of mental health stigma experience worse depression and anxiety symptoms. Further, we investigated the mediating role of internal self-criticism in these relationships and predicted that those who endorse higher levels of self-stigma would report greater depression and anxiety due to an increase in one's tendency to unfairly criticize oneself based on one's idealistic and unattainable standards. Finally, we examined whether interdependent self-construal moderated the influence of internal self-criticism on both depression and anxiety in the context of an interdependent culture like the Philippines.

Anchored on Self-Construal Theory (Markus & Kitayama, 1991), we reasoned that the deleterious impact of internal self-criticism on both depression and anxiety would be weaker among people with higher levels of interdependent self-construal due to the adaptive social function of self-criticism (e.g. adjusting behavior according to norms, maintaining social harmony) in interdependent cultures like the Philippines. On the other hand, we predicted that the inimical influence of internal self-criticism on depression and anxiety would be more substantial among those with lower levels of interdependent self-construal. To our knowledge, this is the first study that examined the mediating role of internal self-criticism on the impact of self-stigma on both depression and anxiety, and the moderating role of interdependent construal on the impact of internal self-criticism on both depression and anxiety in Filipino samples. We believe that looking at the cultural aspect of how self-stigma influences both depression and anxiety is an imperative pursuit given their global nature and prevalence. Simply put, we proposed the following hypotheses:

Hypothesis 1: Higher self-stigma will positively predict greater symptoms of depression and anxiety.

Hypothesis 2: Higher internal self-criticism will mediate the impact of higher self-stigma on greater symptoms of depression and anxiety.

Hypothesis 3: Higher interdependent self-construal will moderate the impact of higher internal self-criticism on greater symptoms of depression and anxiety.

Method

Participants and Procedures

Initial sample size was computed using G*Power 3.1.9.2 (Faul et al., 2009) with $\beta = .99$, $\alpha = .001$, and $f^2 = .15$, which suggested a minimum of 277 respondents. To account for potential errors, additional participants were included resulting in an initial sample size of $n = 319$. Seven invalid and incomplete responses were removed resulting in a total of $n = 312$. Post-hoc power analysis revealed $\beta = .9967$. There were 116 males (37.2%) and 196 females (62.8%) with ages ranging from 18 to 34 years (Mean = 19.62, SD = 2.53). All participants were residing in rural areas in the Philippines. Filipinos who are at least 18 years old were invited to participate in the study. The study was conducted in accordance with the Helsinki Declaration as revised 1989. Ethics and data collection were approved by the administration of Cavite State University-General Trias Campus. After securing the informed consent, the participants completed a paper-and-pencil format questionnaire containing informed consent, demographic questions, and measures for internal self-criticism, relational-interdependent self-construal, self-stigma, depression, and anxiety. All measures were administered in English since Filipinos, especially university students, are bilinguals making them skilled users of both Filipino and English languages (Bernardo, 2005).

Instruments

Self-Stigma of Seeking Help (SSOSH; Vogel et al., 2006)

The SSOSH was used to measure the extent to which the participants internalize and apply stigma toward the self. It is a unidimensional instrument consisting of 10 items measured on a 5-point likert scale (1 = *strongly disagree*; 5 = *strongly agree*), with higher values indicating higher levels of self-stigma. One sample item is, "I would feel worse about myself if I could not solve my own problems." Past studies have used SSOSH as a valid tool in assessing self-stigma using Filipino samples (Tuliao, 2018). Previous studies have confirmed the factor structure of the SSOSH (Vogel et al., 2013), with alpha coefficients ranging from .75 to .81 (Shi et al., 2020; Zuo & Ai, 2011). For the current study, SSOSH yielded an overall reliability of $\alpha = .67$, suggesting adequate reliability.

Levels of Self-Criticism Scale (LOSC; Thompson & Zuroff, 2004)

The LOSC was used to measure the degree of dysfunctional forms of negative evaluation that a person endorses. It comprises the comparative self-criticism (CSC; 12 items) and internal self-criticism (ISC; 10 items) subscales. In the present paper, we used only the ISC subscale to assess the extent to which Filipinos criticize oneself based on an idealistic set of standards. One sample item is, "I am very frustrated when I don't meet the standards I have for myself." Participant responses were measured on a 7-point likert scale (1 = *strongly disagree*; 7 = *strongly agree*), with higher scores indicating greater levels of internal self-criticism. Past studies supported the validity of the internal self-criticism subscale in measuring internally directed negative evaluations across 13 countries (Halamova et al., 2018). More recent research utilized the ISC domain of LOSC to measure internal self-criticism among Filipino adolescents (Aruta et al., 2020). In an earlier study, reliability analyses of the ISC subscale resulted in α = .87 to α = .90 (Castilho et al., 2015; Joeng & Turner, 2015). In the current study, ISC subscale yielded an overall reliability of α = .82, suggesting high internal consistency.

Depression Anxiety and Stress Scale (DASS-42; Lovibond & Lovibond, *1995*)

The DASS-42 was utilized to measure the degree of psychological distress that individuals experience. It consists of the depression, anxiety, and stress subscales containing 14 items per dimension. In the present study, depression and anxiety subscales were used to measure the degree to which the participants experience symptoms of depression and anxiety. Sample items for the depression and anxiety subscales are "I couldn't seem to experience any positive feeling at all" and "I felt scared without any good reason", respectively. Participants indicated the extent to which each item applied to them over the past week and responded on a 4-point likert scale (0 = *did not apply to me at all*; 3 = *applied to me very much or most of the time*), with higher scores indicating greater levels of depression and anxiety symptoms. Previous studies have confirmed the validity of the three-factor structure of the DASS-42 (Habibi et al., 2017), with reliability estimates ranging from α = .89 to α = .95 for depression subscale and α = .85 to α = .90 for anxiety subscale (Adetunji & Ademuyiwa, 2019; Widyana & Safitri, 2020). DASS-42 has been used to assess depression, anxiety, and stress symptoms using Filipino samples (Labrague, 2014). In the present study, depression and anxiety subscales yielded high reliabilities of α = .94 and α = .89, respectively.

Relational Interdependent Self-Construal Scale (RISCS; Cross et al., 2000)

The RISCS was used to assess the extent to which an individual defines oneself as interconnected with social others. It is a unidimensional instrument consisting of 11 items and measured on a 7-point likert scale (1 = *strongly disagree*; 7 = *strongly agree*), with higher values indicating greater degrees of interdependent self-construal. A sample item is, "When I feel very close to someone, it often feels to me like that person is an important part of who I am." Past literature has supported the single-factor structure of RISCS in a Turkish sample (Akın et al., 2010). A recent study employed RISCS to assess the level of interdependent self-construal among Filipino university students (Aruta, 2016), yielding an overall reliability of α = .68. In the current research, the RISCS yielded an alpha coefficient of α = .68, suggesting adequate reliability.

Table 1. Descriptive Statistics and Bivariate Analysis.

Scale	SSOSH	ISC	RISCS	DEP	ANX
SSOSH	–				
ISC	.22***	–			
RISCS	−.02	.30***	–		
DEP	.34***	.38***	.06	–	
ANX	.36***	.32***	.04	.83***	–
M	2.80	4.76	4.97	.95	.94
SD	.43	.95	.67	.68	.57
Alpha	.67	.82	.68	.94	.89

***$p < .001$.

Note: SSOSH = Self-stigma, ISC = Internal self-criticism, RISCS = Interdependent self-construal, DEP = Depression, ANX = Anxiety, M = Mean, SD = Standard deviation.

Data Analysis

Descriptive statistics and bivariate correlations were used as preliminary analyses. Alpha coefficients were used to determine the reliability of the measures. Using structural equation modeling, we conducted a moderated mediation analyses to test our hypotheses through the use of R Statistical Package (R Core Team, 2020), with the packages QuantPsyc (Fletcher, 2012), rockchalk (Johnson, 2019), lavaan (Rosseel, 2012), and semTools (Jorgensen et al., 2020).

Results

Descriptive Statistics and Preliminary Analysis

Descriptive statistics (means and standard deviations) and correlations among the variables are shown in Table 1. Bivariate correlations among the variables show that self-stigma was significantly and positively correlated with internal self-criticism ($r = .22$), depression ($r = .34$), and anxiety ($r = .36$). In addition, internal self-criticism was significantly and positively associated with both depression ($r = .38$) and anxiety ($r = .32$). On the other hand, interdependent self-construal was not related with both depression ($r = .06$) and anxiety ($r = .04$).

Goodness of fit was examined using comparative fit index (CFI), Tucker-Lewis index (TLI), root mean square error approximation (RMSEA), and standardized root mean square residual (SRMR). CFI and TLI values of $\geq .90$ and RMSEA and SRMR values of $\leq .08$ suggest adequate fit, while CFI and TLI values of $\geq .95$ and RMSEA and SRMR values of $\leq .05$ suggest good model fit (Byrne, 2013; Hu & Bentler, 1999). Findings from the initial model indicated poor model fit across several indices ($\chi2 = 306.990$, df $= 10$, $p < .000$, CFI $= .403$, TLI $= −.672$, SRMR $= .098$, RMSEA [90% CI] $= .309$ [.279, .339]). To improve fit, depression and anxiety were allowed to covary. The modified model resulted in a good fit ($\chi2 = 13.981$, df $= 9$, $p < .123$, CFI $= .990$, TLI $= .969$, SRMR $= .033$, RMSEA [90% CI] $= .042$ [.000, .083]).

Moderated Mediation Model

To test our hypotheses, we used structural equation modeling. Figure 1 shows the path analyses indicating a significant and positive direct effect of self-stigma on both

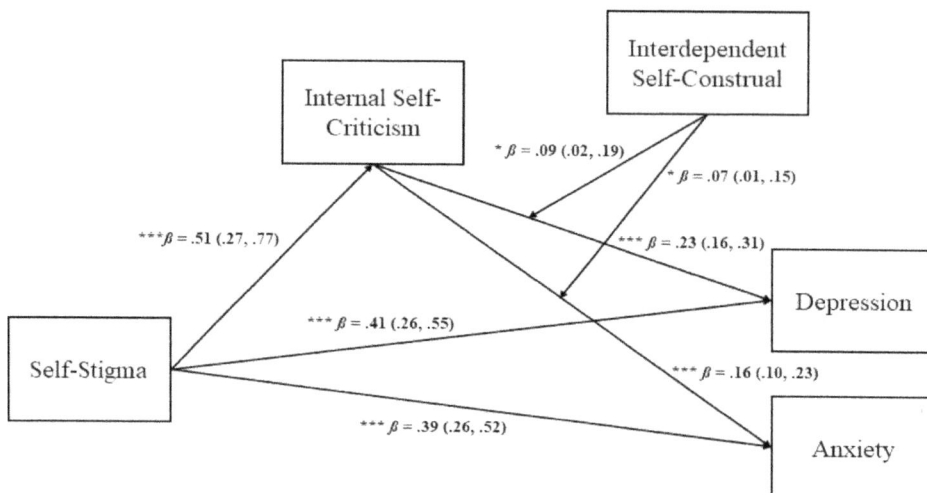

Figure 1. Final moderated mediation model indicating the influence of self-stigma on depression and anxiety in Filipinos.

Table 2. Direct, Indirect, Interaction, and Total Effects on Depression and Anxiety.

	Depression						Anxiety					
					95% CI						95% CI	
Direct effects	ß	SE	t	p	LL	UL	ß	SE	t	p	LL	UL
Self-stigma	.41	.08	5.40	<.001	.26	.55	.39	.07	5.94	<.001	.26	.52
ISCrit	.23	.03	5.95	<.001	.15	.31	.16	.03	4.85	<.001	.09	.23
ISC	−.03	.05	−0.49	.62	−.13	.07	−.02	.04	−0.51	.61	−.11	.07
Indirect effects												
Self-stigma via ISCrit	.05	.03	(z)1.75		.01	.12	.04	.02	(z)1.71		.01	.09
Interaction effects												
ISCrit x ISC	.09	.04	2.13	<.05	.02	.19	.07	.03	2.13	<.05	.01	.15
Total effects	.05	.07	(z)6.09		.31	.60	.43	.06	(z)6.62		.30	.55

Note: ISCrit = internal self-criticism, ISC = interdependent self-construal, CI = confidence interval, LL = lower limit, UL = upper limit.

depression ($ß = .41$, $p < .001$) and anxiety ($ß = .39$, $p < .001$). Moreover, Table 2 presents the mediation analyses indicating significant indirect effects of self-stigma on both depression ($ß = .05$, CI $= .01$, .12) and anxiety ($ß = .04$, CI $= .01$, .09) via internal self-criticism. Specifically, self-stigma significantly and positively influenced internal self-criticism ($ß = .51$, $p < .001$), and internal self-criticism, in turn, significantly and positively predicted both depression ($ß = .23$, $p < .001$) and anxiety ($ß = .16$, $p < .001$). Results yielded significant total effects on depression ($ß = .05$, CI $= .31$, .60) and anxiety ($ß = .43$, CI $= .30$, .55).

Significant positive influence of internal self-criticism on both depression and anxiety were found as stated above. However, we found no direct effects of interdependent self-construal on both depression ($ß = −.03$, $p = .62$) and anxiety ($ß = −.02$, $p = .61$). Interestingly, moderation analyses revealed that there is a significant interaction effects between internal self-criticism and interdependent self-construal on both depression ($ß = .09$, $p < .05$) and anxiety ($ß = .07$, $p < .05$). In particular, Table 3 shows that the conditional impact of internal self-criticism on depression and anxiety vary and remain

Table 3. Conditional Effects of Internal Self-Criticism on Depression and Anxiety Symptoms across the Levels of Interdependent Self-Construal.

	Depression					Anxiety				
				95% CI					95% CI	
Levels of ISC	ß	SE	t	LL	UL	ß	SE	t	LL	UL
−1 SD (low)	.31***	.05	6.49	.22	.41	.22***	.04	5.45	.14	.30
Mean (moderate)	.25***	.04	6.51	.18	.33	.18***	.03	5.37	.11	.25
+ 1 SD (high)	.19***	.04	4.20	.10	.28	.13***	.04	3.34	.05	.20

***$p < .001$.

Note: ISC = interdependent self-construal, CI = confidence interval, LL = lower limit, UL = upper limit, SD = standard deviation.

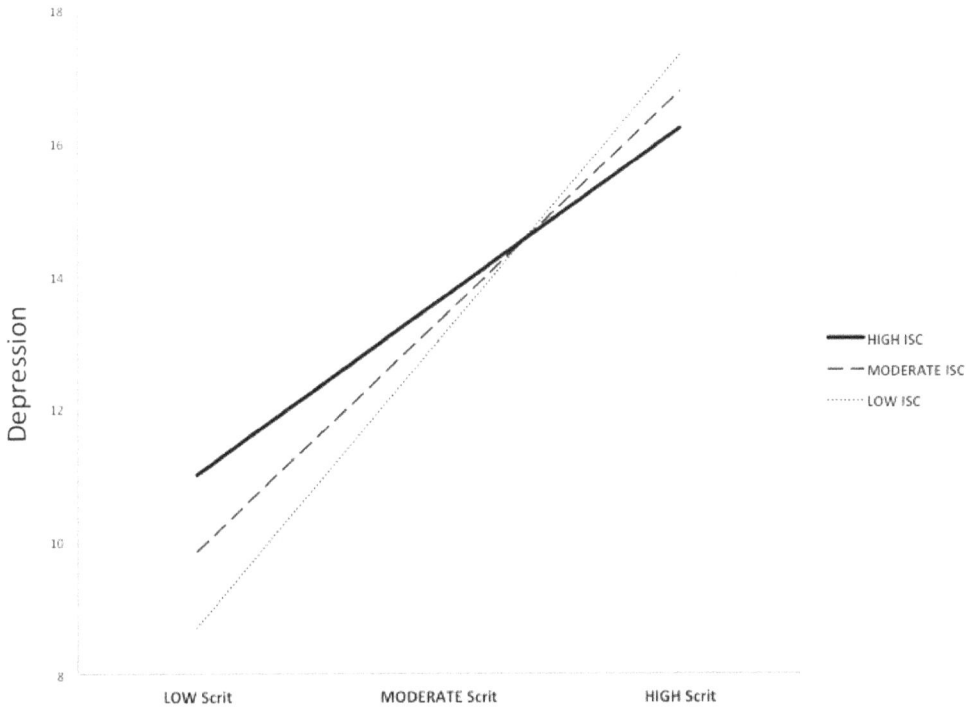

Figure 2. Graphical representation of the interaction effect between internal self-criticism and interdependent self-construal on depression symptoms. Note: Scrit = Internal self-criticism, ISC = Interdependent self-construal.

significant across the different levels of interdependent self-construal as follows: (1) there is a stronger impact of internal self-criticism on both depression ($ß = .31$, $p < .001$) and anxiety ($ß = .22$, $p < .001$) when interdependent self-construal was at lower levels; (2) weaker impact of internal self-criticism on both depression ($ß = .25$, $p < .001$) and anxiety ($ß = .18$, $p < .001$) when interdependent self-construal was at moderate levels, and; 3) weakest impact of internal self-criticism on both depression ($ß = .19$, $p < .001$) and anxiety ($ß = .13$, $p < .001$) when interdependent self-construal was at higher levels. Moreover, Figure 2 and 3 elaborate that depression and anxiety symptoms were greater among individuals with higher levels of internal self-criticism and that the symptoms further increases among those with lower levels of interdependent

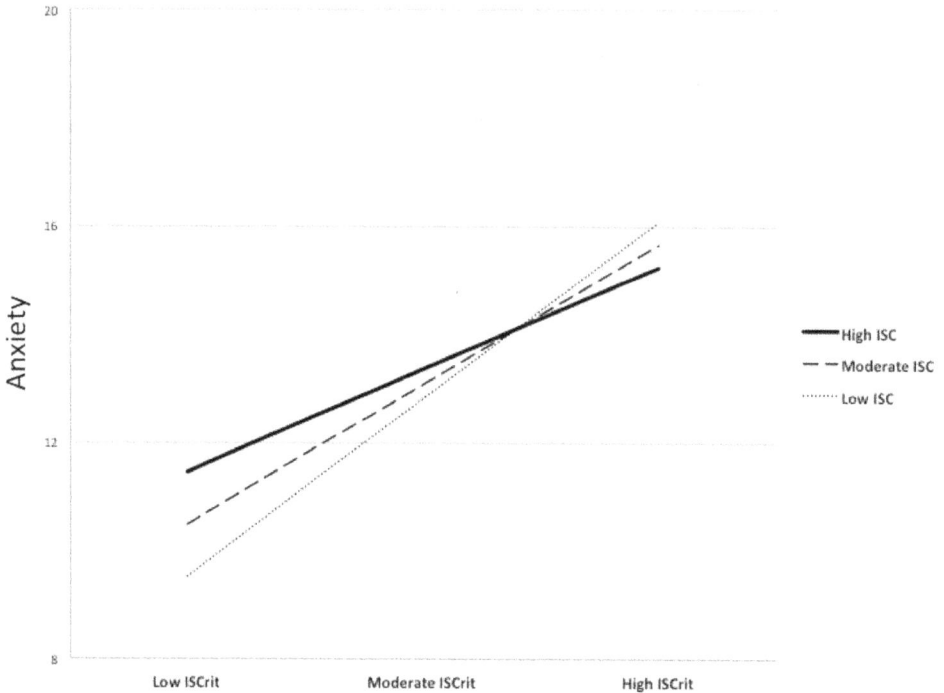

Figure 3. Interaction effect between internal self-criticism and interdependent self-construal on anxiety symptoms. Note: IScrit = internal self-criticism, ISC = interdependent self-construal.

self-construal. On the other hand, depression and anxiety symptoms of highly self-critical individuals tend to be lower among those with higher levels of interdependent self-construal.

Self-stigma, age, and gender accounted for 6%, 1.5%, and .1% of the variance in depression, and 7.7%, .9%, and .2% of the variance in anxiety, respectively. The addition of the internal self-criticism, interdependent self-construal, and the interaction term provided an increase of approximately 8.8%, .06%, and 1.1% of the variance in depression, and 6.1%, .06%, and .2% of the variance in anxiety, respectively. In total, the whole model accounted for 23.67% of the variance in depression and 21.11% of the variance in anxiety. Using Cohen's f^2, moderate effect sizes in depression ($f^2 = .31$) and anxiety ($f^2 = .27$) were achieved. We set age and gender as covariates in order to control for their effects.

Discussion

The overarching goal of the present study was to determine how self-stigma predicts depression and anxiety symptoms among Filipinos. In particular, we examined the mediating role of internal self-criticism in these associations, and whether interdependent self-construal moderates the detrimental impact of internal self-criticism on depression and anxiety. Overall, our findings showed that self-stigma increases depression and anxiety symptoms due to an increase in internal self-criticism. In addition, we also highlight that the extent to which internal self-criticism impacts depression and anxiety vary across people's level of interdependent self-construal.

Key Findings

Detrimental Impact of Self-Stigma on Mental Health

The first notable finding of the present study was that self-stigma positively predicts depression and anxiety, confirming Hypothesis 1. Consistent with previous research (Ali et al., 2015; Cruwys & Gunaseelan, 2016), our findings showed that people who carry internalized stigma about mental health tend to experience worse depressive symptoms, suggesting that applying negative perceptions and attitudes about mental health to oneself could increase one's vulnerability to developing sadness, hopelessness, fatigue, and other depression symptoms. Past findings showed that this detrimental impact of internalized stigma on depression applies even among people with intellectual disabilities (Ali et al., 2015). In addition, stigma was also found to increase suicidal thoughts among South African adolescents with HIV (Casale et al., 2019). Moreover, recent findings showed that self-stigma leads to worse psychological outcomes among Israeli Arabs with depression (Abo-Rass et al., 2020).

Moreover, our findings showed that individuals with higher levels of self-stigma tend to experience greater levels of anxiety symptoms. This finding corroborated with past studies (Ali et al., 2015) demonstrating that people who apply mental health stigma upon themselves are more prone to experiencing excessive worrying and anticipating negative future events. In support to this, a recent systematic review of research findings ($N = 17,066$) showed that individuals with anxiety problems endorsing self-stigma tend to have poorer treatment outcomes (Curcio & Corboy, 2020). Taken together, the findings of the present study provided support to previous research on the deleterious effect of self-stigma on people's mental health. In addition, our findings showed that the influence of self-stigma on both depression and anxiety may also apply in the context of individuals in rural communities in the Philippines.

Impact of Internal Self-Criticism on Mental Health

Extending this line of research, we found that internal self-criticism mediated the impact of self-stigma on both depression and anxiety—confirming Hypothesis 2. In other words, individuals who internalize the negative stereotypes about mental health may develop excessive criticisms toward oneself, which may in turn lead to worse depressive and anxiety symptoms. Both theory and research showed confluence that people who evaluate the self based on one's own idealistic set of standards are more prone to developing depression and anxiety (Abela et al., 2006; Beck, 1983; Joeng & Turner, 2015). Beck (1964, 1983) explained that internally self-critical people have a strong proclivity to selectively process negative things that fit one's problematic self-view. In addition, individuals with greater levels of internal self-criticism tend to blame themselves when outcomes are not in accordance with expectations resulting in higher levels of depression and anxiety (Beck, 1983). Our findings elucidated that people who apply the stigma on mental health upon themselves may develop greater levels of sadness, emotional fatigue, worthlessness, irritability, excessive worrying, and irrational anticipation of future negative events due to the tendency to unfairly criticize oneself and the proclivity to over-emphasize one's shortcomings and limitations.

The Culturally Adaptive Function of Internal Self-Criticism

We highlight that the most critical finding of the present study was that interdependent self-construal attenuate the inimical impact of internal self-criticism on both depression and anxiety among Filipinos, confirming Hypothesis 3. Specifically, our findings explicated that the impact of internal self-criticism on depression and anxiety tends to be stronger in people with lower levels of interdependent self-construal. Furthermore, our findings demonstrated that the impact of internal self-criticism on depression and anxiety tends to be weaker and weakest among people with moderate and higher levels of interdependent self-construal, respectively. Consistent with previous studies (e.g. Yamaguchi et al., 2014), our findings showed that self-reflection and certain levels of emphasis on one's shortcomings could provide personal and social benefits in people in interdependent cultures as self-criticism is necessary for adjusting oneself in accordance to unwritten social norms (Aruta et al., 2020; English & Chen, 2007). Consequently, the fulfillment of social norms and preservation of interpersonal relationships provide a wide ray of psychological benefits including better well-being (Roxas et al., 2019), greater happiness (Hitokoto & Uchida, 2015), and reduced psychological distress (Yamaguchi et al., 2014). Simply put, a certain degree of self-criticism can serve an adaptive function toward self-improvement and preservation of social relationships in a predominantly interdependent culture (Markus & Kitayama, 1991; Yamaguchi et al., 2014; Yamaguchi & Kim, 2013).

There are Filipino values that could explain Filipinos' strong motivation to preserve social harmony through self-reflection and self-criticism. For instance, Filipino values such as *hiya* (embarrassment) or *kahihiyan* (propriety or embarrassment), *pakikipag-kapwa-tao* (together with the person), *pakikiramdam* (sensitivity to others' feelings and situations), and *pakikibagay* (conforming with others) encourage an individual to observe unwritten social expectations and cultural norms (Enriquez, 1986, 1994; Pe-Pua & Protacio-Marcelino, 2000). One's failure to practice these relationship-oriented virtues could lead to interpersonal conflict, negative evaluation from others, and loss of social face, among others. For instance, a person who act inappropriately with the social rules may be called as *walang hiya* (or lacking a sense of propriety) or *kahiya-hiya* (embarrassing), which could damage personal and family reputation (Enriquez, 1986, 1994; Pe-Pua & Protacio-Marcelino, 2000). Furthermore, a person's lack of sensitivity to other people's circumstances and lack of observance of socially acceptable behaviors may be labeled as *walang pakikipagkapwa-tao* (or lack of concern with social others), which could result in social isolation and unfavorable impressions from other people (Reyes, 2015). Through *pagninilay-nilay* (introspection and self-reflection), these Filipino values can be fulfilled by practicing a certain degree of self-criticism (Pe-Pua & Protacio-Marcelino, 2000), allowing a person to adjust one's behavior in accordance to social norms and to preserve social relationships (Aruta et al., 2019). Given the high premium placed on social harmony among people in interdependent cultures like the Philippines (Aruta et al., 2020; Heine, 2003; Heine et al., 1999; Hitokoto & Uchida, 2015; Markus & Kitayama, 1991), it is not surprising why criticizing oneself to maintain social harmony can be functional and beneficial. This finding is consistent with our previous argument that internal self-criticism among people in interdependent cultures may not operate similarly with Western formulations.

However, we clarify that the findings should not be interpreted that internal self-criticism is absolutely adaptive in interdependent cultures. Our findings indicate that in a culture that is predominantly interdependent, internal self-criticism can lead to greater depression and anxiety symptoms among individuals with lower interdependent self-construal suggesting that lack of alignment of personal values with the predominant cultural values might lead to deleterious impact on one's mental health.

Limitations and Future Research

Through its limitations, the present study offers several opportunities for future research. First, the participants were based in rural communities and were mostly adolescents limiting the generalizability of the findings. Future studies may consider using representative samples by involving participants from urban and rural areas across age groups and socioeconomic status. Second, the current study does not claim causal relationships among the variables studied due to the correlational nature of the findings. Researchers in the future may consider conducting controlled experimental studies to establish cause and effect. Third, the study was conducted in one cultural context. Testing the cultural proposition of the present study across countries may provide further insights on how self-stigma and internal self-criticism contribute to depression and anxiety.

Implications

The present study offers several implications to clinical practice through culturally sensitive mental health prevention and intervention, recommending insights on the prevention and reduction of the harmful impact of self-stigma and internal self-criticism on both depression and anxiety in interdependent cultural contexts. Firstly, interventions that aim to reduce self-stigma and other forms of stigma toward mental health should be developed. Our findings indicate that the detrimental impact of self-stigma may also apply in collectivistic cultures like the Philippines. Secondly, our findings showed that the level of internal self-criticism mediates the impact of self-stigma on both depression and anxiety. Clinical interventions that assist clients in combating unfair and biased self-evaluation could help in preventing and reducing symptoms of depression and anxiety. Thirdly, the current research recommends that implementing clinical approaches and programs that emphasize the social and psychological benefits of self-criticism by aiming for self and behavioral improvement is indeed necessary. Our findings indicate that criticizing one's self for the purpose of social harmony may lower one's vulnerability to depression and anxiety in collectivist contexts. Lastly, our findings could inform several mental health professions on the importance of placing the clients' cultural context as an integral part of case conceptualization, assessment, treatment planning, and treatment implementation. Our findings elucidated that there is a protective function of interdependent self-construal against the detrimental impact of self-stigma and internal self-criticism on depression and anxiety among individuals in interdependent cultures like the Philippines.

Acknowledgements

The authors would like to thank Alelie Briones-Diato for the assistance in the data collection.

Disclosure statement

The authors declared that there are no competing interests in the study.

Funding

There is no funding source for this study.

ORCID

John Jamir Benzon R. Aruta ⓘ http://orcid.org/0000-0003-4155-1063

References

Abela, J. R., Webb, C. A., Wagner, C., Ho, M. R., & Adams, P. (2006). The role of self-criticism, dependency, and hassles in the course of depressive illness: A multiwave longitudinal study. *Personality & Social Psychology Bulletin*, *32*(3), 328–338. https://doi.org/doi:https://doi.org/10.1177/0146167205280911

Abo-Rass, F., Shinan-Altman, S., & Werner, P. (2020). Health-related quality of life among Israeli Arabs diagnosed with depression: The role of illness representations, self-stigma, self-esteem, and age. *Journal of Affective Disorders*, *274*, 282–288. https://doi.org/10.1016/j.jad.2020.05.125

Adetunji, A. A., & Ademuyiwa, J. A. (2019). Assessing DASS-42 models among polytechnic staff. *Open Access Library Journal*, *6*, e5334. https://doi.org/10.4236/oalib.1105334

Akı n, A., Eroğlu, Y., Kayı ş, A. R., & Satı cı, S. A. (2010). The validity and reliability of the Turkish version of the relational-interdependent self-construal scale. *Procedia - Social and Behavioral Sciences*, *5*, 579–584. https://doi.org/10.1016/j.sbspro.2010.07.145

Ali, A., King, M., Strydom, A., & Hassiotis, A. (2015). Self-reported stigma and symptoms of anxiety and depression in people with intellectual disabilities: Findings from a cross sectional study in England. *Journal of Affective Disorders, 187,* 224–231. https://doi.org/10.1016/j.jad.2015.07.046

Aruta, J. J. B. (2016). Understanding the structure of autonomy among Filipino adolescents. *Educational Measurement and Evaluation Research, 7,* 37–49.

Aruta, J. J. B. (2020). Connectedness to nature encourages, but materialism hinders, ecological behavior in the Philippines: The higher-order and second-order factors of environmental attitudes as viable mediating pathways. *Ecopsychology.* https://doi.org/10.1089/eco.2020.0053

Aruta, J. J. B., Barretto, D. I., Shin, Y., & Jang, A. (2019). The experience of power in teacher student relationships in collectivistic context. *Psychological Studies, 64*(3), 316–331. https://doi.org/10.1007/s12646-019-00523-0

Aruta, J. J. B. R., Antazo, B., Briones-Diato, A., Crisostomo, K., Canlas, N. F., & Peñaranda, G. (2020). When does self-criticism lead to depression in collectivistic context. *International Journal for the Advancement of Counselling.* https://doi.org/10.1007/s10447-020-09418-6

Bagby, R., Cox, B. J., Schuller, D. R., Levitt, A. J., Swinson, R. P., & Joffe, R. T. (1992). Diagnostic specificity of the dependent and self-critical personality dimensions in major depression. *Journal of Affective Disorders, 26*(1), 59–63. https://doi.org/10.1016/01650327(92)90035-5

Beck, A. T. (1964). Thinking and depression. II. Theory and therapy. *Archives of General Psychiatry, 10,* 561–571. https://doi.org/10.1001/archpsyc.1964.01720240015003

Beck, A. T. (1983). Cognitive therapy of depression: New perspectives. In P. J. Clayton & J. E. Barett (Eds.), *Treatment of depression: Old controversies and new approaches* (pp. 265–284). Raven Press.

Bernardo, A. B. (2005). Bilingual code-switching as a resource for learning and teaching: Alternative reflections on the language and education issue in the Philippines. In D. T. Dayag & J. S. Quakenbush (Eds.), *Linguistics and language education in the Philippines and beyond: A Festschrift in honor of Ma. Lourdes S. Bautista* (pp. 151–169). Linguistic Society of the Philippines.

Blatt, S. J. (1974). Levels of object representation in anaclitic and introjective depression. *The Psychoanalytic Study of the Child, 29*(1), 107–157. https://doi.org/10.1080/00797308.1974.11822616

Blatt, S. J., & Homann, E. (1992). Parent-child interaction in the etiology of dependent and self-critical depression. *Clinical Psychology Review, 12*(1), 47–91. https://doi.org/10.1016/0272-7358(92)90091-L

Brohan, E., Slade, M., Clement, S., & Thornicroft, G. (2010). Experiences of mental illness stigma, prejudice and discrimination: A review of measures. *BMC Health Services Research, 10*(1), 80–11. https://doi.org/10.1186/1472-6963-10-80

Busby Grant, J., Bruce, C. P., & Batterham, P. J. (2016). Predictors of personal, perceived and self-stigma towards anxiety and depression. *Epidemiology and Psychiatric Sciences, 25*(3), 247–254. https://doi.org/10.1017/S2045796015000220

Byrne, B. M. (2013). *Structural equation modeling with LISREL, PRELIS, and SIMPLIS: Basic concepts, applications, and programming.* Psychology Press.

Casale, M., Boyes, M., Pantelic, M., Toska, E., & Cluver, L. (2019). Suicidal thoughts and behaviour among South African adolescents living with HIV: Can social support buffer the impact of stigma? *Journal of Affective Disorders, 245,* 82–90. https://doi.org/10.1016/j.jad.2018.10.102

Castilho, P., Pinto-Gouveia, J., & Duarte, J. (2015). Exploring self-criticism: confirmatory factor analysis of the FSCRS in clinical and nonclinical samples. *Clinical Psychology & Psychotherapy, 22*(2), 153–164. https://doi.org/10.1002/cpp.1881

Chen, S., Burton, C. L., & Bonanno, G. A. (2020). The suppression paradox: A cross-cultural comparison of suppression frequency, suppression ability, and depression. *Journal of Affective Disorders, 274,* 183–189. https://doi.org/10.1016/j.jad.2020.05.126

Corrigan, P., & Matthews, A. (2003). Stigma and disclosure: Implications for coming out of the closet. *Journal of Mental Health, 12*(3), 235–248. https://doi.org/10.1080/0963823031000118221

Corrigan, P. W., Rafacz, J., & Rüsch, N. (2011). Examining a progressive model of self-stigma and its impact on people with serious mental illness. *Psychiatry Research, 189*(3), 339–343. https://doi.org/10.1016/j.psychres.2011.05.024

Corrigan, P. W., & Wassel, A. (2008). Understanding and influencing the stigma of mental illness. *Journal of Psychosocial Nursing and Mental Health Services, 46*(1), 42–48. https://doi.org/10.3928/02793695-20080101-04

Corrigan, P. W., & Watson, A. C. (2002). Understanding the impact of stigma on people with mental illness. *World Psychiatry: Official Journal of the World Psychiatric Association (WPA), 1*(1), 16–20.

Cross, S. E., Bacon, P. L., & Morris, M. L. (2000). The relational-interdependent self-construal and relationships. *Journal of Personality and Social Psychology, 78*(4), 791–808. https://doi.org/10.1037/0022-3514.78.4.791

Cruwys, T., & Gunaseelan, S. (2016). "Depression is who I am": Mental illness identity, stigma and wellbeing. *Journal of Affective Disorders, 189*, 36–42. https://doi.org/10.1016/j.jad.2015.09.012

Curcio, C., & Corboy, D. (2020). Stigma and anxiety disorders: A systematic review. *Stigma and Health, 5*(2), 125–137. https://doi.org/10.1037/sah0000183

Dalida, J. E. D., Aruta, J. J. B., Mercado, I. V., & Poovathinkal, J. R. (2018). Experiences and attitudes of Filipino gay men towards counseling. *The Guidance Journal, 45*(1), 16–28.

Datu, J. A. D. (2017). Sense of relatedness is linked to higher grit in a collectivist setting. *Personality and Individual Differences, 105,* 135–138. https://doi.org/10.1016/j.paid.2016.09.039

English, T., & Chen, S. (2007). Culture and self-concept stability: Consistency across and within contexts among Asian Americans and European Americans. *Journal of Personality and Social Psychology, 93*(3), 478–490. https://doi.org/10.1037/0022-3514.93.3.478

Enriquez, V. G. (1986). Kapwa: A core concept in Filipino social psychology. In A. Aganon & S. M. Assumpta David (Eds.), *Sikolohiyang Pilipino: Isyu, Pananaw, at Kaalaman (New directions 266 ALLWOOD AND BERRY in indigenous psychology)*. National Book Store.

Enriquez, V. G. (1994). *Pagbabangong-dangal: Psychology and cultural empowerment*. Akademya ng Kultura at Sikolohiyang Pilipino.

Faul, F., Erdfelder, E., Buchner, A., & Lang, A. G. (2009). Statistical power analyses using G* Power 3.1: Tests for correlation and regression analyses. *Behavior Research Methods, 41*(4), 1149–1160. https://doi.org/10.3758/BRM.41.4.1149

Fletcher, T. D. (2012). *QuantPsyc: Quantitative psychology tools* (R package Version 1.5). https://CRAN.R-project.org/package=QuantPsyc

Gao, W., Ping, S., & Liu, X. (2020). Gender differences in depression, anxiety, and stress among college students: A longitudinal study from China. *Journal of Affective Disorders, 263*, 292–300.https://doi.org/10.1016/j.jad.2019.11.121

Garg, R., & Raj, R. (2019). A cross-sectional study of self-stigma and discrimination among patients with depression. *Open Journal of Psychiatry & Allied Sciences, 10*(2), 124. https://doi.org/10.5958/2394-2061.2019.00027.2

Göpfert, N. C., Conrad von Heydendorff, S., Dreßing, H., & Bailer, J. (2019). Applying Corrigan's progressive model of self-stigma to people with depression. *PLoS One, 14*(10), e0224418. https://doi.org/10.1371/journal.pone.0224418

Habibi, M., Dehghani, M., Pooravari, M., & Salehi, S. (2017). Confirmatory factor analysis of Persian version of depression, anxiety and stress (DASS-42): Non-clinical sample. *Razavi International Journal of Medicine, 5*(4), e12021. https://doi.org/10.5812/rijm.12021

Halamova, J., Kanovsky, M., & Pacuchova, M. (2018). Slovak validation of the levels of self-criticism scale: An item response theory analysis. *Horizons of Psychology, 27*, 155–166. https://doi.org/10.20419/2018.27.491

Heine, S. J. (2003). An exploration of cultural variation in self-enhancing and self-improving motivations. In V. Murphy-Berman & J. J. Berman (Eds.), *Cross-cultural differences in perspectives on the self* (pp. 118–145). University of Nebraska Press.

Heine, S. J., Lehman, D. R., Markus, H. R., & Kitayama, S. (1999). Is there a universal need for positive self-regard? *Psychological Review, 106*(4), 766–794. https://doi.org/10.1037/0033-295X.106.4.766

Hitokoto, H., & Uchida, Y. (2015). Interdependent happiness: Theoretical importance and measurement validity. *Journal of Happiness Studies, 16*(1), 211–239. https://doi.org/10.1007/s10902-014-9505-8

Hu, L. T., & Bentler, P. M. (1999). Cutoff criteria for fit indexes in covariance structure analysis: Conventional criteria versus new alternatives. *Structural Equation Modeling: A Multidisciplinary Journal, 6*(1), 1–55. https://doi.org/10.1080/10705519909540118

Joeng, J. R., & Turner, S. L. (2015). Mediators between self-criticism and depression: Fear of compassion, self-compassion, and importance to others. *Journal of Counseling Psychology, 62*(3), 453–463. https://doi.org/10.1037/cou0000071

Johnson, P. E. (2019). *rockchalk: Regression estimation and presentation* (R package Version 1.8.144). https://CRAN.R-project.org/package=rockchalk

Jorgensen, T. D., Pornprasertmanit, S., Schoemann, A. M., & Rosseel, Y. (2020). *semTools: Useful tools for structural equation modeling* (R package Version 0.5-3). https://CRAN.R-project.org/package=semTools

Kenny, A., Bizumic, B., & Griffiths, K. (2018). The Prejudice towards people with mental illness (PPMI) scale: Structure and validity. *BMC Psychiatry, 18*(1), 293. https://doi.org/10.1186/s12888-018-1871-z

Kessler, R. C., Stang, P. E., Wittchen, H., Ustun, T. B., Roy-Burne, P. P., & Walters, E. E. (1998). Lifetime panic-depression comorbidity in the national comorbidity survey. *Archives of General Psychiatry, 55*(9), 801–808. https://doi.org/10.1001/archpsyc.55.9.801

Labrague, L. J. (2014). Facebook use and adolescents' emotional states of depression, anxiety, and stress. *Health Science Journal, 8*(1), 80–89.

Lally, J., Samaniego, R. M., & Tully, J. (2019). Mental health legislation in the Philippines: Philippine Mental Health Act. *BJPsych International, 16*(3), 65–67. https://doi.org/10.1192/bji.2018.33

Lovibond, P. F., & Lovibond, S. H. (1995). The structure of negative emotional states: Comparison of the depression anxiety stress scales (DASS) with the Beck depression and anxiety inventories. *Behaviour Research and Therapy, 33*(3), 335–343. https://doi.org/10.1016/0005-7967(94)00075-u

Magtubo, C. (2016). Mental health in the Philippines: By numbers. *MIMS Online.* https://today.mims.com

Markus, H. R., & Kitayama, S. (1991). Culture and the self: Implications for cognition, emotion, and motivation. *Psychological Review, 98*(2), 224–253. https://doi.org/10.1037/0033-295X.98.2.224

Ociskova, M., Prasko, J., & Sedlackova, Z. (2013). Stigma and self-stigma in patients with anxiety disorders. *Activitas Nervosa Superior Rediviva, 55,* 12–18. https://www.researchgate.net/publication/286642493_Stigma_and_selfstigma_in_patients_with_anxiety_disorders

Park, S., & Kim, D. (2020). The centrality of depression and anxiety symptoms in major depressive disorder determined using a network analysis. *Journal of Affective Disorders, 271,* 19–26. https://doi.org/10.1016/j.jad.2020.03.078

Pe-Pua, R., & Protacio-Marcelino, E. (2000). Sikolohiyang Pilipino (Filipino psychology): A legacy of Virgilio G. Enriquez. *Asian Journal of Social Psychology, 3*(1), 49–71. https://doi.org/10.1111/1467-839X.00054

R Core Team. (2020). *R: A language and environment for statistical computing.* R Foundation for Statistical Computing. https://www.R-project.org/.

Rawlings, G. H., & Bains, M. (2020). Experiences of depression in older adults from non-white and ethnic minority groups: A thematic synthesis of qualitative studies. *Journal of Affective Disorders, 266,* 341–348. https://doi.org/10.1016/j.jad.2020.01.165

Reyes, J. (2015). Loob and kapwa: An introduction to a Filipino virtue ethics. *Asian Philosophy, 25*(2), 148–171. https://doi.org/10.1080/09552367.2015.1043173

Ritchie, H., Roser, M. (2018). *Mental health.* Retrieved September 10, 2020, from https://ourworldindata.org/mental-health

Rivera, A., & Antonio, C. (2017). Mental health stigma among Filipinos: Time for a paradigm shift. *Philippine Journal of Health Research and Development, 21*(2), 20–24.

Rosseel, Y. (2012). Lavaan: An R package for structural equation modeling. *Journal of Statistical Software, 48*(2), 1–36. https://doi.org/10.18637/jss.v048.i02

Roxas, M., David, A., & Aruta, J. J. B. (2019). Compassion, forgiveness, and subjective well being among Filipino counseling professionals. *International Journal for the Advancement of Counselling, 41*(2), 272–283. https://doi.org/10.1007/s10447-019-09374-w

Samaniego, R. M. (2017). The evolution of psychiatry and mental health in the Philippines. *Taiwanese Journal of Psychiatry, 31,* 101–114.

Shi, C. R., Zhao, C. X., Cheng, Q., & Ren, Z. H. (2020). Initial validation of the help-seeker stereotype scale in a Chinese cultural context: A bifactor model. *Current Psychology, 39*(3), 821–829. https://doi.org/10.1007/s12144-020-00703-6

Thompson, R., & Zuroff, D. C. (2004). The levels of self-criticism scale: Comparative self-criticism and internalized self-criticism. *Personality and Individual Differences, 36*(2), 419–430. https://doi.org/10.1016/S0191-8869(03)00106-5

Tolentino, U. (2004). The state of mental health in the Philippines. *International Psychiatry, 1*(6), 8–11. https://doi.org/10.1192/S1749367600006950.

Tuliao, A. (2018). *Public stigma, self-stigma, and help-seeking intent: A comparison between a U.S. and Philippines sample.* https://www.researchgate.net/publication/326304573_Public_stigma_selfstigma_and_help-seeking_intent_A_comparison_between_a_US_and_Philippines_sample

Vogel, D. L., Armstrong, P. I., Tsai, P.-C., Wade, N. G., Hammer, J. H., Efstathiou, G., Holtham, E., Kouvaraki, E., Liao, H.-Y., Shechtman, Z., & Topkaya, N. (2013). Cross-cultural validity of the self-stigma of seeking help (SSOSH) scale: Examination across six nations. *Journal of Counseling Psychology, 60*(2), 303–310. https://doi.org/10.1037/a0032055

Vogel, D. L., Wade, N. G., & Haake, S. (2006). Measuring the self-stigma associated with seeking psychological help. *Journal of Counseling Psychology, 53*(3), 325–337. https://doi.org/10.1037/0022-0167.53.3.325

Vogel, D. L., Wade, N. G., & Hackler, A. H. (2007). Perceived public stigma and the willingness to seek counseling: The mediating roles of self-stigma and attitudes towards counseling. *Journal of Counseling Psychology, 54*(1), 40–50. https://doi.org/10.1037/0022-0167.54.1.40

Widyana, R., & Safitri, R. M. (2020). Psychometric properties of internet-administered version of depression, anxiety and stress scales (DASS-42) in sample Indonesian adult. *Talent Development & Excellence, 12*(2), 1422–1434.

Wong, J., & Fisher, J. (2009). The role of traditional confinement practices in determining post-partum depression in women in Chinese cultures: A systematic review of the English language evidence. *Journal of Affective Disorders, 116*(3), 161–169. https://doi.org/10.1016/j.jad.2008.11.002

World Health Organization. (2007). *WHO–AIMS report on mental health system in the* Philippines. https://www.who.int/mental_health/evidence/philippines_who_aims_report.pdf?ua=1

World Health Organization. (2019). *Mental disorders.* https://www.who.int/news-room/fact-sheets/detail/mental-disorders

Yamaguchi, A., & Kim, M. (2013). Effects of self-criticism and its relationship with depression across cultures. *International Journal of Psychological Studies, 5*(1), 1–10. https://doi.org/10.5539/ijps.v5n1p1

Yamaguchi, A., Kim, M. S., & Akutsu, S. (2014). The effects of self-construals, self-criticism, and self-compassion on depressive symptoms. *Personality and Individual Differences, 68,* 65–70. https://doi.org/10.1016/j.paid.2014.03.013

Yen, C., Chen, C., Lee, Y., Tang, T., Yen, J., & Ko, C. (2005). Self-stigma and its correlates among outpatients with depressive disorders. *Psychiatric Services (Washington, D.C.), 56*(5), 599–601. https://doi.org/10.1176/appi.ps.56.5.599

Zahn, R., Lythe, K. E., Gethin, J. A., Green, S., Deakin, J. F., Young, A. H., & Moll, J. (2015). The role of self-blame and worthlessness in the psychopathology of major depressive disorder. *Journal of Affective Disorders, 186,* 337–341. https://doi.org/10.1016/j.jad.2015.08.001

Zuo, B., & Ai, C. (2011). Study on the relation of group identification, self-esteem and stigma of mental illness. *Chinese Journal of Applied Psychology, 17*(4), 299–303.

Language and the Symptoms of Mental Illness Connection via Abstract Representations of the Self and the World

Yaşar Kuzucu, Ömer Faruk Şimşek, and Çiğdem Koşe-Demiray

ABSTRACT
The aim of the present study is to provide additional knowledge about the mediatory processes through which language contributes to the symptoms of mental illness. Although recent studies have provided insight about the relationship between language and the indicators of mental illness, the role of intervening variables in this connection has been ignored. The present investigation tested a structural equation model in which the need for the absolute truth about self and worry mediated the relationship of the gap between inner psychological experience and language with anxiety and depression. The results have provided support for the model and showed that the gap predicts both the need for absolute truth and worry which, in turn, predict the levels of anxiety and depression. The results have been discussed in the light of previous research, and implications for future research have also been considered.

Previous research (e.g. Machado & Gonçalves, 1999; Buck, 1993) has found language to be associated with the indicators of mental illness or ill-being. One of the most important findings of the relevant research is that the disconnect or gap between language and inner psychological experience has critical implications for the study of psychopathology. Studies on Multiple Code Theory (Bucci, 1984; Fertuck, Bucci, Blatt, & Ford, 2004), for example, emphasized that clients with depression do not have a connection between words to denote bodily experiences and those inner experiences themselves; they seem to have a difficulty to use language as an expressive tool for their inner experiences. Bucci (1984) argues that individual efforts for connecting language and psychological experiences make it possible for individuals to make sense of their inner experiences. According to Bucci and Freedman's (1981) findings, low levels of referential activity, inability to verbalize inner psychological experiences with large amounts of concrete detail, was associated with depression. The authors found that most clinically depressed patients have a disconnection between language and emotional experiences and concluded that the levels of referential activity covaried with the levels of depression, both within and between individuals.

Writing paradigm (Pennebaker, 1993) also emphasizes the importance of the representation of traumatic experiences by language in mental health given the finding that the written expression of traumatic experiences were found to be influential in reducing post-traumatic stress disorder symptoms. The basic premise of the Writing Paradigm is that transforming inner psychological experiences, whether it is traumatic or not, into language result in psychological and physical health because such a transformation would help assigning meaning, structure and coherence to these experiences (Pennebaker & Chung, 2011). As indicated by the authors, research findings consistently showed that writing about problematic experiences even for just a couple of days improved mental and physical health, even though the results of the recent meta-analysis concerning the effect of these interventions indicated modest effect sizes (Frattaroli, 2006).

In accordance with the Writing Paradigm and Multiple Code Theory, Şimşek (2010) proposed the concept of 'gap between experience and language' (GAP) referring to the distance between inner psychological experiences and the language used to denote these experiences. GAP refers to an individual perception of a lack of comprehending inner psychological experiences using the linguistic tools available. According to the author, the connection between words denoting personal/phenomenal experience and the experience itself is a critical issue in the construction of the self as well as in the regulation of the problematic emotional experiences. Şimşek defined two basic functions in the context of ordinary language use, the epistemic and the communicative, the lack of which underlies the phenomena of GAP. The epistemic function is related to an individual's belief about the ability of the daily language they use as a reliable means to acknowledge inner psychological experiences. The communicative function, on the other hand, is a personal acknowledgment of this ordinary language as a reliable tool to communicate phenomenal experiences.

Earlier studies have investigated the mediators of the relationship between GAP and the symptoms of mental illness and shown that self-concept clarity (Şimşek & Kuzucu, 2012), self-reflection, self-rumination (Şimşek, 2013) and emotion regulation (Şimşek & Çerçi, 2013) are potential mediators. A more recent study by Bozanoğlu, Şimşek, Altıntaş, and Kocayoruk (in press) showed also that GAP mediated the relationship between adolescents' attachment to their parents and depression they experience. The current study aimed at expanding this line of investigation by emphasizing the mediator role of the abstract representations concerning the self and the outside world in the relationship of GAP with anxiety and depression as the symptoms of mental illness. As stated more clearly below, two inclinations of abstract and repetitive thinking, i.e. need for absolute truth as an inclination to find an abstract representation of the self, and, worry as an abstract representation of the surrounding world, are considered to be the mediators of the relationship between GAP and the indicators of mental illness. In other words, GAP is considered to be closely connected with both an endless search for an absolute truth about self and an abstract conceptualization of the outside world as a combination of possible threats, which in turn contribute negatively to the indicators of mental illness, depression and anxiety, in the present study. We choose these abstract representations as mediators because, as we shall explain in more detail in the next section, they are closely connected to and probably resulted from GAP and contribute to the indicators of mental illness.

Moreover, given that counseling or psychotherapy processes are largely based on the language used by clients, an examination of important mediators in the relationship between GAP and the indicators of mental illness would contribute to the clinical/counseling outcomes. Particularly the need for absolute truth is of special importance in this context since almost every counseling process starts due to a need for finding the truth about the self and gaining self awareness.

The Relationship between Language and Abstract Representations

Recent conceptualizations of self-focus have been underlined that there is both beneficial and detrimental kinds of self-focused attention. Reduced concreteness theory as a leading paradigm in this context advocates that in contrast to abstract thinking, concrete thinking is the main characteristic of repetitive self-focus such as worry and rumination. The reduced concreteness theory operationalize concrete though as "distinct, situationally specific, unequivocal, clear, singular" while abstract thought as "indistinct, cross-situational, equivocal, unclear, aggregated" (Stöber & Borkovec, 2002, p. 92). Research indeed has shown that high-level abstractions (e.g. asking why instead of what or how) could result in mental health problems through their effects on overgeneralizations, lack of affect regulation or problem-solving. For example, Hixon and Swann (1993) demonstrated that "why" questions have a negative effect on mental health. The researchers indicated that when self-focus questions are formulated on an abstract level, they have harmful effects on mental health compared with the concrete forms. Self-focus was shown, on the other hand, to contribute to self-insight, when it focuses on concrete forms by "what" questions. Based on such findings, Watkins and Teasdale (2004) not only emphasized the negative effects of high-level abstract representations on mental health, but also emphasized the benefits of concrete evaluations for problem solving. They stated that self-regulation is easier through less abstract thinking and highlighted that abstract thinking increases the possibility to overgeneralize. As Watkins (2008) indicated, abstract thought is associated with overgeneralization and found to be a common factor in depression. It is clear, then, that to focus on the experiences of the self from a less analytical and concrete perspective (asking how) is more favorable for mental health than a more analytical and abstract focus on causes and meanings (asking why).

It is highly probable at this point that if one cannot find linguistic expressions for inner experiences, the representations of these experiences would suffer from having no concrete referents, which leads to a search for more abstract representations to make sense of them. Pennebaker and Chung (2011) underline the importance of translating emotions into words since such an analog-to-digital process has crucial effects on the way of thinking on these emotions. Indeed, Lyubomirsky and Lepper (1999) found that verbalizing problematic experiences through writing was more helpful than merely thinking about them since such a use of language helps individuals to organize these stressful experiences. The authors indicate that merely thinking about stressful experiences, in contrast to decode them into language, does not provide the content of thought with structure and meaning, leading individuals into repetitive and abstract thinking such as rumination or dwelling. A more recent study also provided findings showing that expressive writing reduced the levels of abstract thinking, i.e. brooding as a kind of maladaptive rumination (Sloan, Marx, Epstein, & Dobbs, 2008).

In light of this literature, we propose that a persistent, i.e. trait, GAP would lead to a search for abstract representations concerning the personal/phenomenal world consisting of both self and the surrounding world. As Segerstrom, Stanton, Alden, and Shortridge (2003, p. 909) indicated, repetitive thought is the "process of thinking attentively, repetitively or frequently about one's self and one's world," GAP, thus, could be expected to result in an inclination to a repetitive search for abstract representations, of which we focus on the two critical phenomena having crucial implications for mental illness: the need for absolute truth and worry.

Inspired by the works of Watkins and Teasdale (2004), Şimşek (2013) introduced the need for absolute truth (NAT) as a kind of self-analysis aimed to acquire absolute knowledge about the self. As a very new conceptualization in the self-consciousness literature, it refers to a repetitive search for stable, constant and objective knowledge, which is highly associated with a higher-order thinking capacity (Şimşek, Ceylandağ, & Akcan, 2013). NAT is a powerful wish for an abstract type of self-knowledge and self-relevant information as a rigid and inflexible conceptualization of the self, which aims to capture knowledge about personal experiences and the self. It refers to the absolute knowledge beyond personal experiences valid every time and for every situation, that is an overgeneralized truth. It represents, thus, one of the highest level representations about the self and was found to be positively related to psychopathology indicators such as depression, anxiety and self-rumination while negatively related to the mental health indicators such as self-concept clarity, self-esteem, and insight (Şimşek, 2013; Şimşek et al., 2013).

The effects of the GAP on the NAT, as indicated above, seem to be clear given that language is the main tool for making highly fluid inner experiences concrete and assigning meaning to them. The functions of language, in this respect, are the means through which the individual acknowledges inner psychological experiences. Words help to categorize and develop meaning (Owen, 1991) and especially figurative language enables insight and knowledge about the self (Barlow, Pollio, & Fine, 1977). According to Şimşek (2010), as the epistemic function increases, the levels of GAP decrease and what is felt becomes known for individuals. Communicative function of GAP is also about self-knowledge since sharing inner experiences helps people to gain knowledge about the self through emotional understanding (Howe, Aquan-Assee, Bukowski, Lehoux, & Rinaldi, 2001). Indeed, epistemic and communicative functions of language were shown to have a close connection with self-knowledge (Şimşek, 2010, Şimşek, 2013). An increase in the levels of GAP, consequently, could result in decreased levels of concrete thought, which probably leads to higher levels of abstract thought about the self and experiences. Thus, it is possible to argue that when language does not represent phenomenal experiences, these experiences become more problematic and coercive to individual and s/he would probably in need of an insistent search for higher-order or abstract conceptualizations about the self.

Second, GAP has also implications for worry given that worry has a close connection directly with language as well as abstract thinking. The most convincing support for the importance of language and abstract thinking comes from reduced concreteness theory.

According to Borkovec, Robinson, Pruzinsky, and DePree (1983, p. 10), worry "represents an attempt to engage in mental problem-solving on an issue whose outcome is uncertain but contains the possibility of one or more negative outcomes" Research findings provide strong evidence that the quality of the engagement, i.e. abstract verbal elaborations of or reduced concreteness concerning the problem, could be one of the main causes of worry (Stöber, 1998; Stöber & Borkovec, 2002). The main argument of Stöber and Borkovec is that individuals prefer using a verbal articulation of the worrying situation in order to escape aversive imagery related to it. Abstract verbal content, thus, eliminate the vivid representation of the worrying situation and resulted in a better emotional processing at the earlier periods of phenomenal worry experience. Later, however, such a manipulation would lead to poor problem solving strategies since there exists no concrete elements concerning the situation, which resulted in higher levels of worry. Dual-level information theory, on the other hand, underlines the detrimental effects of abstract thinking in worry (Sibrava & Borkovec, 2006). According to the theory, the schematic (or implicational) level consists of abstracted information from past emotional experiences and is not accessible to consciousness. The propositional level, however, is consciously accessible and contains concrete, episodic information. Research based on the manipulation of these two emotional processing levels found that dealing with information abstractly results in valenced emotion and low levels of emotional processing than does dealing with the information at the propositional level. It is clearly possible, then, to argue that the functions of language contribute to the concrete processing as it provides individuals with the ability to label and organize experiences into a self-system. To put it another way, a decrease in the levels of the functions of language could be connected to an increase in the inclination to think abstractly, which in turn could possibly contributes to heightened worry.

Present Study

Based on the literature mentioned above, the present research suggests that the relationship of GAP with the indicators of psychopathology is mediated by both NAT and worry that are repetitive and abstract representations concerning self and the world, respectively. In order to clarify the processes by which GAP is associated with symptoms of mental health, it seems important to illuminate the role of the need for absolute truth and worry. According to the model depicted, GAP is related to both NAT and worry, which in turn connected to the ill-being latent variable defined by the most important indicators of mental illness such as depression and anxiety in the present research. We tested this hypothesis by using a structural equation model (Figure 1).

Method

Participants and Procedure

The number of 390 individuals participated in the study in Turkey. Participant was voluntary and following the data screening procedure (Normality of each variable, missing-value pattern and presence of outliers) a sample of 374 was used for analyses. Mean age of the sample was 25.12 (SD = 8.55) ranging from 18 to 67 years. Of the participants,

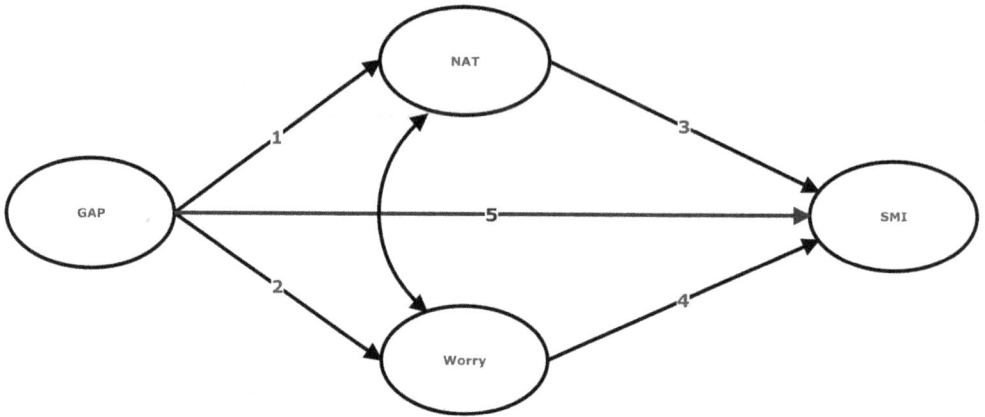

Figure 1. The proposed model of the relationships among GAP, NAT, Worry and Mental Health. Notes: GAP = The gap between experience and language; NAT = Need for absolute truth; SMI = Symptoms of Mental Illness; observed variables are not shown in the model.

249 were female (66.9%) and 123 were male (33.1%). The data were collected from a non-clinical sample. The age distribution of the samples is unbalanced. A preparatory analysis should be conducted on the effect of age using statistical methods.

A battery of self-report measures was administered to the participants with an overall administration time of approximately 30 min. All participants completed a written informed consent form. Participants were volunteers and no incentive was given to them. No personal identifying information was collected. Participants were asked to complete questionnaires including the measures of beliefs about the functions of language, need for absolute truth, worry and mental health.

Variables and Measures

The Gap between Experience and Language

Beliefs about the Functions of Language Scale (BAFL, Şimşek, 2010) was developed in Turkish to assess subjects' perception of association between language and inner experiences by six studies. Likert-type scale has twelve items with acceptable internal consistencies, $\alpha =.70$ and $\alpha =.83$, respectively, and good test-retest reliability ($r = .82$). Internal consistency of the present study is $\alpha =. 87$. Factorial validity studies indicated that the scale consisted of the two factors with acceptable reliability estimates. Items had at least .46 factor loadings and the correlation between factors was found to be .38. Five of the items include epistemic factor such as "I believe that the real meaning of my experiences is beyond language" and "I think there is a gap between my feelings and the corresponding words". The rest, seven items, reflect communicative function such as "I do not feel people can fully understand the words I use to express myself" and "I feel words can reflect my feelings exactly to other people". Validity studies reported moderate or strong correlations with many mental illness indicators such as depression ($r = .50$), anxiety (.53), and somatization (.41) as well as empathic tendency ($-.37$) and self-concept clarity ($-.47$).

Need for Absolute Truth (NAT)

NAT (Şimşek, 2013) was developed in Turkish and used to measure the desire to have absolute knowledge about the self. The NAT has been found to have an acceptable internal consistency ($\alpha = .75$) and good test-retest reliability ($r = .72$). Five-point Likert-type scale has one factor and five items such as "I always try to find "the facts" about me" and "I always think about "the facts" about me". This factor accounted for 51% of the variance with an eigenvalue of 2.56. According to the confirmatory factor analysis findings, factor loadings ranged from .55 to .89 and yielded t-values ranging from 9.19 to 22.62. The scores on the NAT Scale were found to be moderately correlated with mental health indicators such as depression ($r = .51$), anxiety ($r = .47$), self-concept clarity ($r = .58$) and self-esteem ($r = .42$) as well as with some measures of self-focus such as self-rumination ($r = 54$), self-reflection ($r = .63$), and insight ($-.28$).

Worry

Penn State Worry Questionnaire (PSWQ; Meyer, Miller, Metzger, & Borkovec, 1990) was used to measure subjects' level of worry. Scale was developed to assess the proneness to worry in terms of uncontrollability of trait like worry, frequency and intensity. It is a five-point Likert-type scale with 16 items. In the present study, the Turkish version of the questionnaire that was adapted by Boysan, Keskin, and Beşiroğlu (2008) was administered. Internal consistency of the questionnaire was $\alpha = .88$. Correlation between PSWQ total scores and Beck Depression Inventory was $r = 0.45$. PSWQ is significantly correlated with Beck Anxiety Inventory $r = 0.46$. The correlation between PSWQ and Rosenberg Self Esteem Scale was $r = -0.36$. Internal consistency of the present study is $\alpha = .91$.

Symptoms of Mental Illness

Depression and anxiety sub-scales of Brief Symptom Inventory (BSI) were used to measure individuals' depression and anxiety symptoms. Of the 53 item scale 12 items were related to depression and 13 items were related to anxiety. It is a 5-point Likert-type scale. The scale has a good internal consistency reliability ranging from .71 to .85. It is developed by Derogatis (1992) and adapted to Turkish by Şahin and Durak (1994). The adapted Turkish version has five subscales; anxiety, depression, negative self, somatization and hostility. In the present study, Alpha coefficients for depression and anxiety sub-scale were found to be .87 and .84, respectively.

Strategy of Analysis

Following Anderson and Gerbing's method (1988), the measurement model is estimated prior to the structural model. After the descriptive statistics and correlation analysis, measurement model was tested before the full structural model. As SEM is used for theory testing, alternative models must be considered in order to detect whether the proposed model fits the data better (Green, 2015). Therefore, two alternative models were also tested against the proposed model in order to ensure that the model fitted the data due to its theoretical soundness, not because of a statistical coincidence.

Table 1. Means, Standard Deviations, Intercorrelations of Observed Variables.

Observed variables	M	SD	1	2	3	4	5	6	7	8	9	10	11
GAP													
1. Epis	15.14	4.15	–										
2. Com	19.94	5.92	.69**	–									
Worry													
3. Worry 1	13.77	3.88	.23**	.28**	–								
4. Worry 2	17.51	4.35	.23**	.28**	.83**	–							
5. Worry 3	13.50	3.84	.15**	.25**	.78**	.81**	–						
SMI													
6. Depression	30.01	8.61	.43**	.44**	.51**	.55**	.48**	–					
7. Anxiety	27.08	7.94	.42**	.47**	.56**	.56**	.49**	.80**	–				
Need For Truth													
8. N1	3.51	1.04	.27**	.22**	.15**	.10	.09	.20**	.20**	–			
9. N2	3.40	1.15	.36**	.40**	.27**	.29**	.22**	.40**	.36**	.21**	–		
10. N3	3.88	1.36	.28**	.27**	.20**	.16**	.09	.24**	.25**	.35**	.54**	–	
11. N4	3.88	1.14	.30**	.32**	.22**	.19**	.16**	.30**	.33**	.47**	.43**	.58**	–
12. N5	3.29	1.02	36**	.33**	.19**	.14**	.12*	.30**	.28**	.42**	.25**	.31**	.53**

Notes: $N = 374$, GAP = Gap between language and experience; NFT = The Need for Absolute Truth; NFT1-5 = Five parcels from the Need for Absolute Truth Scale; Worry 1, 2 and 3 = Three parcels from the Worry Scale; SMI = Symptoms of Mental Illness.
$*p < .05; **p < .01$.

Results

Preliminary Analyses

Means, standard deviations, and zero-order correlations for the 12 measured variables are shown in Table 1.

The distribution of the variables was scanned by using skewness (an index of steepness of score distribution) and kurtosis (an index of asymmetry of distribution) value. All values were less than 1.5, ranging from -0.092 to -1.35 for skewness and from -0.68 to 3.65 for kurtosis, indicating that there was no problem with normal distribution for any variable and all variables are normally distributed in the sample. In addition to the skewness and kurtosis analyses, Kolmogorov-Smirnov test was used and the results ($p > .05$) supported the normality.

In order to test the multivariate normality of the distribution of a group of variables the Mardia based Kappa curtosis index was calculated. Multivariate kurtosis was investigated with the normalized estimate of Mardia's (1970) kappa and there was evidence of kurtosis. Values > 1.96 mean there is significant kurtosis, which shows that there is no multivariate normality. Mardia's coefficient (8.23) indicated no multivariate normality. The data suggested the use of the LISREL WLS estimation method for ordinal variables (Jöreskog & Sörbom, 2003) polychoric correlations matrix and the asymptotic covariance matrix were used as input for data analysis. Therefore, appropriate estimation procedures were applied in both measurement and structural models.

The gender and age distribution of the samples is unbalanced. A preparatory analysis conducted on the effect of gender and age using statistical methods (t-test and measures of central tendency). Findings indicated that there weren't any gender differences. For each observed variables, the differences between mean scores of groups were examined and t values revealed no significant differences, values changed between 1.21 ($p > .05$) and 2.51 ($p > .05$). The measures of central tendency was also supported this finding.

Table 2. Correlations among the Latent Variables with (above diagonal) and without (below diagonal) Control Variable.

Latent variable	1	2	3	4
GAP	–	.44**	.29**	.50**
Need for truth	.46**	–	.25**	.39**
Worry	.30**	.25**	–	.60**
SMI	.50**	.41**	.60**	–

Notes: N = 374.
**p < .001. SMI = symptoms of mental illness.

The age effect was also checked. The structural equations model was tested by taking AGE as a control variable, paths from AGE to all observed variables of the other latent constructs were added, while the covariance of latent AGE constructs with other latent constructs was constrained to be zero (Johnson, Rosen & Djurdjevic, 2011). Additionally, the variance of AGE was set to 1.00 in order to achieve identification.

As seen in Table 2, mental illness symptoms had positive correlations with each factor of GAP, parcels of worry and parcels of the Need for Truth. Parcels of the Need for Truth, except the parcel N1, had a moderate correlation with mental illness factors and worry parcels.

Test of the Measurement Model

SEM is a multivariate strategy of analysis including the test of measurement and structural models. Before a structural equation model is tested, the confirmatory factor analysis is conducted to examine whether a measurement model provides an acceptable fit to the data. Since the measurement model which has the greatest number of free parameters is the least restricted model, it is impossible for any structural model having a mediational hypothesis to fit the data better than a measurement model.

In this study, the measurement model was estimated by using the Maximum-Likelihood Method in the LISREL 8.8 program (Jöreskog & Sörbom, 2003). The Maximum-Likelihood estimation method created fit indices that are less likely to be influenced by sample size and distribution than the methods such as Weighted Least Squares or Unweighted Least Squares (Hu & Bentler, 1998). Moreover, the non-convergent values of the factor loadings in the measurement and structural models have been considered problematic in model testing, which is called interpretational confounding by Anderson and Gerbing (1988). The indicators, or the measured variables, in the model were defined according to a priori factor structures of the constructs demonstrated by the earlier research.

The measurement model specified the posited relations of the observed variables to their underlying constructs allowed to intercorrelate freely. Four latent variables were used in the structural equation model testing: The gap between experience and language (GAP), need for absolute truth (NAT), worry and mental illness symptoms. The latent construct GAP was defined by the sum scores of its sub-scales, namely communicative and epistemic functions. The sum scores on Depression and Anxiety sub-scales of the Brief Symptom Inventory defined the latent construct "symptoms of mental illness" (SMI). The NAT Scale is a one-dimensional measure with five items that are used as observed variables. Finally, three parcels created by the items of PSWQ to define the latent variable worry. Item parceling is a method that normalizes the distribution of observed variables and increases the reliability of these indicators (Little, Cunningham, Shahar, & Widaman, 2002).

Before the measurement model tested, the correlations between all latent variables in the model were checked and found all statistically significant ($p < .01$, see Table 2). After the control variable, there are still moderate correlation between the variables. The correlations among the constructs (Table 2) indicated very small changes.

The test of the measurement model resulted in an acceptable fit to the data, as indicated by the following goodness of fit statistics: $\chi^2(47, N = 374) = 116.38$; $\chi^2/df = 2.46$; GFI $= 0.99$; CFI $= 0.99$; SRMR $= 0.060$; RMSEA $= 0.063$ (90 percent confidence interval for RMSEA $= 0.048$–0.077). All loadings of the measured variables on the latent constructs were large and statistically significant (standardized values ranged from 0.26 to 0.87, $p < .01$).

The measurement model was tested once more, this time with the AGE construct as a control variable. The model produced better fit to the data: $\chi^2(47, N = 374) = 99.57$; $\chi^2/df = 2.11$; GFI $= 0.99$; CFI $= 0.99$; SRMR $= 0.057$; RMSEA $= 0.055$ (90 percent confidence interval for RMSEA $= 0.040$–0.070). As Table 3 demonstrates, all loadings of the measured variables on the latent constructs were large and statistically significant (standardized values ranged from 0.31 to 0.89, $p < .01$).

Test of the Structural Models

The mediational hypotheses were tested by examining the fit of a series of structural models to the data. Figure 1 summarizes the full number of hypothesized relations between the latent variables. The numbers on the figure refer to the relationship of GAP to SMI with the mediatory role of NAT and worry (1, 2, 3, and 4) or without such mediation (5).

Table 3. Factor Loadings, Standard Errors, and t-Values for the Measurement Model.

Measure and variable	Unstandardized factor loading	SE	t	Standardized factor loading
GAP				
Epis	0.73	0.03	19.17	0.67
Com	0.80	0.03	20.79	0.80
SMI				
Dep	0.65	0.03	16.62	0.80
Anx	0.75	0.03	20.31	0.87
Worry				
WP1	0.73	0.03	23.09	0.84
WP2	0.76	0.03	24.02	0.89
WP3	0.71	0.03	21.96	0.78
Need For Truth				
NFT1	0.56	0.04	13.84	0.31
NFT2	0.53	0.04	12.10	0.39
NFT3	0.67	0.03	18.67	0.46
NFT4	0.88	0.02	32.56	0.79
NFT5	0.66	0.03	18.51	0.46

Notes: $N = 374$, Epis = Epistemic Function; Com = Communicative Function; Dep = Depression; Anx = Anxiety. Worry 1, 2 and 3 = Three parcels created from the Worry scale; NFT1–NFT5 = Five items from the Need for Absolute Truth Scale; SMI = Symptoms of Mental Illness.

With the AGE construct as a control variable, the tests of mediation were performed by examining whether there were differences between the partially mediated model represented in Figure 1, which includes the direct effect from GAP to Mental Health (path 5), and the full mediation model in which this path is omitted.

Testing the mediation effect of worry and NAT with respect to SMI where the path 5 was set to zero, resulted in the following goodness of fit statistics: $\chi^2(49, N = 374) = 117.92$; $\chi^2/df = 2.40$; GFI =.99; CFI=.99; SRMR= 0.073; RMSEA = 0.061 (90 percent confidence interval for RMSEA = 0.047–0.076).

Test of the partial mediated model resulted in an acceptable fit to the data as indicated by the following goodness of fit statistics: $\chi^2(47, N = 374) = 100.62$; $\chi^2/df = 2.14$; GFI = .99; CFI = .99; SRMR = 0.058; RMSEA = 0.054 (90 percent confidence interval for RMSEA = 0.039–0.069). These results show that the partial mediation model worked better than the full mediation model because the chi-square difference test (0.17, 2: $p < .001$) indicated a difference between the models, and the path from GAP to SMI is required to achieve a better fit to the data.

Standardized estimates for the paths in the model are represented in Figure 2. As can be seen from Figure 2, the estimation of the total effect of GAP on SMI is 0.60 (SE:0.06) and after the mediators is included in the model, direct effect of GAP on SMI reduced to .31 (SE:0.05)

Compared to the saturated model, lower values of AIC and ECVI indicate a better model fit (Jöreskog & Sörbom, 1993). The AIC and ECVI statistics were 200.32 and 0.54, respectively, and they supported the model in which the path is retained. It is clear

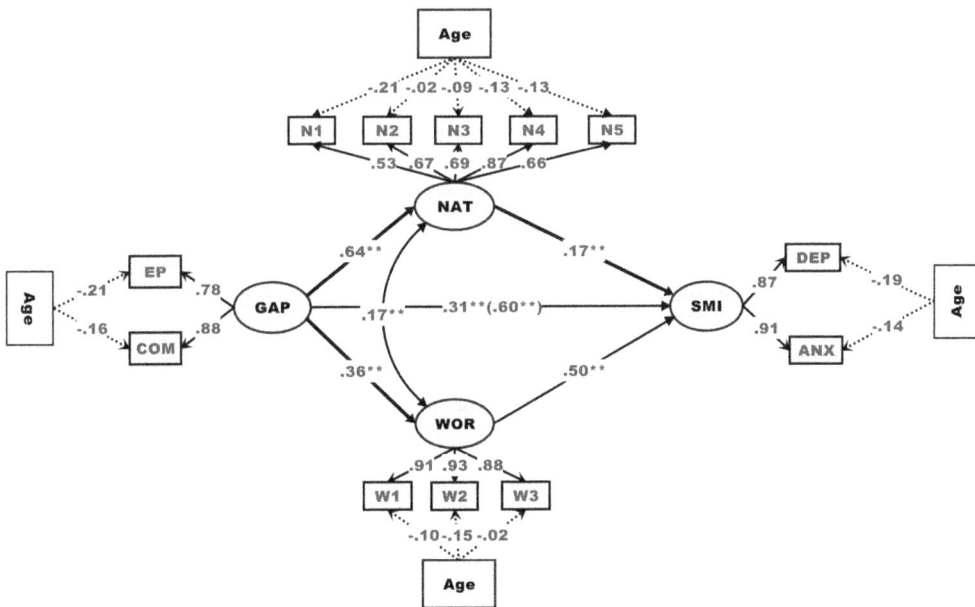

Figure 2. Standardized parameter estimates for the mediation model with age controlled for.
Notes: EP = Epistemic function, COM = Communicative function, GAP = Gap between experience and language, N1-N5 = The items of the Need for Absolute Truth Scale, NAT = Need for absolute truth, W1-W3 = Parcels created from the PSWQ, WOR = Worry, SMI = Symptoms of Mental Illness, DEP = Depression, ANX = Anxiety. Dashed lines refers to the effect of age on the observed variables.

from the findings that the relationship between GAP and SMI is partially mediated by NAT and worry.

According to the findings, 41% of the variance in NAT was explained by GAP, 13% of the variance in Worry was explained by GAP. GAP, NAT and worry in turn, accounted for 63% of the variance in SMI. Clearly, LISREL estimates for the indirect effects of GAP (0.31, $p < .01$) on SMI through NAT and worry verified the partially mediator role in the model.

Although the structural model resulted in a good fit to the data, the mediation hypotheses were examined by calculating bootstrap confidence intervals. The bootstrapping procedure is used to determine whether or not the indirect pathways were significantly different from zero (Shrout & Bolger, 2002). This method is based on testing the significance of the indirect paths from the independent variable (GAP) to the mediators (WORRY and NAT) and from the mediators to the dependent variable (SMI). Bootstrapping produces a large number of samples from the dataset and uses them to obtain estimates of the standard errors. In the present study, 10,000 bootstrap samples were drawn. The interval confidence of these standard errors is considered when testing the significance of indirect effects. These standard errors were used to calculate the 95% confidence interval (CI) for each indirect effect. Significant mediation is indicated when the upper and the lower limits of the 95% CI do not include zero. The final model excluded zero at both the 95% confidence intervals (the mediation role of worry between GAP and Mental Health = .42–.83; the mediation role of NAT between GAP and Mental Health = .38–.91). Confidence intervals for the indirect effects provided support for the mediation hypotheses. More specifically, there was a statistically significant indirect effect of GAP on Mental Health, through both NAT and Worry. That is, NAT and Worry mediates the relationship between GAP and mental health.

Discussion

The structural equation model tested in the present research provided preliminary support for the mediator roles of worry and NAT in the relationship of the gap between language and experience with the symptoms of mental illness in a non-clinical sample. The basic assumption of the present study was that GAP contributes to higher-order thinking processes through which individuals try to construe their internal and external world using abstract representations. Such a process through these repetitive representations, in turn, was expected to contribute to mental illness indicators such as depression and anxiety. The results of the present study supported these expectations and showed that NAT and worry mediated the relationship between GAP and these basic indicators of mental illness. Adding age of the participants into the structural equation model as a control variable did not change the whole picture.

As formulized by Şimşek (2010), GAP refers to experiencing language as a lack of means of representing personal reality to the individual her/himself (epistemic function) and to others (communicative function). Given that language serves as one of the basic mediums by which personal reality is constructed and reconstructed (Neimeyer & Mahoney, 1995), an experienced gap between a problematic experience and language is expected to have an effect on repetitive thinking such as NAT and worry in searching for certainty about self and the surrounding world. Research findings (Engels et al., 2007) support such inclinations and show that individuals exhibited greater activation of the left inferior frontal gyrus, a brain region playing an important role in language and speech production, when exposed to a problematic situation. Moreover, research also provided evidence that brain activity associated with speech production decreased in individuals with generalized anxiety disorder after receiving either pharmacological (Hoehn-Saric, Schlund, & Wong, 2004) or non-pharmacological treatment (Borkovec, Ray, & Stober, 1998). These findings indicate that problematic experiences urge individuals to use language as a means of elaborating the situation and thus making sense of it. Finally, support for the effects of language on repetitive thinking comes from a recent study (Francis, Hawes, Abbott, & Costa, 2018) providing evidence that the verbal ability of the children aged 9 to 15 years has an indirect effect on worry *via* intolerance of uncertainty. In other words, high verbal intelligence negatively associated with intolerance of uncertainty which, in turn, positively correlated with worry.

Morin (2006) argues with the findings of neuroimaging studies that the personal use of language, i.e. inner speech, helps individuals to have a rich and well articulated self-knowledge and higher-levels of self-awareness, an intrapersonal model of self-information acquisition. Moreover, the author indicates that inner speech has also an indirect effect on self-knowledge through interpersonal conversations. Accordingly, individuals are influenced by the significant others' appraisals, which affect one's inner speech about her/himself, which is called interpersonal mode of self-information acquisition.

Similarly, Dimaggio, Vanheule, Lysaker, Carcione, and Nicolo (2009) indicate that language as the only means for inner speech or discourse provides individuals with the capacity to form an integrated view of self by making them able to form questions and answers both intra and interpersonal processes. The authors, then, presents findings from brain imaging studies indicating that the damage in language areas are correlated with the quality of inner speech which in turn contributes to poor self-reflection. Morin (2006) similarly differentiate basic levels of self-consciousness like sensorimotor awareness or awareness of other individuals from higher-levels of self-awareness or meta self-awareness and indicate that the latter requires language.

It is clear, then that the GAP has a special importance at this point given that language has been considered to be the basic tool for making highly fluid inner experiences concrete and accessible to consciousness (Şimşek, 2010). Human beings are distinguished from other organisms by a sophisticated language and its complex relations with inner psychological experiences. Şimşek (2010) used Russell's (1912) distinction between "knowledge by acquaintance" and "knowledge by description" as a useful model in order to understand the (dis)connect between language and inner experiences. From this perspective, the knowledge by acquaintance refers to the direct and the immediate nature of bodily experiences; it is the pure presentation of experiences from senses without any judgment. Knowledge by description, on the other hand, represents formation of linguistic symbols for felt experiences.

Although Russell considered knowledge by acquaintance a more direct and genuine kind of truth, this is hardly viable when the issue is inner psychological experiences. Such experiences are hard to capture by the individual since there is no concrete referents corresponding for these experiences and this is especially true for the problematic emotional experiences. Musacchio (2002) call subjective experiences phenomenal knowledge which is language-independent representations although they are absolute requirement for developing propositional knowledge, or knowledge by description. The author insists that the phenomenal and the propositional knowledge are dependent on fundamentally different neurobiological processes, which results in an inevitable gap between them.

Consequently, as Buck (1993) stated, such phenomenal experiences are not so easy to acknowledge and individuals should educate themselves concerning putting subjective experiences such as emotions, feelings, and desires (knowledge by acquaintance) into words. Indeed, people obtain information about their experiences and become competent to think about their mental states by language (Buck, 1993; Ivey, 1986; Morin, 2006). In other words, creation of meaning can only be possible through knowledge by description both in the therapeutic processes (Clarke, 1989) and in the daily life. Bucci (1984) makes similar categorizations and names the two processes as symbolic and subsymbolic representations. Sub-symbolic representations, just like the knowledge by acquaintance, are the information from five senses, while symbolic representations refer to the symbolizations of sub-symbolic representations just like the knowledge by description.

Such a lack of self-information would have an effect on a need for self-knowledge, i.e. NAT as a kind of repetitive, higher-order thinking. Consistently, earlier research found that GAP and having a clear picture of the attributes of the self (self-concept clarity) are strongly and negatively correlated (Şimşek & Kuzucu, 2012). Şimşek (2013) indicates that NAT is probably the highest-order thinking about the self given that it refers to a kind of abstract thinking that aims to capture overgeneralizations about the self and rules about personal behavior that are independent from the situation. The results of the present study showed that higher levels of GAP experienced by the individual is associated with higher levels of NAT. It is an expected result given that having no words corresponding to the concrete aspects of the experience would contribute to an obsessive need for finding more abstract and higher-order representations of the self, that is, NAT.

Second, GAP was also found to be strongly associated with worry in the present research. The findings of the present research indicated that higher levels of worry could result from GAP experienced by individuals. As individuals are prone to or have a lack of concrete verbalizations concerning threats, they are more likely to experience higher levels of worry, which leads to depression and anxiety. Worry can be conceptualized as concerns about the perceived threat (Zuellig & Borkovec, 1996) and verbalization has been used as a strategy for abstraction, disengagement, and inhibition of emotional arousal associated with feared stimuli (Tucker & Newman, 1981). Abstract thought in response to feared stimuli decreases emotional arousal. Thus, worry related thought contains words and sentences of lowered concreteness (Stöber, 1998, Stöber, Tepperwien, & Staak, 2000). Consistent with this assumption, research showed that concrete words elucidate more concrete and vivid imagery (Paivio & Marschark, 1991). Conceptualizing outside world without such a concreteness would be more likely to result in worry, since worry and problem elaboration tasks are found to be inversely associated as Stöber (1998) clearly indicated. It is plausible to argue that finding corresponding verbalizations for inner psychological experiences also means finding referents that are concrete and easy to elaborate. Consequently, as GAP increases concrete thinking decreases, which brings about high-level, pathological worry.

The findings provided by the present research have important implications for mental health interventions. The last decade of research has provided valuable insights into the role of language in mental health by focusing on the benefits of expressive writing. Research findings clearly showed that expressive writing for just three sessions contribute to mental and physical well-being (Pennebaker & Chung, 2011). However, the most recent meta-analysis showed that the effects of emotional disclosure were modest, and its efficacy was affected by a number of variables (Frattaroli, 2006).

The findings of the present research imply that the main contribution of using language as an expressive agent, might be through making problematic inner experiences, which is ineffable in most cases, more concrete, lower-level constructions. Indeed, Pennebaker and Graybeal (2001) assume that expressive writing contributes to mental health by changing the way individuals thought about the event. It is probable to argue that two kinds of higher-order thinking, NAT and worry, could be considered as mediators for the effectiveness of expressive writing procedures. O'Connor, Walker, Hendrickx, Talbot, and Schaefer (2013), in this respect, indicated that the reason for their findings showing no effectiveness of writing protocol might be individuals' propensity to engage in perseverative thinking about stressful events. Indeed, Gortner, Rude, and Pennebaker (2006) found that the effectiveness of expressive writing on the levels of depression is mediated by brooding.

Future research may test the hypothesis that GAP might be a moderator for the effectiveness of expressive writing. That is, the effectiveness of expressive writing might be moderated by the levels of GAP experienced by the individual. Past research showed that expressive writing might not be beneficial for the individuals who are already expressing their emotions in daily life. Gortner et al. (2006) mention the research findings indicating that the individuals with high levels of alexithymia, fear of social rejection, and suppression benefited more from expressive writing. The authors indicate that expressive writing might be most beneficial for those who are not able or willing to express their emotions. Expressive writing, thus had little added value for such individuals. It is highly probable then to argue that individuals with lower levels of GAP might not be benefited from expressive writing since these individuals may already be sharing their problems with close others. Future research should tested this hypothesis given that GAP is highly associated with empathic tendency as well as interpersonal sensitivity.

Although we used advanced statistical procedures to examine direct and indirect effects of GAP on the symptoms of mental illness through NAT and worry in the present study, several limitations should be noted. The current study is based on nonclinical samples; thus the findings cannot be generalized to clinical populations. Another important limitation is that the data is obtained using self-report measures. Future research should use multi-trait multi-method analysis with multi-informant data in order to assure the validity and to control bias in the measurement. Although the present research has contributed a new explanation to the literature, the hypotheses were tested by cross-sectional data. Future research should test the hypotheses using experimental or longitudinal data.

Conflict of Interest

On behalf of all authors, the corresponding author states that there is no conflict of interest.

References

Anderson, J. C., & Gerbing, D. W. (1988). Structural equation modeling in practice: A review and recommended two-step approach. *Psychological Bulletin, 103*(3), 411–423. doi:10.1037//0033-2909.103.3.411

Barlow, J. M., Pollio, H. R., & Fine, H. J. (1977). Insight and figurative language in psychotherapy. *Psychotherapy: Theory, Research & Practice, 14*, 212–222. doi:10.1037/h0086530

Borkovec, T., Robinson, E., Pruzinsky, T., & DePree, J. (1983). Preliminary exploration of worry: Some characteristics and processes. *Behaviour Research and Therapy, 21*(1), 9–16. doi:10.1016/0005-7967(83)90121-3

Borkovec, T. D., Ray, W. J., & Stober, J. (1998). Worry: A cognitive phenomenon intimately linked to affective, physiological, and interpersonal behavioral processes. *Cognitive Therapy and Research, 22*(6), 561–576.

Boysan, M., Keskin, S., & Beşiroğlu, L. (2008). Penn State Endişe Ölçeği Türkçe formunun hiyerarşik faktör yapısı, geçerlik ve güvenilirliği (Assessment of hierarchical factor structure, reliability and validity of Penn State Worry Questionnaire Turkish version.). *Klinik Psikofarmakoloji Bülteni (Bulletin of Clinical Psychopharmacology), 18*(3), 174–182.

Bozanoğlu, İ., Şimşek, Ö. F., Altıntaş, & Kocayörük, E. (in press). Revisiting attachment to parents and depression link in adolescence: The importance of language use and emotion regulation. *Current Psychology*. doi:10.1007/s12144-017-9714-5

Bucci, W. (1984). Linking words and things: Basic processes and individual variation. *Cognition, 17*(2), 137–153. doi:10.1016/0010-0277(84)90016-7

Bucci, W., & Freedman, N. (1981). The language of depression. *Bulletin of the Menninger Clinic, 45*(4), 334–358.

Buck, R. (1993). What is this thing called subjective experience? Reflections on the neuropsychology of qualia. *Neuropsychology, 7*(4), 490–499. doi:10.1037/0894-4105.7.4.490

Clarke, K. M. (1989). Creation of meaning: An emotional processing task in psychotherapy. *Psychotherapy: Theory, Research, Practice, Training, 26*(2), 139–148.

Derogatis, L. R. (1992). *The Brief Symptom Inventory-BSI administration, scoring and procedures manual-II.* Clinical Pscyhometric Research Inc.

Dimaggio, G., Vanheule, S., Lysaker, P. H., Carcione, A., & Nicolo, G. (2009). Impaired self-reflection in psychiatric disorders among adults: A proposal for the existence of a network of semi independent functions. *Consciousness and Cognition*, *18*(3), 653–664. doi:10.1016/j.concog.2009.06.003

Engels, A. S., Heller, W., Mohanty, A., Herrington, J. D., Banich, M. T., Webb, A. G., & Miller, G. A. (2007). Specificity of regional brain activity in anxiety types during emotion processing. *Psychophysiology*, *44*(3), 352–363. doi:10.1111/j.1469-8986.2007.00518.x

Fertuck, E. A., Bucci, W., Blatt, S. J., & Ford, R. Q. (2004). Verbal representation and therapeutic change in anaclitic and introjective inpatients. *Psychotherapy: Theory, Research, Practice, Training*, *41*(1), 13–25. http://dx.doi.org/10.1037/0033. doi:10.1037/0033-3204.41.1.13

Francis, R., Hawes, D. J., Abbott, M. J., & Costa, D. S. (2018). Cognitive mechanisms for worry in early adolescence: Re-examining the role of high verbal intelligence. *Personality and Individual Differences*, *120*, 179–184. doi:10.1016/j.paid.2017.08.04

Frattaroli, J. (2006). Experimental disclosure and its moderators: A meta-analysis. *Psychological Bulletin*, *132*(6), 823–865. doi:10.1037/0033-2909.132.6.823

Gortner, E. M., Rude, S. S., & Pennebaker, J. W. (2006). Benefits of expressive writing in lowering rumination and depressive symptoms. *Behavior Therapy*, *37*(3), 292–303. doi:10.1016/j.beth.2006.01.004

Green, T. (2015). A methodological review of structural equation modelling in higher education research. *Studies in Higher Education*, 1–31. doi:10.1080/03075079.2015.1021670

Hixon, J. G., & Swann, W. B. (1993). When does introspection bear fruit? Self-reflection, self-insight, and interpersonal choices. *Journal of Personality and Social Psychology*, *64*(1), 35–43. doi:10.1037/0022-3514.64.1.35

Hoehn-Saric, R., Schlund, M. W., & Wong, S. H. Y. (2004). Effects of citalopram on worry and brain activation in patients with generalized anxiety disorder. *Psychiatry Research: Neuroimaging*, *131*(1), 11–21. doi:10.1016/j.pscychresns.2004.02.003

Howe, N., Aquan-Assee, J., Bukowski, W. M., Lehoux, P. M., & Rinaldi, C. M. (2001). Siblings as confidants: Emotional understanding, relationship warmth, and sibling self-disclosure. *Social Development*, *10*(4), 439–454. doi:10.1111/1467-9507.00174

Hu, L., & Bentler, P. M. (1998). Fit indices in covariance structure modeling: Sensitivity to under-paremeterized model misspecification. *Psychological Methods*, *3*(4), 424–453. doi:10.1037/1082-989X.3.4.424

Ivey, A. E. (1986). *Developmental therapy: Theory into practice*. San Francisco, CA: Jossey-Bass.

Jöreskog, K. G., & Sörbom, D. (1993). *LISREL 8: Structural equation modeling with the SIMPLIS command language*. Lincolnwood, IL: Scientific Software International, Inc.

Jöreskog, K. G., & Sörbom, D. (2003). Lisrel (Version 8.54) [Computer software]. Chicago: Scientific Software.

Johnson, R. E., Rosen, C. C., & Djurdjevic, E. (2011). Assessing the impact of common method variance on higher order multidimensional constructs. *Journal of Applied Psychology*, *96*(4), 744–761. doi:10.1037/a0021504

Little, T. D., Cunningham, W. A., Shahar, G., & Widaman, K. F. (2002). To parcel or not to parcel: Exploring the question, weighing the merits. *Structural Equation Modeling: A Multidisciplinary Journal*, *9*(2), 151–173. doi:10.1207/S15328007SEM0902_1

Lyubomirsky, S., & Lepper, H. S. (1999). A measure of subjective happiness: Preliminary reliability and construct validation. *Social Indicators Research*, *46*, 137–155.

Machado, P. P., & Gonçalves, O. F. (1999). Introduction: Narrative in psychotherapy: The emerging metaphor. *Journal of Clinical Psychology*, *55*(10), 1175–1177.

Mardia, K. V. (1970). Measures of multivariate skewness and kurtosis with applications. *Biometrika*, *57*, 519–530.

Meyer, T. J., Miller, M. L., Metzger, R. L., & Borkovec, T. D. (1990). Development and validation of the Penn State Worry Questionnaire. *Behaviour Research and Therapy*, *28*(6), 487–495. doi:10.1016/0005-7967(90)90135-6

Morin, A. (2006). Levels of consciousness and self-awareness: A comparison and integration of various neurocognitive views. *Consciousness and Cognition*, *15*(2), 358–371. doi:10.1016/j.concog.2005.09.006

Musacchio, J. M. (2002). Dissolving the explanatory gap: Neurobiological differences between phenomenal and propositional knowledge. *Brain and Mind, 3*(3), 331–365.

Neimeyer, R. A. & Mahoney, M. J. (Eds.). (1995). *Constructivism in psychotherapy.* Washington, D.C.: American Psychological Association.

O'Connor, D. B., Walker, S., Hendrickx, H., Talbot, D., & Schaefer, A. (2013). Stress-related thinking predicts the cortisol awakening response and somatic symptoms in healthy adults. *Psychoneuroendocrinology, 38*, 438–446.

Owen, I. R. (1991). Using the sixth sense: The place and relevance of language in counseling. *British Journal of Guidance & Counselling, 19*(3), 307–320. doi:10.1080/03069889108260394

Paivio, A., & Marschark, M. (1991). Integrative processing of concrete and abstract sentences. In A. Paivio (Ed.), *Images in the mind: The evolution of a theory* (pp.134–154). New York, NY: Harvester Wheatsheaf.

Pennebaker, J. W. (1993). Putting stress into words: Health, linguistics, and therapeutic implications. *Behaviour Research and Therapy, 31*(6), 539–548. http://dx.doi.org/10.1016/0005-7967.(93)90105-4. doi:10.1016/0005-7967(93)90105-4

Pennebaker, J. W., & Chung, C. K. (2011). Expressive writing and its links to mental and physical health. In H. S. Friedman (Ed.), *Oxford handbook of health psychology* (pp. 417–437). New York, NY: Oxford University Press.

Pennebaker, J. W., & Graybeal, A. (2001). Patterns of natural language use: Disclosure, personality, and social integration. *Current Directions in Psychological Science, 10*(3), 90–93. doi:10.1111/1467-8721.00123

Russell, B. (1912). *The problems of philosophy.* New York, NY: Galaxy.

Segerstrom, S. C., Stanton, A. L., Alden, L. E., & Shortridge, B. E. (2003). A multidimensional structure for repetitive thought: What's on your mind, and how, and how much?. *Journal of Personality and Social Psychology, 85*(5), 909–921. doi:10.1037/0022-3514.85.5.909

Sibrava, N. J., & Borkovec, T. D. (2006). The cognitive avoidance theory of worry. In G. C. L. Davey, & A. Wells (Eds.), *Worry and its psychological disorders: Theory, assessment, and treatment* (pp. 239–256). West Sussex, UK: John Wiley.

Shrout, P. E., & Bolger, N. (2002). Mediation in experimental and nonexperimental studies: New procedures and recommendations. *Psychological Methods, 7*(4), 422–445. doi:10.1037/1082-989X.7.4.422

Sloan, D. M., Marx, B. P., Epstein, E. V., & Dobbs, J. L. (2008). Expressive writing buffers against maladaptive rumination. *Emotion, 8*(2), 302–306. doi:10.1037/1528-3542.8.2.302

Stöber, J. (1998). Worry, problem solving, and suppression of imagery: The role of concreteness. *Behaviour Research and Therapy, 36*(7-8), 751–756.

Stöber, J., & Borkovec, T. D. (2002). Reduced concreteness of worry in a generalized anxiety disorder: Findings from a therapy study. *Cognitive Therapy and Research, 26*(1), 89–96.

Stöber, J., Tepperwien, S., & Staak, M. (2000). Worry leads to reduced concreteness of problem elaborations: Evidence for the avoidance theory of worry. *Anxiety, Stress, and Coping, 13*(3), 217–227. doi:10.1080/10615800008549263

Şahin, N. H., & Durak, A. (1994). Kısa Semptom Envanteri: Türk gençleri için uyarlanması (Brief Seymptom Inventory: Adaptation for the Turkish Youth). *Türk Psikoloji Dergisi, 9*(31), 44–56.

Şimşek, Ö. F. (2010). Language and the inner: Development of the Beliefs about Functions of Language (BAFL) Scale. *European Psychologist, 15*(1), 68–79. doi:10.1027/1016-9040/a000005

Şimşek, Ö. F., & Kuzucu, Y. (2012). The gap that makes us desperate: Paths from language to mental health. *International Journal of Psychology, 47*(6), 467–477. doi:10.1080/00207594.2011.645479

Şimşek, Ö. F. (2013). The relationship between language use and depression: Illuminating the importance of self-reflection, self-rumination, and the need for absolute truth. *The Journal of General Psychology, 140*(1), 29–44. doi:10.1080/00221309.2012.713407

Şimşek, Ö. F., Ceylandağ, A. E., & Akcan, G. (2013). The need for absolute truth and self-rumination as basic suppressors in the relationship between private self-consciousness and mental health. *Journal of General Psychology, 140*(4), 294–310.

Şimşek, Ö. F., & Çerçi, M. (2013). Relationship of the gap between experience and language with mental health in adolescence: The importance of emotion regulation. *The Journal of Psychology, 147*(3), 293–309. doi:10.1080/00223980.2012.691914

Tucker, D. M., & Newman, J. P. (1981). Verbal versus imaginal cognitive strategies in the inhibition of emotional arousal. *Cognitive Therapy and Research, 5*(2), 197–202. doi:10.1007/BF01172527

Watkins, E. (2008). Constructive and unconstructive repetitive thought. *Psychological Bulletin, 134*(2), 163–206. doi:10.1037/0033-2909.134.2.163

Watkins, E., & Teasdale, J. D. (2004). Adaptive and maladaptive self-focus in depression. *Journal of Affective Disorders, 82*(1), 1–8. doi:10.1016/j.jad.2003.10.006

Zuellig, A. R., & Borkovec, T. D. (1996, November). Predominance of thoughts and images during trauma recall and worry. Poster presented at the meeting of the Association for Advancement of Behavior Therapy, New York, NY.

Personality Trait Interactions in Risk for and Protection against Social Anxiety Symptoms

Patryk Łakuta

ABSTRACT

Previous attempts to identify personality traits that enhance inclination to social anxiety (SA) have been limited by a tendency to focus on selected traits in isolation, rather than examining their interactions. Additional research is needed to better understand whether and how these dimensions are linked to SA. In a prospective study, it was examined how interactions between the Big Five personality factors predict SA symptoms. A total of 135 individuals, aged 18–50 years, were recruited. Personality traits were measured at baseline, and SA symptoms were assessed one month later. Results showed that low emotional stability was an independent predictor of higher levels of SA. Additionally, two significant interactions emerged: the interactions between extraversion and openness, and between openness and agreeableness predicted SA symptoms. At high openness, higher extraversion was associated with significantly lower levels of SA, suggesting that the interaction provides incrementally greater protection against SA. Thus, extraverts are likely to be protected against social anxiety symptoms, but more so the more open they are. Moreover, at high levels of agreeableness, low openness has been shown to be uniquely predictive for higher levels of SA symptoms, indicating that the combined effect of openness with agreeableness may be more important to SA than either trait in isolation. These findings highlight the importance of testing interaction effects of personality traits on psychopathology.

Personality includes multiple traits, and these might not always work in isolation with one another. Although personality research adopting a more holistic and interactive perspective on personality has provided evidence that traits work together and interact in meaningful ways in affecting psychological and behavioral outcomes (cf. Bardi & Ryff, 2007; Eliasz & Klonowicz, 2001; King, George, & Hebl, 2005; Marszał-Wiśniewska, 2001; Shoss & Witt, 2013; Strelau, 1998, 2008; Zalewska, 2011), studies on interactive approach to personality–psychopathology associations are still sparse. Indeed, prior studies on personality and social anxiety have predominantly focused on the main effects of personality traits (see Kotov, Gamez, Schmidt, & Watson, 2010). The present research rectifies this paucity by examining the interaction effects of personality traits – testing whether social anxiety symptoms might be predicted by interactions among personality traits (e.g., interaction effects that can lead to an internal incongruence among personality mechanisms or produce amplification effects). As growing evidence supports, an examination of multiple personality traits, and their interactions, has the potential to provide rich insight into unique patterns of thoughts, beliefs, and behaviors (cf. Allen et al., 2018; Vasey et al., 2013, 2014). Furthermore, it appears that links between personality traits are of considerable practical and theoretical importance, and thus deserve greater attention in this literature.

According to the five-factor model (FFM) of personality (Digman, 1990; McCrae & Costa, 1999, 2013), the full range of personality traits can be well defined in terms of five basic dimensions: Extraversion, Neuroticism (vs. Emotional Stability), Agreeableness, Conscientiousness, and Openness to Experience (also known as Openness, Imagination, Intellect, or Culture). Research on personality and psychopathology (see Kotov et al., 2010) has led to a growing recognition that many psychiatric disorders represent maladaptive variations on normative traits. Much of this work has been conducted within the framework of the FFM, which is currently the most widely used model of personality (McCrae & Costa, 2013). However, the attempts to identify personality traits that enhance inclination to social anxiety (SA) have been limited by a tendency to focus on selected traits in isolation, rather than examining their interactions (e.g., synergistic effects in risk for and protection against social anxiety symptoms). Moreover, prior research (see Kotov et al., 2010) has frequently been focused on one specific domain of social anxiety disorder (SAD), namely the features of fear and avoidance, rather than the full dimension of social anxiety symptoms (cf. Clark, 2001; Heimberg, Brozovich, & Rapee, 2014; Modini & Abbott, 2017; Norton & Abbott, 2016; Penney & Abbott, 2014), which could limit their ability for detecting links between SAD and personality traits. Additional research is therefore needed to enhance our understanding of effects of the Big Five trait dimensions[1] on SAD. Examining whether traits moderate one another to predict the nature and severity of social anxiety symptoms, including negative self-views; anticipatory and post-event rumination; self-focused attention; somatic and cognitive symptoms; and safety behaviors (cf. Clark, 2001; Heimberg et al., 2014; Modini & Abbott, 2017; Norton & Abbott, 2016; Penney & Abbott, 2014), may help elucidate etiological mechanisms, help to inform psychological assessment and treatment planning, and provide clinicians and other professionals with information about the personality traits (and their combinations) that are more intertwined with SAD.

The accumulating data indicate that with regard to the higher-order personality traits of the Big Five, main effects clearly exist between SAD and Extraversion and Neuroticism (for a meta-analysis, see Kotov et al., 2010; see also Levinson, Kaplan, & Rodebaugh, 2014). Extraversion and Neuroticism are consistently linked with emotional functioning (cf. Watson, 2000; Watson & Clark, 1992). Extraversion (called positive emotionality) determines a tendency to take up activity (tasks and social interactions) and the level of energy (McCrae & Costa, 1991). It also makes predisposition to positive experiences and emotions connected with sensitivity to attractive stimuli (cf. DeNeve & Cooper, 1998; Diener & Lucas, 1999). Neuroticism is by far the trait most strongly linked to negative affectivity (Watson, 2000; Watson & Clark, 1992). High neuroticism is associated with tending to be emotional, insecure, impulsive, and susceptible to psychological distress (cf. Diener & Lucas, 1999; McCrae & Costa, 1991) – predisposes one to negative experiences and emotions because of higher levels of sensitivity to aversive stimuli. The two dimensions of personality typically emerge as the strongest independent predictors of SAD (Bienvenu, Hettema, Neale, Prescott, & Kendler, 2007; Kotov et al., 2010). Thus, in keeping with previous findings from research on personality – SAD (cf. Kotov et al., 2010), it was hypothesized that Extraversion and Neuroticism would be the strongest predictors of social anxiety symptoms.

The remaining Big Five personality traits — Agreeableness, Conscientiousness, and Openness to Experience — have been less studied in research on SAD, and evidence of links between SAD and the other personality traits is mixed (cf. Kotov et al., 2010). However, there are good theoretical reasons to believe that these traits would be important in predicting SA symptoms. Importantly, these traits may interact and produce attenuation or amplification effects with other traits (e.g., a trait may be significantly related to SA symptoms only at positive values of another trait). Following McCrae and Costa (1991) and other personality researchers (cf. Bardi & Ryff, 2007; Eliasz, 2006; Eliasz & Klonowicz, 2001; King et al., 2005; Marszał-Wiśniewska, 2001; Shoss & Witt, 2013; Strelau, 1998, 2008; Zalewska, 2011), personality traits can moderate one another and lead to attenuate/amplify one's detrimental/beneficial effects. Specifically, person's cognitive and affective evaluations, behavior patterns, social adaptation, and susceptibility to disorders may result from interaction effects between traits.

For example, as proposed by McCrae and Costa (1991), high Openness can amplify emotional reactions, e.g., positive emotionality of high Extraversion. Thus, Extraverts are likely to experience positive affect, but more so the more open they are. Similarly, enhanced psychological distress may result from combination of high Neuroticism with higher levels of Openness. Based on theoretical accounts and growing research literature on the Big Five trait dimensions, another hypothesized interaction can be proposed, namely interaction of Openness with Agreeableness. Given the interpersonal nature of Agreeableness (e.g., positivity of interpersonal motivations and behaviors and increased affective reactivity in response to interpersonal conflicts; see Costa & McCrae, 1992; Graziano & Eisenberg, 1997; Graziano, Bruce, Sheese, & Tobin, 2007a; 2007b Jensen-Campbell et al., 2002; Jensen-Campbell, Gleason, Adams, & Malcolm, 2003; Suls, 2001) and motivations and cognitive styles associated with low Openness (e.g., low tolerance for different worldview or lifestyles, prejudiced, "seizing and freezing" process when judging how threatening the world seems to be; see DeYoung, 2015; McCrae, 1987, 1996; Onraet, Van Hiel, Roets, & Cornelis, 2011; Perry & Sibley, 2013), high Agreeableness with low Openness may produce intra-individual inconsistency. Another effect, it has been shown that combination of high Neuroticism and low Conscientiousness contributes to higher levels of stress and dysfunctional patterns of coping (Grant & Langan-Fox, 2006; Vollrath & Torgersen, 2000). Accordingly, it is important to take into account that combinations of personality factors may display differential influences on psychological functioning, including affect, behavior, and cognition. In terms of research on links between personality and SAD, interaction effects between personality traits may contribute to a more complex understanding of how and when different personality traits may or may not be related to social anxiety, e.g., may help explain equivocal links observed in past research (cf. Kotov et al., 2010).

In sum, consistent with prior literature, one of the explanatory hypotheses for the associations between personality traits and psychopathology is the cumulative risk hypothesis (extension of the predisposition/vulnerability hypothesis; see Andersen & Bienvenu, 2011; Clark, 2005; see also Strelau, 1998, 2008), stating that certain personality factors interact to magnify the overall risk of a negative outcome (e.g., high SA), such that the resulting risk status is higher than would follow from the sum of the individual factors (e.g., Allen et al., 2018; Atkinson et al., 2015). The inverse of this hypothesis is that certain trait interactions confer protection against the development of psychological disorders (Masten & Wright, 1998), e.g., lessen the chance of negative outcomes by moderating levels of the undesired trait; see Kaplan, Levinson, Rodebaugh, Menatti, & Weeks, 2015). In line with the interactive approach, to advance our understanding of associations between social anxiety and personality, it was examined how interactions between the Big Five personality traits predict SA symptoms. In this study, therefore, interaction effects of personality traits in risk for and protection against SA symptoms were tested.

Method

Participants and Procedure

The study used a prospective design. The hypotheses in the present study were tested using two measurement points. Thus, personality traits were measured at Time 1 (T1) and social anxiety symptoms at Time 2 (T2; one month later). Participants' data across each time points were anonymized and matched across time points using a unique code identifier.

Based on the research applying the FFM that has typically identified medium- to large-sized effects of personality variables on SAD after controlling for neuroticism (see Kotov et al., 2010), the minimum sample size was estimated. G*Power (Faul, Erdfelder, Lang, & Buchner, 2007) was used to calculate the required sample size to detect medium-sized moderating effects with 80% power using multiple linear regression. A potential 30% dropout rate (at Time 2) was considered. Consequently, the minimum sample size of $N= 120$ would be required. A total of 135 nonclinical individuals participated in the study at T1, aged 18–50 years ($M= 24.92$ years, $SD = 5.66$). At T1, participants were requested to complete measure of the Big-Five personality traits; among them 80% were women; 59.3% were students; and 39.3% of the participants were full-time employees. Approximately one month later, at T2 the measure assessing SA symptoms was administered. In this sample, the age of participants ranged from 18 to 43 years ($M= 24.85$, $SD = 5.01$), 72 (81.8%) were women, 38.6% of the individuals were full-time employees. The dropout rate from T1 to T2 was 34.8%. Completers constituting the final sample did not differ from those who dropped out at T2 (see below).

The study was conducted in accordance with the Codes of Ethics and conduct specified by the Helsinki Declaration. An informed consent was obtained. Participants were provided with an assurance of their anonymity in participation and were free to withdraw from the study at any time. All individuals received the same questionnaires and no clinical or experimental treatment.

Measures

Ten Item Personality Measure (TIPI)

Personality traits were assessed via the widely used 10-item Personality Inventory (Gosling, Rentfrow, & Swann, 2003) that bases on the FFM (McCrae & Costa, 1999). The questionnaire begins with the phrase: "I see myself as ... ," followed by 10 pairs of adjectives (e.g., for extraversion "extraverted, enthusiastic"; for openness "open to new experiences, complex"). Answers are provided on a 7-point scale, ranging from 1 (*disagree strongly*) to 7 (*agree strongly*). The score for each of the five personality dimensions (Extraversion, Emotional Stability, Openness, Conscientiousness, and Agreeableness) is the mean score of two items (after recoding the reverse-scored items), and higher scores indicate stronger intensity of a trait. Good reliability and good validity of the measure have been supported in many studies (cf. Furnham, 2008; Gosling et al., 2003).

Social Anxiety Questionnaire (SAQ)

The SAQ is a 10-item self-report measure assessing social anxiety symptoms according to Clark and Wells's (1995; Clark, 2001) model. The measure captures five aspects of social anxiety: negative self-processing; self-focused attention and self-monitoring; safety behaviors; somatic and cognitive symptoms; and anticipatory and post-event rumination. Items are rated on a 5-point Likert-type scale, ranging from 1 (*strongly disagree*) to 5 (*strongly agree*). Sample items for the SAQ are "Anxiety which I feel in social situations significantly disrupts my occupational or academic functioning, or social activities or relationships" and "I try not to attract attention for fear of being negatively evaluated by other people." Total scores range from 10 to 50, with higher scores reflecting higher levels of social anxiety symptoms. Research has shown good psychometric properties of the SAQ in terms of internal consistency, temporal stability, as well as convergent and divergent validity (Łakuta, 2018). In the present study, Cronbach's α-value for the SAQ was .90.

Statistical Analyses

To examine whether the Big Five factors of personality and their interactions predict SA symptoms a hierarchical multiple regression analysis controlling for age and gender was conducted. All variables were standardized before being entered into the equation. Interactions were probed using Hayes's (2013) PROCESS macro for SPSS.

Results

Preliminary Analyses

Attrition analysis showed no significant differences between completers and dropouts in age, $t(133)=0.25$, $p=.806$; education, $\chi^2(1)=1.53$, $p=.216$; and gender, $\chi^2(1)=0.522$, $p=.470$.

Descriptive Statistics

Means, standard deviations, and bivariate correlations for the study variables are presented in Table 1. Negative correlations between social anxiety and Extraversion (r=-0.62, p<.001) and Emotional Stability (r=-0.50, p<.001) emerged. Moreover, low but significant correlations were found between the SAQ scores and Openness to Experience and Conscientiousness, and there were, however, no correlations between the SAQ and Agreeableness.

The Big Five Personality Traits and Their Interactions as Predictors of Social Anxiety

The results of a hierarchical regression analysis examining whether personality traits and their interactions predict SA are presented in Table 2. Age and sex as control variables were entered as a first step. In Step 2, personality traits were entered accounting for 54% of the variance in social anxiety symptoms. Sex, Extraversion, and Emotional Stability all significantly predicted scores on SA. In Step 3, Emotional Stability and Extraversion remained significant as predictors of SA. Importantly, a significant interaction between Extraversion and Openness, and interaction between Openness and Agreeableness yielded a significant increase in R^2 (p<.05), accounting for an additional 11% of variance in the outcome variable.

As shown in Table 2, Extraversion was significantly related to social anxiety and Openness significantly moderated this relationship. The interaction was probed by testing the conditional effects of Extraversion at three levels of Openness, one standard deviation below the mean, at the mean, and one standard deviation above the mean. As shown in Figure 1, the estimated simple slopes were negative and statistically significant at all values of Openness (all ps<.05); the simple slopes became increasingly negative as levels of Openness increased. Indeed, the Johnson-Neyman technique (see Hayes, 2013) showed that the conditional effects of Extraversion emerged when Openness was higher than -1.44 SDs. Specifically, high Extraversion at high Openness was strongly predictive of lower levels of social anxiety symptoms measured one month later (b=-.70, 95% CI [-.93, -.47], SE=.12, t=-6.08, p<.001). Individuals low in Extraversion appeared at higher risk of social anxiety symptoms. However, note that low Extraversion combined with high Openness has been found to predict the most severe symptoms (see Figure 1).

Table 1. Means (M), Standard Deviations (SD), and Correlations Between the Study Variables at T1 and T2.

	M (SD)	1.	2.	3.	4.	5.	6.
1. Social anxiety (T2)	30.15 (8.97)	–	-0.62***	-0.16	-0.36***	-0.50***	-0.28**
2. Extraversion (T1)	4.34 (1.42)		–	0.11	0.24*	0.31**	0.39***
3. Agreeableness (T1)	5.10 (1.05)			–	0.18	0.34***	0.03
4. Conscientiousness (T1)	5.01 (1.43)				–	0.33**	0.01
5. Emotional stability (T1)	3.51 (1.46)					–	0.10
6. Openness (T1)	5.01 (1.23)						–

Note. T1 – Time 1, baseline; T2 – Time 2, 1-month follow-up.
***p<.001;
**p<.01;
*p<.05.

Table 2. Hierarchical Multiple Regression With Personality Traits and Their Interactions on Social Anxiety.

	β	SE	F	R^2	ΔR^2	$F\Delta R^2$
Step 1			0.48	0.01	0.01	0.48
Age	−0.10	0.11				
Gender (men)	0.07	0.11				
Step 2			14.23***	0.55	0.54	19.52***
Age	−0.10	0.08				
Gender (men)	0.25**	0.09				
Extraversion	−0.50***	0.09				
Emotional stability	−0.40***	0.09				
Conscientiousness	−0.05	0.09				
Openness	−0.07	0.08				
Agreeableness	0.06	0.08				
Step 3			8.16***	0.66	0.11	2.29*
Age	−0.13	0.08				
Gender (men)	0.23*	0.09				
Extraversion	−0.52***	0.08				
Emotional stability	−0.31**	0.09				
Conscientiousness	−0.15	0.09				
Openness	−0.17	0.08				
Agreeableness	0.07	0.08				
Emotional stability × Agreeableness	−0.06	0.09				
Openness × Agreeableness	−0.29**	0.09				
Conscientiousness × Agreeableness	−0.02	0.08				
Extraversion × Emotional stability	−0.12	0.09				
Extraversion × Openness	−0.19*	0.08				
Extraversion × Conscientiousness	−0.05	0.08				
Extraversion × Agreeableness	0.17	0.10				
Conscientiousness × Emotional stab.	−0.03	0.08				
Conscientiousness × Openness	0.15	0.09				
Emotional stability × Openness	0.02	0.10				

Note.
***$p < .001$;
**$p < .01$;
*$p < .05$.

Furthermore, despite no significant main effects of Openness or Agreeableness, a significant interaction was emerged between these traits on social anxiety levels (see Table 2). This interaction is illustrated in Figure 2. Simple slopes analysis showed that Openness was significantly related to social anxiety symptoms when Agreeableness was one standard deviation above the mean ($b = -.43$, 95% CI [−.69, −.18], SE$= .13$, $t = -3.36$, $p = .001$), but not when Agreeableness was one standard deviation below the mean ($p = .34$). Accordingly, a combination of high Agreeableness and high Openness is likely to protect against social anxiety symptoms. However, at high levels of Agreeableness, low Openness is significantly related to higher levels of SA symptoms (Figure 2).

Discussion

This project explored personality trait interaction patterns as plausible factors in social anxiety symptoms. Previous studies on personality – SAD associations focused primarily on the two of the Big Five traits – Extraversion and Neuroticism. Moreover, the findings on the remaining personality factors – Conscientiousness, Agreeableness, and Openness – have been mixed (cf. Kotov et al., 2010). Based on the literature documenting the potential role of trait interactions in internalizing psychopathology (cf. Allen

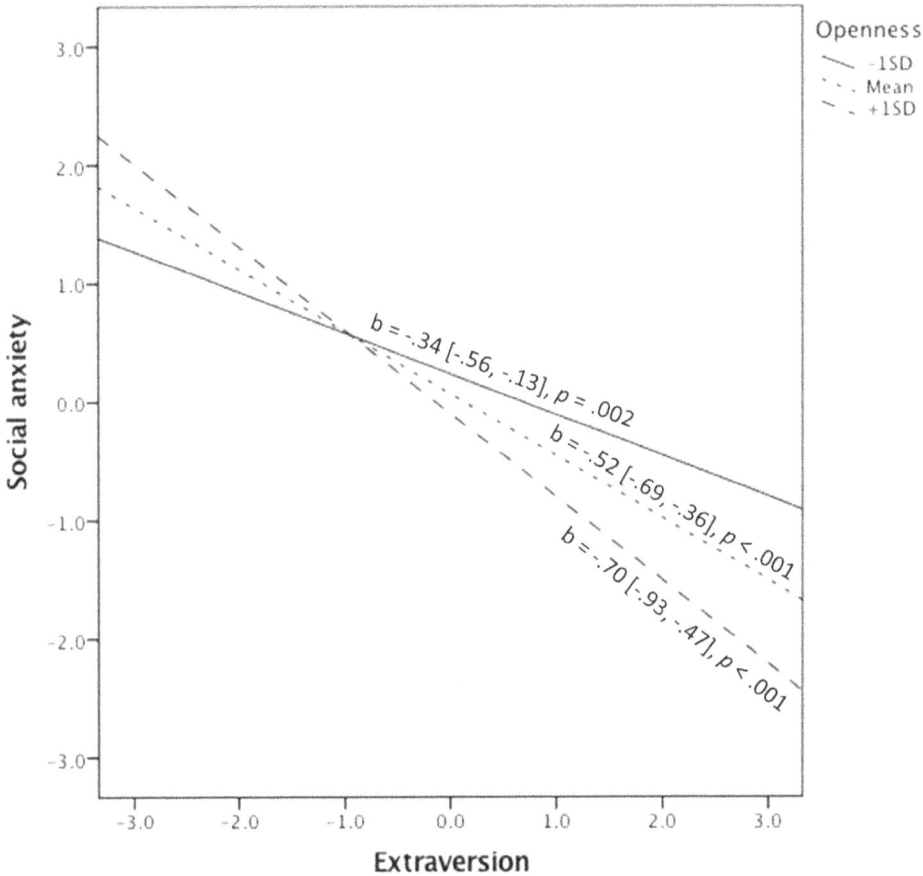

Figure 1. A visual depiction of significant 2-way interaction ($b=-.18$, 95% CI [$-.33$, $-.03$], $p=.02$) between Extraversion and Openness in predicting social anxiety symptoms. *Note.* Both the X and Y axes represent standardized values. Brackets denote upper and lower boundaries of 95% confidence intervals.

et al., 2018; Kaplan et al., 2015; Vasey et al., 2013, Vasey, 2014; see also Andersen & Bienvenu, 2011; Strelau, 1998, 2008), it was proposed that personality traits can moderate one another and lead to attenuate or amplify one's effects (e.g., synergistic effects in risk for and protection against social anxiety symptoms). Thus, in the present research, a key question was whether social anxiety symptoms might also be predicted by interactions among personality traits. As expected from past research (cf. Bienvenu et al., 2007; see also Kotov et al., 2010; Levinson et al., 2014), Extraversion and Neuroticism were found to act as key determinants of social anxiety symptoms measured at one-month follow-up. However, one of the main contributions is to show that personality trait interactions did, indeed, significantly predict social anxiety symptoms, suggesting that personality traits can work synergistically to contribute to the etiology of social anxiety.

First, the results revealed a significant interaction effect of Openness and Extraversion on SA. High Extraversion at high Openness was strongly predictive of lower levels of social anxiety symptoms, and interaction of these traits seems to provide incrementally greater protection against SA. The interaction illustrates personality synergies in

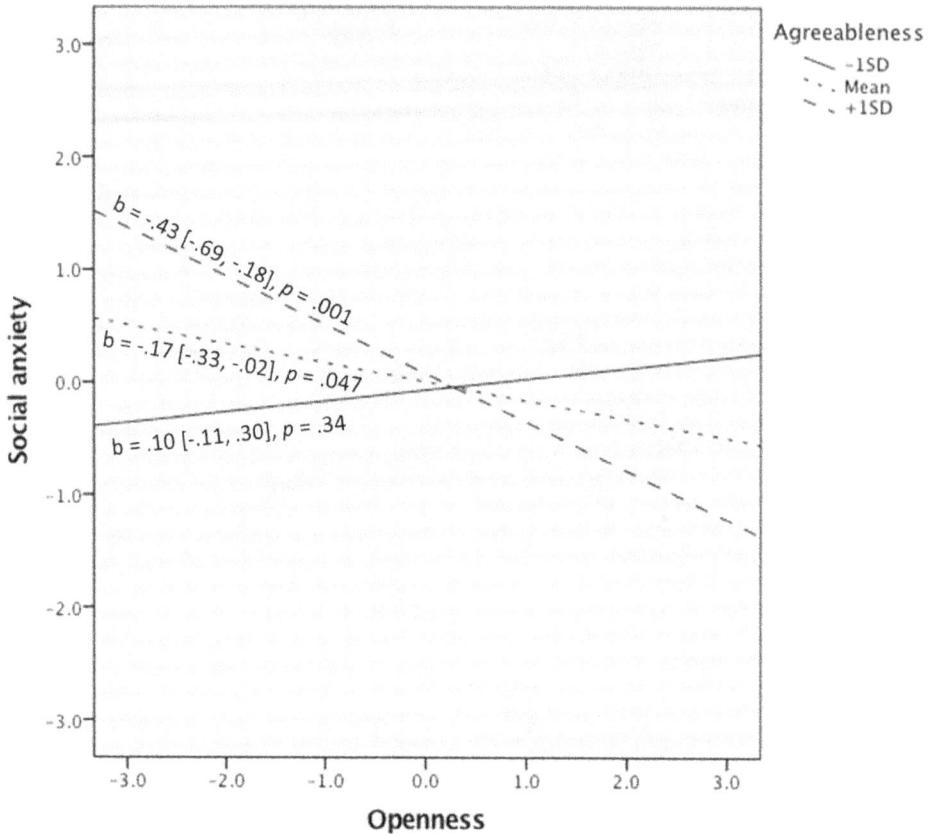

Figure 2. A visual depiction of significant 2-way interaction ($b=-.26$, 95% CI [$-.43$, $-.10$], $p=.002$) between Openness and Agreeableness in predicting social anxiety symptoms. *Note.* Both the X and Y axes represent standardized values. Brackets denote upper and lower boundaries of 95% confidence intervals.

protection against social anxiety so that high Openness seems to amplify beneficial effects of positive emotionality of high Extraversion. Conversely, individuals low in Extraversion appeared at higher risk of social anxiety symptoms. However, the most severe symptoms were associated with low Extraversion combined with high Openness. This pattern of findings confirms the hypothesis that follows directly from McCrae and Costa's (1991) suggestion regarding the amplification effects of Openness.

The present findings contribute to a more complex understanding of effects of personality traits on SAD. Previous research has shown Extraversion, in particular, has the strongest links to SAD (Kotov et al., 2010). There is also some evidence suggesting links between Openness to Experience and SAD (e.g., Hummelen, Wilberg, Pedersen, & Karterud, 2007). According to the obtained results, the most beneficial effects may be expected from a combination of high Openness and high Extraversion. Extraverts tend to have a strong tendency for positive affect (DeNeve & Cooper, 1998; Diener & Lucas, 1999; McCrae & Costa, 1991, 1999), and they have considerably more positive experiences (Heady & Wearing, 1989; Magnus, Diener, Fujita, & Pavot, 1993). Thus, it is not surprising that this is the Five-Factor trait most consistently and negatively linked to

SAD (cf. Kotov et al., 2010). However, based on the results, the effect of Extraversion can be moderated by Openness, and these two personality traits can work synergistically to contribute to lower risk of SA. Openness amplifying extroverted tendencies, including the basic emotional tendency of Extraversion for positive effect, seems to provide incrementally greater protection against SA. More broadly, at high levels of Extraversion that encompasses broad tendencies toward sociability and positive emotionality (McCrae & Costa, 1999, 2013), high Openness may provoke engaging in novel situations (including social ones) and being more receptive to new input from other people and surroundings, and thus, an individual can benefit from the naturalistic exposure provided by everyday interactions with other people and maximize opportunities for disconfirming negative beliefs by direct observation of the social situation, rather than oneself (cf. Clark, 2001; Heimberg et al., 2014; Norton & Abbott, 2016). Thus, Extraverts are likely to be protected against social anxiety symptoms, but more so the more open they are, however, future research is needed to test a direct mechanism by which these traits interaction may protect against social anxiety.

The results of the present research also showed another theoretically meaningful and interesting interaction. The interaction between Openness and Agreeableness yielded a significant increase in prediction of SA symptoms. Simple slopes analysis showed that the role of Openness was more salient at higher levels of Agreeableness – Openness was significantly related to social anxiety symptoms when Agreeableness was one standard deviation above the mean, but not when Agreeableness was one standard deviation below the mean. Specifically, at high levels of Agreeableness, low Openness was related to higher levels of social anxiety. The interaction pattern was uniquely predictive for higher risk of SA symptoms. Again, the interaction highlights the importance of considering combined effects of personality traits, demonstrating that the combined effect of the traits is more important to SA than either trait in isolation. Importantly, the current research extends our understanding of the link between social anxiety and Agreeableness and Openness, and helps to explain equivocal links observed in past research (cf. Kotov et al., 2010).

Agreeableness is one of the major dimensions of personality that is most relevant to interpersonal functioning (Costa & McCrae, 1992; McCrae & Costa, 1991), i.e., positivity of interpersonal motivations and behaviors (Graziano et al., 2007a, 2007b Graziano & Eisenberg, 1997; Jensen-Campbell & Graziano, 2001). Agreeable people, compared with individuals low in Agreeableness, tend to be warm, pleasant, and harmonious in relationships with others (Graziano, Jensen-Campbell, & Hair, 1996; Jensen-Campbell et al., 2002), tend to experience greater distress in the face of interpersonal stressors (Suls, Martin, & David, 1998), they are particularly adverse to interpersonal conflict (Jensen-Campbell et al., 2003; Suls, 2001). In conceptual contrast, low openness as has been shown in past research to be associated with right-wing authoritarianism (e.g., Cohrs, Kämpfe-Hargrave, & Riemann, 2012; Sibley & Duckitt, 2008), religious fundamentalism (e.g., Saroglou, 2002), and other conservative values (e.g., Jost, Glaser, Kruglanski, & Sulloway, 2003), all of which are consistently linked with prejudice and discrimination (e.g., see Brandt & Reyna, 2010, 2014; Cohrs et al., 2012; Hall, Matz, & Wood, 2010; Jost, Nosek, & Gosling, 2008; Sibley & Duckitt, 2008). People low in

Openness are not only more conventional but also more likely to be anchored by threat-relevant cues and tend to seize and freeze on their opinions and attitudes (DeYoung, 2015; McCrae, 1987, 1996; Onraet et al., 2011). Importantly, they also tend to engage in a seizing and freezing process when judging how threatening the world seems to be (Perry & Sibley, 2013). In this case, cognitive and motivational tendencies associated with low Openness, and the positivity of interpersonal motivations and behaviors related to high Agreeableness, reviewed above, stand in contradiction and may lead to within-person functional inconsistency that results in patterns related to SA. This finding accords with previous studies (Kashdan, Elhai, & Breen, 2008) demonstrating social anxiety severity as associated with experiencing greater approach–avoidance conflicts. Future studies on social anxiety can draw from the work to carry a step further and strengthen knowledge of mechanisms by which interactions among these traits influence social anxiety.

Limitations and Directions for Future Research

The results of this study demonstrate the importance of testing interactions between traits that combine in theoretically meaningful ways to predict SAD. The current findings contribute to a growing body of literature examining personality trait interactions on psychopathology; however, as with most research, this study is not without limitations. First, personality traits were assessed using a relatively brief self-report measure. Although many studies have adopted the TIPI demonstrating its good validity across diverse samples (cf. Furnham, 2008; Gosling et al., 2003), estimation through a standard multi-item instrument (e.g., NEO-PI-R; Costa & McCrae, 1992) would be more accurate. Further, measurement of social anxiety symptoms through a self-report measure is also a limitation; corroboration through clinician assessments and self-ratings may provide more accurate estimates of the outcome. Moreover, additional research is needed to test the generalizability of the findings across a more diverse range of samples. It should also be recognized that relations among the personality traits measured at T1 and SA symptoms measured at T2 (one-month follow-up) did not permit inferences of directionality or causation. Finally, future studies could also aim to examine trait interactions located at a level of the personality hierarchy below the five factors.

Conclusions

Taken together, the results underscore the need for greater focus on examining trait interactions in affecting social anxiety. Findings from the current research demonstrate that only a comprehensive consideration of the interrelations among personality traits may provide an in-depth understanding of the contribution of personality traits to SAD (i.e., understanding of how these dimensions are linked to social anxiety symptoms). The current study shows that Neuroticism and the combined effects of Extraversion and Openness, and Openness and Agreeableness significantly predict social anxiety symptoms. This pattern of findings supports the importance of synergistic effects of personality traits in risk for and protection against SAD.

Note

1. Although the labels the Big-Five and the FFM are often used interchangeably to refer to the consensus on their importance as major constructs of personality, they derive from different research traditions (see, e.g., Johnson, 2017).

Acknowledgements

The author wishes to thank Professor Anna M. Zalewska for helpful comments on an earlier draft of this paper.

Declarations of interest

There are no conflicts of interest to declare.

Funding

This research did not receive any specific grant from funding agencies in the public, commercial, or not-for-profit sectors.

References

Allen, T. A., Carey, B. E., McBride, C., Bagby, R. M., DeYoung, C. G., & Quilty, L. C. (2018). Big five aspects of personality interact to predict depression. *Journal of Personality, 86*(4), 714–725. doi:10.1111/jopy.12352

Andersen, A. M., & Bienvenu, O. J. (2011). Personality and psychopathology. *International Review of Psychiatry, 23*(3), 234–247. doi:10.3109/09540261.2011.588692

Atkinson, L., Beitchman, J., Gonzalez, A., Young, A., Wilson, B., Escobar, M., … Villani, V. (2015). Cumulative risk, cumulative outcome: A 20-year longitudinal study. *PLoS One, 10*(6), e0127650. doi:10.1371/journal.pone.0127650

Bardi, A., & Ryff, C. D. (2007). Interactive effects of traits on adjustment to a life transition. *Journal of Personality, 75*(5), 955–984. doi:10.1111/j.1467-6494.2007.00462.x

Bienvenu, O. J., Hettema, J. M., Neale, M. C., Prescott, C. A., & Kendler, K. S. (2007). Low extraversion and high neuroticism as indices of genetic and environmental risk for social phobia, agoraphobia, and animal phobia. *American Journal of Psychiatry, 164*(11), 1714–1721. doi:10.1176/appi.ajp.2007.06101667

Brandt, M. J., & Reyna, C. (2010). The role of prejudice and the need for closure in religious fundamentalism. *Personality and Social Psychology Bulletin, 36*(5), 715–725. doi:10.1177/0146167210366306

Brandt, M. J., & Reyna, C. (2014). To love or hate thy neighbor: The role of authoritarianism and traditionalism in explaining the link between fundamentalism and racial prejudice. *Political Psychology, 35*(2), 207–223. doi:10.1111/pops.12077

Clark, D. M. (2001). A cognitive perspective on social phobia. In W. R. Crozier, & L. E. Alden (Eds.), *International handbook of social anxiety: Concepts, research and interventions relating to the self and shyness* (pp. 405–430). New York, NY: John Wiley & Sons.

Clark, D. M., & Wells, A. (1995). A cognitive model of social phobia. In R. G. Heimberg, M. Liebowitz, D. A. Hope, & F. R. Schneier (Eds.), *Social phobia: Diagnosis, assessment, and treatment* (pp. 69–93). New York, NY: Guilford Press.

Clark, L. A. (2005). Temperament as a unifying basis for personality and psychopathology. *Journal of Abnormal Psychology, 114*(4), 505–521. doi:10.1037/0021-843X.114.4.505

Cohrs, J. C., Kämpfe-Hargrave, N., & Riemann, R. (2012). Individual differences in ideological attitudes and prejudice: Evidence from peer-report data. *Journal of Personality and Social Psychology, 103*(2), 343–361. doi:10.1037/a0028706

Costa, P. T., & McCrae, R. R. (1992). *Revised NEO personality inventory (NEO-PI-R) and NEO five- factor inventory (NEO-FFI) professional manual.* Odessa, FL: PAR.

DeYoung, C. G. (2015). Openness/intellect: A dimension of personality reflecting cognitive exploration. In M. Mikulincer, P. R. Shaver, M. L. Cooper, & R. J. Larsen (Eds.), *APA handbook of personality and social psychology, Vol. 4: Personality processes and individual differences* (pp. 369–399). Washington, DC: American Psychological Association. http://dx.doi.org/10.1037/14343-017

DeNeve, K. M., & Cooper, H. (1998). The happy personality: A meta-analysis of 137 personality traits and subjective well-being. *Psychological Bulletin, 124*(2), 197–229. http://doi.org/10.1037/0033-2909.124.2.197

Diener, E., & Lucas, R. E. (1999). Personality and subjective well-being. In D. Kahneman, E. Diener, & N. Schwarz (Eds.), *Well-being: The foundations of hedonic psychology* (pp. 213–229). New York, NY: Russell Sage Foundation.

Digman, J. M. (1990). Personality structure: Emergence of the five-factor model. *Annual Review of Psychology, 41*(1), 417–440. https://doi.org/10.1146/annurev.ps.41.020190.002221

Eliasz, A. (2006). Internal incongruence among personality mechanisms as a constant 'sore point'. *European Health Psychologist, 8*, 5–7. doi:10.1146/annurev.ps.41.020190.002221

Eliasz, A., & Klonowicz, T. (2001). Top-down and bottom-up approaches to personality and their application to temperament. In A. Eliasz & A. Angleitner (Eds.), *Advances in research on temperament* (pp. 14–42). Lengerich, Germany: Pabst.

Faul, F., Erdfelder, E., Lang, A.-G., & Buchner, A. (2007). G*Power 3: A flexible statistical power analysis program for the social, behavioral, and biomedical sciences. *Behavior Research Methods, 39*(2), 175–191. doi:10.3758/BF03193146

Furnham, A. (2008). Relationship among four big five measures of different length. *Psychological Reports, 102*(1), 312–316. doi:10.2466/pr0.102.1.312-316

Gosling, S. D., Rentfrow, P. J., & Swann, W. B. (2003). A very brief measure of the Big Five personality domains. *Journal of Research in Personality, 37*(6), 504–528. https://doi.org/10.1016/S0092-6566(03)00046-1 doi:10.1016/S0092-6566(03)00046-1

Grant, S., & Langan-Fox, J. (2006). Occupational stress, coping and strain: The combined/interactive effect of the Big Five traits. *Personality and Individual Differences, 41*(4), 719–732. doi:10.1016/j.paid.2006.03.008

Graziano, W. G., Bruce, J., Sheese, B. E., & Tobin, R. M. (2007a). Attraction, personality, and prejudice: Liking none of the people most of the time. *Journal of Personality and Social Psychology, 93*(4), 565–582. doi:10.1037/0022-3514.93.4.565

Graziano, W. G., & Eisenberg, N. (1997). Agreeableness: A dimension of personality. In R. Hogan, J. Johnson, & S. Briggs (Eds.), *Handbook of personality psychology* (pp. 795–824). San Diego, CA: Academic Press.

Graziano, W. G., Habashi, M. M., Sheese, B. E., & Tobin, R. M. (2007b). Agreeableness, empathy, and helping: A person x situation perspective. *Journal of Personality and Social Psychology, 93*(4), 583–599. doi:10.1037/0022-3514.93.4.583

Graziano, W. G., Jensen-Campbell, L. A., & Hair, E. C. (1996). Perceiving interpersonal conflict and reacting to it: The case for agreeableness. *Journal of Personality and Social Psychology, 70*(4), 820–835. doi:10.1037/0022-3514.70.4.820

Hall, D. L., Matz, D. C., & Wood, W. (2010). Why don't we practice what we preach? A meta-analytic review of religious racism. *Personality and Social Psychology Review, 14*(1), 126– 139. doi:10.1177/1088868309352179

Hayes, A. F. (2013). *Introduction to mediation, moderation, and conditional process analysis: A regression based approach.* New York, NY: Guilford Press.

Heady, B., & Wearing, A. (1989). Personality, life events, and subjective wellbeing: Toward a dynamic equilibrium model. *Journal of Personality and Social Psychology, 57,* 731–739. doi: 10.1037/0022-3514.57.4.731

Heimberg, R. G., Brozovich, F. A., & Rapee, R. M. (2014). A cognitive-behavioral model of social anxiety disorder. In S. G. Hofmann & P. M. DiBartolo (Eds.), *Social anxiety: Clinical, developmental, and social perspectives* (pp. 705–728). London, UK: Academic Press. https://doi.org/10. 1016/B978-0-12-394427-6.00024-8

Hummelen, B., Wilberg, T., Pedersen, G., & Karterud, S. (2007). The relationship between avoidant personality disorder and social phobia. *Comprehensive Psychiatry, 48*(4), 348–356. doi: 10.1016/j.comppsych.2007.03.004

Jensen-Campbell, L. A., Adams, R., Perry, D. G., Workman, K. A., Furdella, J. Q., & Egan, S. K. (2002). Agreeableness, extraversion, and peer relations in early adolescence: Winning friends and deflecting aggression. *Journal of Research in Personality, 36*(3), 224–251. doi:10.1006/ jrpe.2002.2348

Jensen-Campbell, L. A., Gleason, K. A., Adams, R., & Malcolm, K. T. (2003). Interpersonal conflict, agreeableness, and personality development. *Journal of Personality, 71*(6), 1059–1086. doi: 10.1111/1467-6494.7106007

Jensen-Campbell, L. A., & Graziano, W. G. (2001). Agreeableness as a moderator of interpersonal conflict. *Journal of Personality, 69*(2), 323–361. doi:10.1111/1467-6494.00148

Johnson, J. A. (2017). Big-Five model. In V. Zeigler-Hill, T.K. Shackelford (Eds.), *Encyclopedia of personality and individual differences* (pp. 1–16). New York, NY: Springer. doi:10.1007/978-3-319-28099-8_1212-1

Jost, J. T., Glaser, J., Kruglanski, A. W., & Sulloway, F. J. (2003). Political conservatism as motivated social cognition. *Psychological Bulletin, 129*(3), 339–375. http://doi.org/10.1037/0033-2909.129.3.339

Jost, J. T., Nosek, B. A., & Gosling, S. D. (2008). Ideology: Its resurgence in social, personality, and political psychology. *Perspectives on Psychological Science, 3*(2), 126–136. doi:10.1111/ j.1745-6916.2008.00070.x

Kaplan, S. C., Levinson, C. A., Rodebaugh, T. L., Menatti, A., & Weeks, J. W. (2015). Social anxiety and the Big Five personality traits: The interactive relationship of trust and openness. *Cognitive Behaviour Therapy, 44*(3), 212–222. doi:10.1080/16506073.2015.1008032

Kashdan, T. B., Elhai, J. D., & Breen, W. E. (2008). Social anxiety and disinhibition: An analysis of curiosity and social rank appraisals, approach-avoidance conflicts, and disruptive risk-taking behavior. *Journal of Anxiety Disorders, 22*(6), 925–939. doi:10.1016/j.janxdis.2007.09.009

King, E. B., George, J. M., & Hebl, M. R. (2005). Linking personality to helping behaviors at work: An interactional perspective. *Journal of Personality, 73*(3), 585–607. doi:10.1111/j.1467-6494.2005.00322.x

Kotov, R., Gamez, W., Schmidt, F., & Watson, D. (2010). Linking "big" personality traits to anxiety, depressive, and substance use disorders: A meta-analysis. *Psychological Bulletin, 136*(5), 768–821. doi:10.1037/a0020327

Levinson, C. A., Kaplan, S. C., & Rodebaugh, T. L. (2014). Personality: Understanding the socially anxious temperament. In J. Weeks (Ed.), *The Wiley Blackwell handbook of social anxiety disorder* (pp. 111–132). Chichester, UK: Wiley.

Łakuta, P. (2018). Social Anxiety Questionnaire (SAQ): Development and preliminary validation. *Journal of Affective Disorders, 238,* 233–243. doi:10.1016/j.jad.2018.05.036

Magnus, K., Diener, E., Fujita, F., & Pavot, W. (1993). Extraversion and neuroticism as predictors of objective life events: A longitudinal analysis. *Journal of Personality and Social Psychology, 65*(5), 1046–1053. doi:10.1037/0022-3514.65.5.1046

Marszał-Wiśniewska, M. (2001). Self-regulatory abilities, temperament, and volition in everyday life situations. In H. Brandstätter, A. Eliasz (Eds.), *Persons, situations, and emotions: An ecological approach* (pp. 74–94). New York, NY: Oxford University Press.

Masten, A. S., & Wright, M. O. (1998). Cumulative risk and protection models of child maltreatment. *Journal of Aggression, Maltreatment & Trauma, 2,* 7–30. doi:10.1300/J146v02n01_02

McCrae, R. R. (1987). Creativity, divergent thinking, and openness to experience. *Journal of Personality and Social Psychology, 52*(6), 1258–1265. doi:10.1037/0022-3514.52.6.1258

McCrae, R. R. (1996). Social consequences of experiential openness. *Psychological Bulletin, 120*(3), 323–337. http://doi.org/10.1037/0033-2909.120.3.323 doi:10.1037//0033-2909.120.3.323

McCrae, R. R., & Costa, P. T. Jr. (1991). Adding liebe und arbeit: The full five-factor model and well-being. *Personality and Social Psychology Bulletin, 17*(2), 227–232. doi:10.1177/014616729101700217

McCrae, R. R., & Costa, P. T. Jr. (1999). A five-factor theory of personality. In L. A. Pervin & O. P. John (Eds.), *Handbook of personality theory and research* (pp. 139–153). New York, NY: Guilford Press.

McCrae, R. R., & Costa, P. T. (2013). Introduction to the empirical and theoretical status of the five-factor model of personality traits. In T. A. Widiger & P. T. Costa (Eds.), *Personality disorders and the five-factor model of personality* (3rd ed., pp. 15–27). Washington DC: American Psychological Association.

Modini, M., & Abbott, M. J. (2017). Negative rumination in social anxiety: A randomised trial investigating the effects of a brief intervention on cognitive processes before, during, and after a social situation. *Journal of Behavior Therapy and Experimental Psychiatry, 55,* 73–80. doi: 10.1016/j.jbtep.2016.12.002

Norton, A. R., & Abbott, M. J. (2016). Self-focused cognition in social anxiety: A review of the theoretical and empirical literature. *Behaviour Change, 33*(01), 44–64. doi:10.1017/bec.2016.2

Onraet, E., Van Hiel, A., Roets, A., & Cornelis, I. (2011). The closed mind: 'Experience' and 'cognition' aspects of openness to experience and need for closure as psychological bases for right-wing attitudes. *European Journal of Personality, 25*(3), 184–197. doi:10.1002/per.775

Penney, E. S., & Abbott, M. J. (2014). Anticipatory and post-event rumination in social anxiety disorder: A review of the theoretical and empirical literature. *Behaviour Change, 31*(2), 79–101. doi:10.1017/bec.2014.3

Perry, R., & Sibley, C. G. (2013). Seize and freeze: Openness to experience shapes judgments of societal threat. *Journal of Research in Personality, 47*(6), 677–686. doi:10.1016/j.jrp.2013.06.006

Saroglou, V. (2002). Religion and the five factors of personality: A meta-analytic review. *Personality and Individual Differences, 32*(1), 15–25. http://doi.org/10.1016/S0191-8869(00)00233-6 doi:10.1016/S0191-8869(00)00233-6

Sibley, C. G., & Duckitt, J. (2008). Personality and prejudice: A meta-analysis and theoretical review. *Personality and Social Psychology Review, 12*(3), 248–279. doi:10.1177/1088868308319226

Shoss, M. K., & Witt, L. A. (2013). Trait interactions and other configural approaches to personality. In N. D. Christiansen & R. P. Tett (Eds.), *Handbook of personality at work* (pp. 392–418). New York, NY: Routledge.

Strelau, J. (1998). *Perspectives on individual differences. Temperament: A psychological perspective.* New York, NY: Plenum Press.

Strelau, J. (2008). *Temperament as a regulator of behavior: After fifty years of research.* Clinton Corners, NY: Eliot Werner Publications.

Suls, J. (2001). Affect, stress and personality. In J. P. Forgas (Ed.), *Handbook of affect and social cognition* (pp. 392–409). Mahwah, NJ: Lawrence Erlbaum.

Suls, J., Martin, R., & David, J. P. (1998). Person-environment fit and its limits: Agreeableness, neuroticism, and emotional reactivity to interpersonal conflict. *Personality and Social Psychology Bulletin, 24*(1), 88–98. doi:10.1177/0146167298241007

Vasey, M. W., Harbaugh, C. N., Fisher, L. B., Heath, J. H., Hayes, A. F., & Bijttebier, P. (2014). Temperament synergies in risk for and protection against depressive symptoms: A prospective replication of a three-way interaction. *Journal of Research in Personality*, *53*, 134–147. doi: 10.1016/j.jrp.2014.09.005

Vasey, M. W., Harbaugh, C. N., Lonigan, C. J., Phillips, B. M., Hankin, B. L., Willem, L., & Bijttebier, P. (2013). Dimensions of temperament and depressive symptoms: Replicating a three-way interaction. *Journal of Research in Personality*, *47*(6), 908–921. doi:10.1016/j.jrp.2013.09.001

Vollrath, M., & Torgersen, S. (2000). Personality types and coping. *Personality and Individual Differences*, *29*(2), 367–378. http://doi.org/10.1016/S0191-8869(99)00199-3 doi:10.1016/S0191-8869(99)00199-3

Watson, D. (2000). *Mood and temperament*. New York, NY: The Guilford Press.

Watson, D., & Clark, L. A. (1992). On traits and temperament: General and specific factors of emotional experience and their relation to the five-factor model. *Journal of Personality*, *60*(2), 441–476. doi:10.1111/j.1467-6494.1992.tb00980.x

Zalewska, A. M. (2011). Relationships between anxiety and job satisfaction - Three approaches: "Bottom-up", "top-down" and "transactional." *Personality and Individual Differences*, *50*(7), 977–986. doi:10.1016/j.paid.2010.10.013

Insecure Attachment and Subclinical Depression, Anxiety, and Stress: A Three-Dimensional Model of Personality Self-Regulation as a Mediator

Ahmad Valikhani, Zahra Abbasi, Elham Radman, Mohammad Ali Goodarzi, and Ahmed A. Moustafa

ABSTRACT
Although the effects of insecure attachment on vulnerability, incidence, and developing mental disorders have been confirmed by many studies, the mechanism of this effect is still unknown. Therefore, the main aim of this study was to investigate the mediating and moderating role of the three-dimensional model of personality self-regulation in the relationship between insecure attachment and subclinical depression, anxiety, and stress. Four hundred Iranian students at Shiraz University were recruited and completed the following scales: the Revised Adult Attachment, Depression Anxiety Stress, Integrative Self-Knowledge, Mindful Attention Awareness, Self-Control, and Self-Compassion. Results showed that there was a moderate correlation among all the variables under study in the expected directions. Multiple mediating models analyses indicated that regarding the relationship between insecure attachment and depression, the components of integrative self-knowledge, self-control, and self-compassion functioned as mediators. However, regarding the relationship between insecure attachment and anxiety and stress, the components of integrative self-knowledge, mindfulness, and self-compassion relatively functioned as mediators. Further, our results showed that only mindfulness and self-compassion were identified as moderators in the relationship between insecure attachment and depression. It is concluded that insecure attachment may cause psychological damage due to deficiency in the components of the three-dimensional model of personality self-regulation, and that mindfulness and self-compassion may play a protective role in the relationship between insecure attachment and depression.

There is a high prevalence of emotional disorders (e.g., depression and anxiety) among students, compared to the general population (Dyrbye, Thomas, & Shanafelt, 2006; Eisenberg, Gollust, Golberstein, & Hefner, 2007; Ibrahim, Kelly, Adams, & Glazebrook, 2013). In Iran, almost half of the students are affected by some form of mental and physical disorders (depression, anxiety, somatic symptoms, and social dysfunction)

(Mokhtari et al., 2013). Another study has shown that the rates of physical complains, anxiety, social dysfunction, and depression in college students were 46.2, 50.2, 65.7, and 33.1%, respectively (Rahmati, Rahmani, Akbarzadeh Baghban, Fathollahzadeh, Gharibnavaz, 2015). However, other studies have reported different rates. One study has shown that 28.1 (Dadkhah, Mohammadi, & Mozaffari, 2006) and 31.6% (Dibajnia & Bakhtiari, 2002) of college students suffer from some kind of a mental disorder. To sum up, according to one study that reviewed 12 articles published using data from Iran using the General Health Questionnaire-28, the prevalence of mental disorders among college students was between 22.7 and 52.3% (Alizadeh-Navaei, & Hosseini, 2014). Compared to American students, it seems that the prevalence of mental disorders among Iranian college students is high. In the USA, studies have shown that the estimated rate of depressive or anxiety disorder was 15.6% for undergraduates and 13.0% for graduate students (Eisenberg et al., 2007). In another study, the rates of mental disorders were as follows:17.3% for depression, 4.1% for panic disorder, 7.0% for generalized anxiety, 6.3% for suicidal ideation, and 15.3% for non-suicidal self-injury (Eisenberg, Hunt, & Speer, 2013).

In addition, studies have shown that depression and anxiety are more likely to be related to other disorders such as self-harm (Gollust, Eisenberg, & Golberstein, 2008). Hence, due to the high prevalence of depression, anxiety, and stress with other mental disorders (e.g., self-harm) among students, it is necessary to identify the risk factors associated with depression and anxiety. In this regard, it has been indicated that individuals who experienced negative events during childhood and adolescence have reported a higher rate of mental disorders (Facundes & Ludermir, 2005). Therefore, it is possible that one factor underlying the development of mental disorders is related to the type of interaction children and adolescent have with their primary caregiver.

Culture and Mental Disorders and Attachment

According to Keyes (2005), mental health has two separate but correlating axes: one referring to the presence or absence of mental disorders, and the other to a high level of positive mental health to a low level of positive mental health. The results of the study by Gilmour (2014) supported Keyes' two continuous model, which is the percentages of Canadians aged 15 or older classified as having flourishing, moderate or languishing mental health were 76.9, 21.6, and 1.5%, respectively. Compared with estimates in other countries, a higher percentage of Canadians were flourishing. However, one study conducted in Iran revealed that about 16% of students were flourishing, 20% were languishing, and 64% were relatively mentally healthy (Nosratabadi, Joshanloo, Mohammadi, & Shahmohammadi, 2010). Similarly, another study showed that Iranian university students scored significantly lower than those in the Netherlands and South Africa on emotional, social, and psychological well-being (Joshanloo, Wissing, Khumalo, & Lamers, 2013). One study showed that Iranian participants considered the absence of mental disorder as a prerequisite for mental health and no one considered absence of mental disorder and positive mental health as two distinguished notions. In fact, those participants from Iran reported no difference between positive mental health (i.e., mental well-being) and mental health (Mirabzadeh et al., 2018). To investigate the role of different feelings in differentiating health from disease in Iranian collectivistic culture and Swedish individualistic culture, in one study, of a group of Iranian students and of a group of Swedish students showed that in the Iranian society there was a relationship between the mental health and balance affect while in the Swedish society there was a more significant relationship between the mental health and positive effect, indicating that Iranians see mental health as a balance affect between negative and positive affect (Farahani & Kormi Nouri, 2016).

The concept of mental health is interpreted differently in different cultures with respect to its expression and significance (Vaingankar et al., 2012). Along these lines, sadness is central to the Iranian character, history, and culture (Ebrahimnejad, 2002). In addition, Iranian people may interpret and present their depression and distress as somatic illness (Dejman, 2010).

One reason why attitude to an expression of mental disorders and well-being is different between Iran and Western nations can be explained by the concept of collectivism versus individualism, as Iranian culture tends to be collectivist. In addition, the higher prevalence of possible cases of mental disorders can be attributed to the impact of social, political, financial, and cultural problems, which have occurred in Iran (Noorbala et al., 2017). Because Iran differs from Western countries in terms of sociopolitical structures, level of economic development, and cultural and religious traditions (Cicognani et al., 2008).

Schmitt et al. (2004) conclude that individuals in East Asia show a more preoccupied attachment style than individuals in other cultural regions. In fact, when compared to North American populations, Asian populations are more insecurely attached in adulthood (DiTommaso, Brannen, & Burgess, 2005). In Iran, there is no systematic research to review the attachment process in the context of Iran's culture, but it seems that insecure attachment may be more common than secure attachment at least among university students (Haghshenas et al., 2016). In sum, findings from previous studies suggest that when compared to North American populations, Asian populations are more insecurely attached in adulthood (Friedman, 2010). Although the attachment process functions in largely the same manner across cultures, cultural context probably plays some role in the attachment process (van Ijzendoorn & Sagi, 1999). However, Rothbaum et al. (2000) showed that much of the work on infant attachment is very biased by assumptions made by researchers in Western cultures (for example, the role of infant autonomy as a sign of attachment security) that might not apply to other cultures, such as Japan.

Attachment, Self-Regulation, and Psychopathology

Bowlby (1973) has stressed the attachment plays a key role in understanding normal development and psychopathology. He assumed that attachment experiences have lasting effects throughout one's life and are the determining factors in the structure of personality and psychological disorders (Blatt & Levy, 2003). In this regard, insecure attachment has been found to be associated with depression, anxiety, and stress (Blatt & Levy, 2003; Bowlby, 1973; Fonagy & Target, 2002).

Self-regulation is one of the variables which is related to both attachment and psychopathology. Self-regulation is a process in which an individual adjusts their behavior by controlling their thoughts, feelings, impulses, and performance in order to achieve their goals (Baumeister, Gailliot, DeWall, & Oaten, 2006; Papies & Aarts, 2011). In fact, self-regulation involves continuous adaptation, decision making, knowledge to obtain information, and a proper understanding of each situation, the state of reflection about what needs to be done, what is being done, or what has already been done in life (de Acedo Lizarraga, Ugarte, Cardelle-Elawar, Iriarte, & de Acedo Baquedano, 2003).

The growth of self-regulation is heavily dependent on parent-child interactions and attachment style (Delker, Noll, Kim, & Fisher, 2014; Drake, Belsky, & Fearon, 2014; Sroufe, Duggal, Weinfield, & Carlson, 2000; Whitebread & Basilio, 2012). To date, attachment theory has been the main psychological theory explaining the emergence and development of self-regulation in children. This relationship is very strong such that even the new theory of modern attachment which is derived from the classical theory of attachment, considers attachment theory as the theory of self-regulation (Schore & Schore, 2008). Along these lines, insecure attachment reduces the child's effort to self-regulate in a coherent and flexible manner (Vondra, Shaw, Swearingen, Cohen, & Owens, 2001).

The growth of self-regulation in childhood and adolescence predicts important psychological consequences during life (Delker et al., 2014; Fonagy & Target, 2002). Baumeister and Heatherton (1996) claim that self-regulation failure can lead to crime, teenage pregnancy, alcoholism, drug addiction, sexually transmitted diseases, educational failure, gambling, and domestic violence. Previous studies have also shown that self-regulation has a negative correlation with different types of psychopathology such as neuroticism (Ibánez, Ruipérez, Moya, Marqués, & Ortet, 2005), negative affect, depression, anxiety, and stress (Diehl, Semegon, & Schwarzer, 2006; Luszczynska, Diehl, Gutiérrez-Doña, Kuusinen, & Schwarzer, 2004; Valikhani, Goodarzi, & Hashemi, 2017).

The Three-Dimensional Model of Personality Self-Regulation

A review of theoretical and empirical studies indicates that effective self-regulation requires three basic components: (1) self-knowledge processes (integrative self-knowledge and mindfulness) which include abilities, capacities, and goals as well as evaluating and monitoring behaviors with respect to a certain goal in the process of self-knowledge; (2) self-control which involves the ability to ignore and remove undesirable responses to a specific goal and the tendency to perform effectively in order to achieve that goal; and finally (3) self-compassion which is characterized by a kind response to self when there is a pressure and when a failure occurs. Below, we will provide a detailed description of the model and its relationship with self-regulation.

Baumeister and Heatherton (1996) and Vohs and Baumeister (2011) emphasized that self-control or willpower is related to self-regulation, However, Fishbach and Converse (2011) argued that self-control and self-knowledge are more intimately related to self-regulation. Self-regulation involves continuous awareness about the current time (mindfulness) and continuous self-knowledge (Ghorbani, Watson, Farhadi, & Chen, 2014). Therefore, self-knowledge involves adaptive effort of 'self' to understand one's experiences over time which enables a person to identify and adapt their thoughts and emotions by recognizing and selecting optimal activities that lead to desired outcomes (Asghari & Besharat, 2011). After that, 'self' should be able to have self-control in order to be able to adapt behaviors according to the internal standards (Ghorbani et al., 2014). Self-regulation especially in times of suffering and failure, also needs self-compassion, as self-compassion in the face of negative life events can improve self-regulation by reducing defensive and emotional behaviors and self-blame which interfere with self-regulation (Terry & Leary, 2011).

Self-control helps to prevent doing certain behaviors that stop one from achieving their main objective (Tangney, Baumeister, & Boone, 2004), which in turn results in achieving long-term goals (Rachlin, 1974). Therefore, self-control aims to eliminate the tendency to practice on automatic pilot and directs behavior in the desired direction (Bauer & Baumeister, 2011). On the other hand, metacognitive abilities are the basic cognitive components of self-regulation (Whitebread & Basilio, 2012). According to Bandura's social cognitive theory of self-regulation (1991), the human capacity for foresight, reflective self-evaluation, and self-reaction are essential components of self-regulation. By using foresight, people direct their actions in an initially predicted way. In fact, people have self-reflection and self-reaction capacities that enable them to exercise control over their thoughts, feelings, motivations, and actions (Bandura, 1991). In this respect, self-knowledge and mindfulness are key elements of self-regulation (Brown & Ryan, 2003; Ghorbani et al., 2014; Ghorbani, Watson, Bing, Davison, & LeBreton, 2003).

In fact, self-knowledge determines the direction of self-regulation (Bandura, 1991). In addition, self-compassion has been known as a self-regulation strategy to cope with negative emotions (Vettese, Dyer, Li, & Wekerle, 2011). Self-compassion has been recommended as a potential mechanism to reduce poor emotional self-regulation (Loess & Waltz, 2014) and as an effective emotional strategy (Warren, 2015). People with low self-compassion; mostly treat themselves critically and unkindly when they experience negative events. Hence, self-compassion should facilitate self-regulation and lead to effective self-regulation (Kelly, Zuroff, Foa, & Gilbert, 2010; Terry & Leary, 2011).

A review of theoretical and empirical research studies indicates a strong relationship between the three components of the personality self-regulation model and attachment. The internal working models have been defined as inner dynamic representations of the relationships between cognitive and emotional components, and that self-knowledge is related to the cognitive component of the internal working model (Pipp, Easterbrooks, & Brown, 1993; Pipp, Easterbrooks, & Harmon, 1992). In fact, the first feeling about our identity is created through our initial interactions in early childhood (Morf & Koole, 2012), such that secure attachment is related to self-recognition in infants (Fonagy & Targate, 2002). In order to understand how mindfulness and self-compassion develop, the parent-child interaction and attachment style should be taken into consideration (see, Hackmann, 2011; Pepping, Davis, & O'Donovan, 2013; Snyder, Shapiro, & Treleaven, 2012). Self-care representations result from the internalization of the soothing qualities of sensitive, careful, and available attachment which in turn helps the person to cope with stress-inducing situations (Moreira, Gouveia, Carona, Silva, & Canavarro, 2015).

Attachment figures as well as their soothing, comforting, and supportive aspects are embodied in self-care and self-compassion. The representations of attachment figures thus become a real part of one's self (Shaver, Lavy, Saron, & Mikulincer, 2007). Further, attachment experiences are related to certain emotional cognitive patterns. Impaired emotional cognitive patterns in insecurely attached individuals may reduce their capacity for openness, flexibility, and non-judgmental awareness of their inner and outer world (Caldwell & Shaver, 2013). Empirical research have shown that secure and insecure attachment have a positive and negative correlation with mindfulness (Pepping, O'Donovan, & Davis, 2014; Pepping, O'Donovan, Zimmer-Gembeck, & Hanisch, 2015; Walsh, Balint, Fredericksen, & Madsen, 2009) and a negative correlation with self-compassion (Moreira et al., 2015; Pepping, Davis, O'Donovan, & Pal, 2015; Raque-Bogdan, Ericson, Jackson, Martin, & Bryan, 2011), respectively. It appears that attachment to the primary caregiver is a necessary step in the development of self-control (Heydari, Teymoori, & Nasiri, 2015). According to Gottfredson and Hirschi's (1990) self-control theory, self-control is derived from parental exercises (Gibbs, Giever, & Martin, 1998). Empirical and cross-cultural studies have shown that self-control is positively correlated with secure attachment but negatively correlated with insecure attachment (Li, Delvecchio, Lis, Nie, & Di Riso, 2015; Tangney et al., 2004).

The relationship between the components of the three-dimensional model of personality self-regulation and emotional disorders has been the subject of many studies. These studies have shown that mindfulness is negatively correlated with emotional abuse and morbid symptoms of internalization (English, 2012), emotional distress and difficulty in emotional self-regulation (Marsh Pow, 2014; Pepping et al., 2013), eating disorders and neuroticism (Pidgeon & Grainger, 2013), suppression of thought, rumination, and poor attentional control (Caldwell & Shaver, 2013), suppressed excitement and poor emotional regulation (Caldwell & Shaver, 2015), and depression and anxiety (Martin, 2009). Integrative self-knowledge has a negative correlation with perceived stress, depression, and anxiety (Ghorbani et al., 2014; Ghorbani, Watson, Chen, & Norballa, 2012; Valikhani & Goodarzi, 2017) and damaged mental activities, rumination, repression, and social anxiety (Ghorbani, Watson, & Hargis, 2008). Self-control is also negatively correlated with behavior problems (Moon & Han, 2009), depression symptoms (Li et al., 2015), perceived stress, anxiety, and depression (Ghorbani et al., 2014; Valikhani et al., 2017). Further, self-compassion is negatively correlated with depression and anxiety (Ju & Lee, 2015), childhood abuse, poor emotional regulation, intensity of drug and alcohol addiction, and the level of psychological symptoms (Vettese et al., 2011).

This Study

To date, numerous studies have reported the effect of insecure attachment on vulnerability, incidence, and increase of mental disorders but the mechanism of this effect is still unknown. However, as indicated in the above-mentioned studies, attachment plays a causal role in the development and growth of self-regulation in general and is related to every component of the three-dimensional model of personality self-regulation (self-knowledge, including mindfulness; self-control; and self-compassion). Therefore, in this study, it is assumed that insecure attachment causes the incidence or at least, vulnerability to developing mental disorders by disrupting the processes of self-knowledge, self-control, and self-compassion. Hence, the main aim of this study was to investigate the mediating role of the components of the three-dimensional model of personality self-regulation in the relationship between insecure attachment and psychopathology (depression, anxiety, and stress). Further, the moderating role of the components of the three-dimensional model of personality self-regulation in the relationship between insecure attachment and psychopathology was investigated. Further, mindfulness and self-knowledge were investigated separately as variable components.

Method

Participants and Procedure

Participants included 400 (193 females, 199 males, and 8 missing data) students at undergraduate, graduate, and post-graduate levels from Shiraz University, Iran who were recruited through random sampling. The mean age of the participants was 24.75 years (SD = 3.74), and in the 18–41 age range. Of the total number of participants, 150 were enrolled in undergraduate, 171 in master's, and 65 in doctoral programs. Sixteen individuals did not identify their educational status. Students volunteered and consented to participate in the study. Prior to the administration of the questionnaires (which we describe below), all participants were informed in detail about their voluntary participation, confidentiality of their information, and how to respond to the questionnaires. All the questionnaires were administered in the same manner to all participants. It took between 30 and 40 min to complete the study. This study was approved by the Ethics Committee of Shiraz University.

Measurement

Revised Adult Attachment Scale: To measure insecure attachment, the revised adult attachment scale was utilized. This revised scale (Collins, 1996) was designed by developing the adult attachment scale originally proposed by Collins and Read (1990). This scale consists of 18 statements which are scored on a five-point Likert scale from 1 (never) to 5 (very much). It measures one's general feeling as related to important and close relationships in their life. In this scale, scoring can be done in two ways. First, the scale assesses the three proximity, dependence, and anxiety modes. Second, scoring is done on two dimensions: anxious attachment and avoidant attachment. In this study, we used an insecure attachment variable with sum of the scores of avoidant attachment and anxious insecure attachment. In order to avoid false correlation scores, scores obtained for each dimension were first converted to z scores and then summed up. In Iran, this scale has been translated and validated by Pakdaman (2001) by conducting it to high school students and this version was used in this study. In this study, the scale showed high internal consistency (Cronbach's alpha = 0.80).

    Depression Anxiety Stress Scale-21: Depression Anxiety Stress Scale-21 (DASS-21) is the shorter version of DASS-42 (Lovibond & Lovibond, 1995) which measures three clinical symptoms of depression, anxiety, and stress on a 4-point range (0 = not at all to

3 = high). A Persian version of this scale was validated in Iran. The convergent validity of the scale with the Beck Depression Scale was 0.70, and with Zung Anxiety Scale was 0.67. In Iran, this scale has been translated and validated by Sahebi, Asghari, and Salari (2005), and indicated that its Cronbach's alpha coefficients were adequate, which internal consistency of the subscales of depression, anxiety, and stress were 0.77, 0.79, and 0.78, respectively. In this study, the subscales of depression, anxiety, and stress showed high internal consistency (Cronbach's alpha = 0.86, 0.76, and 0.83, respectively).

Integrative Self-Knowledge Scale: The Integrative Self-Knowledge Scale (ISK) consists of 12 items which is scored on a 5-point Likert scale (0 = mostly false to 4 = mostly true). High score on this scale is an indication of high integrative self-knowledge of the person. Ghorbani et al. (2008) developed this scale and validated it in a study conducted on 723 Iranian and 900 American individuals in order to measure the temporally integrated understanding of the self. The results of the study indicated that the integrated self-knowledge scale had internal reliability as well as criterion and convergent validity. Cronbach's alpha coefficients of the scale in the Iranian and American samples were 0.82 and 0.78, respectively. In this study, the scale showed high internal consistency (Cronbach's alpha = 0.82).

Mindful Attention Awareness Scale: Mindful Attention Awareness Scale (MAAS) was designed by Brown and Ryan (2003) to measure the mindfulness trait. MAAS has 15 statements scored by the participants using a 5-point Likert-type scale (from 1 = almost always to 5 = almost never) with the highest score indicating an individual's high mindfulness trait. The scale is of good inter-rater reliability and the internal consistency of 0.82 has been reported for that. The convergent and divergent correlations of the scale were confirmed (Brown & Ryan, 2003). This scale has been validated and translated by Ghorbani, Watson, and Weathington (2009) in Iran with a Cronbach's alpha coefficient of 0.82. The convergent and divergent validity of the scale was confirmed. As a result, the scale has high reliability and validity and is considered as an appropriate tool for administration in different cultures (Ghorbani et al., 2009). In this study, the scale showed high internal consistency (Cronbach's alpha = 0.81).

Self-Control Scale: The short form of the self-control scale, designed by Tangney et al. (2004), contains 13 statements. Responses are scored on a five-point range (from 1 = not at all to 5 = very much). A high score on this scale is an indication of individual's high self-control. Tangney et al. (2004) showed that the divergent and convergent validity of the scale was confirmed. In the first study, the alpha coefficient was 0.83 and in the second study, it was 0.85. In addition, the reliability value of the re-test over a three-week interval was estimated at 0.89. This scale has been translated by Ghorbani et al. (2014) to Farsi and conducted on a large sample of college students, the Cronbach's alpha of 0.72 was obtained. In this study, the scale showed high internal consistency (Cronbach's alpha = 0.84).

Self-Compassion Scale: Self-compassion scale is a scale with 12 statements with three bipolar dimensions: self-kindness versus self-judgment, common humanity versus isolation, and mindfulness versus over-identification. This scale is assessed on a five-point scale from 1 (almost never) to 5 (almost always). Higher scores on this scale indicate a person's high self-compassion. In this study, the total scale score was used for analysis. The scale is a short form of self-compassion scale with 26 items (Neff, 2003) which was developed by Raes, Pommier, Neff, and Van Gucht (2011). The short form of self-compassion scale was validated on three groups of the population, the results of which showed that both the short and original long form have high correlation coefficients ($r > 0.97$; Raes et al., 2011). In Iran, the original form has likewise been used in several studies. This scale has been translated by Kord and Pashasharifi (2014) to Farsi, their study result's Cronbach's alpha coefficient of the total scale was 0.77 and the coefficient of the two parts was 0.76. In another study conducted on 619 students, Cronbach's alpha of the total scale was reported at 0.76 (Khosravi, Sadeghi, & Yabande, 2014). In this study, this scale had relatively high internal consistency (Cronbach's alpha $= 0.76$).

Data Analysis

Data analysis was conducted using SPSS 21.0 and macro SPSS software (SPSS Inc., Chicago, IL). First, to examine the relationship between the variables under study, several Pearson correlations were performed. To examine the relationship between three-dimensional model of personality self-regulation (self-knowledge, including mindfulness; self-control; and self-compassion) and insecure attachment and psychopathology (depression, anxiety, and stress), the multiple mediation analysis proposed by Preacher and Hayes (2008) was used. Unlike Baron and Kenny's (1986), simple mediation analysis which is limited and inapplicable to mediation analyses which contain more than one variable, multiple mediation analysis can analyze several variables simultaneously. Multiple mediation models do not only provide the total indirect effects by combining multiple mediation variables, but also computes specific indirect effect of every mediation variable. In fact, the specific indirect effect indicates the ability of that the variable as a mediator for mediating the effect of the independent variable (X) on the criterion variable (Y) by controlling all the other mediation variables. There are several different approaches to measure the significance of total and specific indirect effects in multiple mediation models. One of these methods is Sobel test in which the significance level is computed according to standardized normal distribution. However, the use of standardized normal distribution for indirect effect has some limitations because sampling distribution of the models' paths is usually normal only in large samples. Bootstrapping nonparametric re-sampling method is a strategy which does not limit the assumptions of the normal distribution sampling. In this study, this method is preferred to other methods of assessing indirect effects. Currently, it is often used in studies with mediation analyses. Bootstrapping is a strong computational method that involves repeated sampling of dataset and estimation of the indirect effect on a dataset which has been re-sampled (Preacher & Hayes, 2008). This procedure is not sensitive to the assumptions of regression models and structural equations such as univariate or multivariate normality of data and sample size.

As suggested by Preacher and Hayes (2008), the multiple mediation model has two stages tasks: (1) it investigates the total indirect effect or identifies whether or not the mediation variables, transfer the effect of X to Y; and (2) it investigates the specific indirect effect related to any mediating variables. Nevertheless, the significance of the total indirect effect is not a prerequisite for investigating the specific indirect effect, and sometimes it is possible to obtain the significance of the specific indirect effect in light

TABLE 1. Mean, Standard Deviation, and Pearson Correlation Coefficients among the Variables under Study ($n = 400$).

Measures	1	2	3	4	5	6	7	8
1. Insecure attachment	–	–	–	–	–	–	–	–
2. Depression	0.48	–	–	–	–	–	–	–
3. Anxiety	0.49	**0.57**	–	–	–	–	–	–
4. Stress	**0.52**	**0.71**	**0.61**	–	–	–	–	–
5. Self-knowledge	−0.53	−0.54	−0.55	−0.53	–	–	–	–
6. Mindfulness	−0.48	−0.38	−0.53	−0.45	**0.55**	–	–	–
7. Self-control	−0.38	−0.44	−0.36	−0.42	**0.58**	0.44	–	–
8. Self-compassion	−0.47	−0.57	−0.45	−0.53	**0.61**	0.41	**0.50**	–
Mean	2.62	.76	.61	1.12	3.75	3.63	3.41	3.26
SD	.58	.66	.50	.65	.65	.56	.68	.60

All correlation coefficients are significant (two-tailed; $p < .001$). High correlation coefficients are bolded.

of the total indirect effect. The assumption that whether the two indirect effects are equal is tested. Since, in this method, it was not possible to enter multiple criterion variables such as the predicting variable (unlike the mediation variables), all the analyses in relation to the criterion variables were conducted separately. Analyzing the total and specific indirect effects was done using the bootstrapping method with 5000 re-sampling of the original data with 95% bias-corrected bootstrapped confidence interval (Preacher & Hayes, 2008). In order to investigate the two-way interaction of insecure attachment with every component of the three-dimensional model of personality self-regulation in predicting depression, anxiety, and stress, the regression analysis was used separately. That is, in the first step, the scores of the insecure attachment and one of the components of the three-dimensional model were inserted into the first block of the regression equation, and in the second step, their interaction was inserted in the equation. To avoid creating false correlations when obtaining the variables' interaction score, the variables were first centered and then their results were multiplied.

Results

Preliminary Analyses

The results of Pearson correlation coefficients among the variables under study are shown in Table 1. There was at least a moderate correlation among all the variables. So, insecure attachment had a moderate positive correlation with depression and anxiety, and a strong positive correlation with stress. In addition, insecure attachment had a strong negative correlation with integrative self-knowledge, and a moderate negative correlation with mindfulness, self-control, and self-compassion. Depression and stress had a strong negative correlation with integrative self-knowledge and self-compassion and a moderate negative correlation with mindfulness and self-control. Anxiety has a strong negative relationship with integrative self-knowledge and mindfulness, and a moderate negative correlation with self-control and self-compassion.

Meditation Analyses

The analysis of the mediation model of insecure attachment on depression was significant considering the mediating role of the components of the three-dimensional model

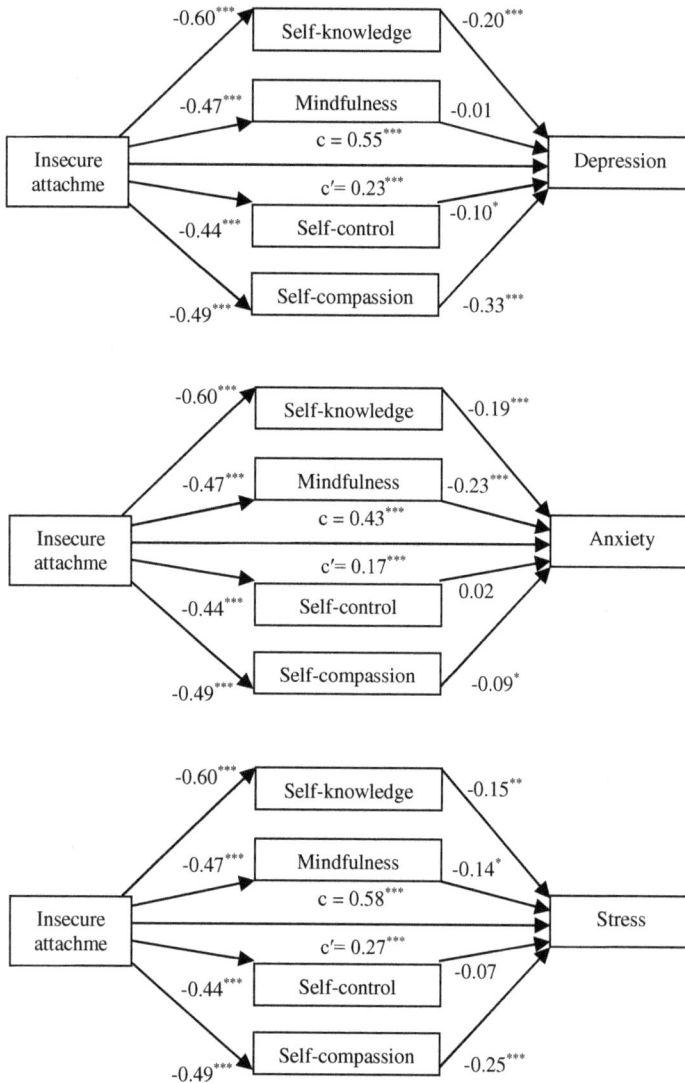

Figures 1–3. Statistical graphs of multiple mediation model for the mediating role of the three-dimensional model of personality self-regulation in the relationship between insecure attachment and depression (Figure 1), anxiety (Figure 2), and stress (Figure 3), respectively ($n = 400$). Note: The path values are non-standard regression coefficients; c is insecure attachment total effect on depression/anxiety/stress (the sum of the direct effect and all specific effects), whereas c' shows its direct effect by controlling the mediating variables on depression/anxiety/stress. $*p < .05$, $**p < .01$, $***p < .001$.

of personality self-regulation ($F_{(5,394)} = 56.98$, $p < .001$) and explained 42% of the variance of depression. The total direct effect of the insecure attachment on depression was significant. The total indirect effect through mediating variables was also significant (PE $= 0.33$, CI$_{95\%} = 0.2540$–0.4097). Specific indirect effects of the integrative self-knowledge (PE $= 0.12$, CI$_{95\%} = 0.0368$–0.1999), self-control (PE $= 0.04$, CI$_{95\%} = 0.0046$–0.0855), and self-compassion (PE $= 0.16$, CI$_{95\%} = 0.1041$–0.2369) variables were significant. However, the specific indirect effect of mindfulness (PE = 0.01, $CI_{95\%}$ = −0.0499–0.0580) was not significant. Similarly, results of pairwise contrasts showed that the indirect effect of integrative self-knowledge was significantly higher than that of mindfulness (PE = 0.11, $CI_{95\%}$ = 0.0031–0.2280); and indirect effect of self-compassion was significantly higher than that of mindfulness (PE = −0.16, $CI_{95\%}$ = −0.2563 − 0.0765), and self-control (PE = −0.12, $CI_{95\%}$ = −0.2055–0.0411). These results indicate that of the components of the three-dimensional model of personality self-regulation, components of integrative self-knowledge, self-control, and self-compassion are moderate mediators in the relationship between insecure attachment and symptoms of depression, and the role of self-compassion and integrative self-knowledge, respectively, was more than the role of self-control (see Figure 1).

The analysis of the mediation model of insecure attachment on anxiety was significant considering the mediating role of the components of the three-dimensional model of personality self-regulation ($F_{(5,394)}$ = 54.68, $p < .001$) and explained 41% of the variance of anxiety. The total direct effect of the insecure attachment on anxiety was significant. Its total indirect effect through the mediating variables was also significant (PE = 0.26, $CI_{95\%}$ = 0.1986–0.3237). Specific indirect effects of the integrative self-knowledge (PE = 0.11, $CI_{95\%}$ = 0.0577–0.1794), mindfulness (PE = 0.11, $CI_{95\%}$ = 0.0646–0.1626), and self-compassion (PE = 0.05, $CI_{95\%}$ = 0.0038–0.0897) variables were significant. However, the specific indirect effect of self-control (PE = −0.01, $CI_{95\%}$ = −0.0405–0.0186) was not significant. Similarly, results of pairwise contrasts showed that the indirect effect of integrative self-knowledge was significantly higher than that of self-control (PE = 0.12, $CI_{95\%}$ = 0.0558–0.2021); and indirect effect of mindfulness was significantly higher than that of self-control (PE = 0.12, $CI_{95\%}$ = 0.0610–0.1803). These results indicate that of the components of the three-dimensional model of personality self-regulation, components of integrative self-knowledge, mindfulness, and self-compassion are moderate mediators in the relationship between insecure attachment and symptoms of anxiety, and the role of integrative self-knowledge and mindfulness, respectively, was more than the that of self-compassion (see Figure 2).

The analysis of the mediation model of insecure attachment on stress was significant considering the mediating role of the components of the three-dimensional model of personality self-regulation ($F_{(5,394)}$ = 55.77, $p < .001$) and explained 41% of the variance of stress. The total direct effect of the insecure attachment on stress was significant. The total indirect effect through the mediating variables was also significant (PE = 0.31, $CI_{95\%}$ = 0.2372–0.3816). Specific indirect effects of the integrative self-knowledge (PE = 0.09, $CI_{95\%}$ = 0.0178–0.1700), mindfulness (PE = 0.07, $CI_{95\%}$ = 0.0134–0.1194), and self-compassion (PE = 0.12, $CI_{95\%}$ = 0.0696–0.1832) variables were significant. However, self-control had no significant specific indirect effect (PE = 0.03, $CI_{95\%}$ = −0.0057–0.0742). Similarly, results of pairwise contrasts showed that the indirect effect of self-compassion was significantly higher than that of self-control (PE= −0.09, $CI_{95\%}$ = −0.1683−−0.0200). These results indicate that of the components of the three-dimensional model of personality self-regulation, components of integrative self-knowledge, mindfulness, and self-compassion were moderate mediators in the relationship between insecure attachment and symptoms of stress, and the role of self-compassion was more than that of the other components (see Figure 3).

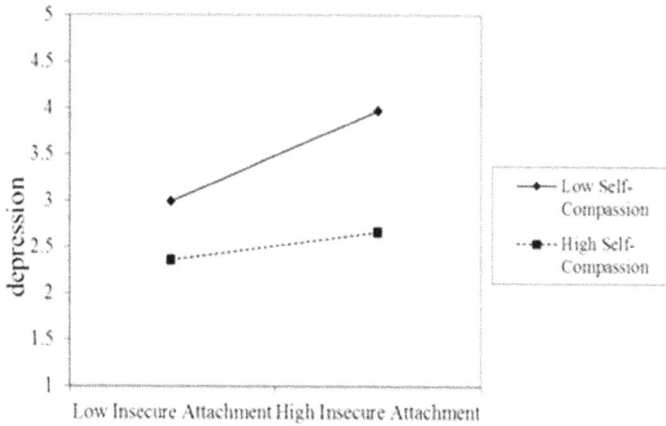

Figure 4. Two-way interaction between insecure attachment and mindfulness in predicting depression.

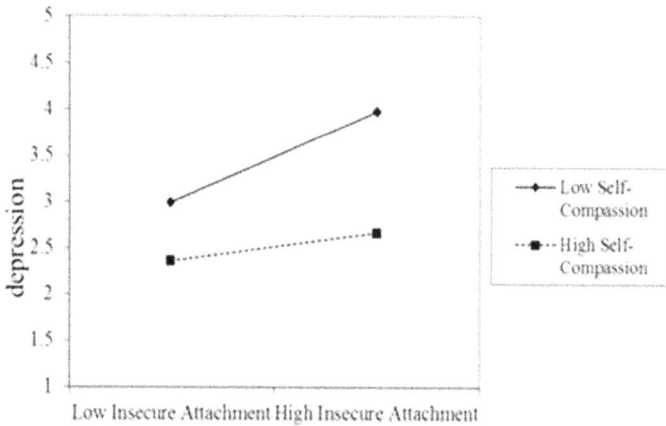

Figure 5. Two-way interaction between insecure attachment and self-compassion in predicting depression.

Moderation Analyses

A two-way interaction between insecure attachment and mindfulness was significant in predicting depression ($\Delta R^2 = 0.01$, $\Delta F = 5.14$, $\beta = -0.10$, $p = .024$). Thus, as shown in Figure 4, individuals who reported a low level of mindfulness and a high level of insecure attachment were more likely to have high levels of depression. This indicates that a high level of mindfulness may prevent or reduce the impact of insecure attachment on depression.

Two-way interaction between insecure attachment and self-compassion was significant in predicting depression ($\Delta R^2 = 0.01$, $\Delta F = 5.23$, $\beta = -0.10$, $p = .023$). Therefore, individuals who reported a low level of self-compassion and a high level of insecure attachment were identified with higher depression. This indicates that a high level of self-compassion may prevent or reduce the impact of insecure attachment on depression (see Figure 5).

The results of the two-way interactions between insecure attachment and each component of the three-dimensional model of personality self-regulation in predicting depression, anxiety, and stress were not significant, and thus were not reported here.

Discussion

This study investigated both the mediating role, and the moderating role of the components of the three-dimensional model of personality self-regulation in the relationship between insecure attachment and depression, anxiety, and stress. Overall, our results support the assumption that insecure attachment affects depression, anxiety, and stress through the components of the three-dimensional model of personality self-regulation. These findings show that the pillars of self-regulation (self-knowledge processes; self-control; and self-compassion) relatively act as a mechanism by which the insecure attachment is related to psychopathology. Given that the context of the emergence and development of self-regulation depends on the attachment created between early caregivers and child (see Schore & Schore, 2008; Sroufe et al., 2000; Whitebread & Basilio, 2012), insecure attachment may affect the child's dysfunction of self-regulation system and causes the 'self' not to be able to regulate cognition, emotion and behavior. This, at least partially, affects the emergence of mental disorders. Generally, it appears that interfering with the processes of attachment leads to a development of cognitive, emotional, and behavioral disorder.

On the other hand, our results indicated that insecure attachment has a direct influence on mental disorders (depression, anxiety, and stress). This finding is consistent with Bowlby's idea that attachment experiences have lasting effects throughout one's life and are the determining factors in the structure of personality and psychological disorders (Blatt & Levy, 2003), and also, that insecure attachment is associated with psychopathology, particularly depression, and anxiety (Bowlby, 1973). In fact, both theoretically and empirically, the relationship between attachment structure and psychopathology has been reported in several studies (Nakash-Eisikovits, Dutra, & Westen, 2002; Westen, Nakash, Thomas, & Bradley, 2006). Individual differences in the initial attachments include motivational, emotional, and behavioral regulation patterns which function as a prototype for the individual's personality (Sroufe et al., 2000).

The results of this study indicated that insecure attachment was a negative predictor of all the components of self-knowledge, self-control, and self-compassion in the three-dimensional model of personality self-regulation. Insecure attachment was a negative predictor of self-knowledge. This finding is consistent with the limited literature available in this area of study (Pipp et al., 1992; Pipp et al., 1993). We often have our first interaction with our primary caregiver who is usually our mother. The first feeling of our identity develops through these initial interactions in infancy (Morf & Koole, 2012). Moreover, the internal working models have been defined as internal dynamic representations of the relationships which contain cognitive (self-knowledge) and emotional components (Pipp et al.,1992). As a result, it appears that insecurely attached individuals are not clear about internal working models which are shaped during their initial relationships with their caregivers. As a result, self-knowledge and persistent visualization of 'self' as a main feature of integrative self-knowledge (Shahmohammadi,

Ghorbani, & Besharat, 2007) are not formed in insecurely attached individuals or has a limited capacity. In fact, s children, we knew ourselves, others, and the world through relationship with others. Hence, when the relationship that we have with our caregivers is damaged (i.e., having insecure attachment), then our knowledge of ourselves, others, and the world is likely to be distorted.

On the contrary, secure attachment provides a stable ground in which a child can explore their watchful mind, and thereby, learns about their own and others' mental states (Fonagy, 2000). Further, we found that insecure attachment was a negative predictor of mindfulness, which is consistent with the findings of prior studies (Jones, Welton, Oliver, & Thorburn, 2011; Marsh Pow, 2014; Pepping et al. 2013; Pepping et al., 2015; Walsh et al., 2009;). Attachment experiences are associated with specific cognitive emotional patterns that may contribute to mindfulness. Damaged cognitive emotional patterns formed in insecure attachment relationships by insecurely attached individuals may reduce one's capacity for openness and flexibility about the inner and outer world (Caldwell & Shaver, 2013). Instead of viewing experiences through the filter of beliefs and expectations, mindfulness involves direct observation of them.

Previous studies are in agreement with the findings of this study and suggest that insecure attachment has a negative correlation with self-control (e.g., Tangney et al., 2004; Valikhani, Sarafraz, & Moghimi, 2018). It is likely that attachment to a primary caregiver is a necessary step for the development of self-control (Heydari et al., 2015). According to self-control theory, self-control is derived from exercising parenting (Gottfredson & Hirschi, 1990, cited in Gibbs et al., 1998). Indeed, an insecure individual cannot integrate different aspects of the 'self' properly due to impaired cognitive emotional patterns and this can lead to self-control failure.

In addition, in line with our findings, previous studies also showed that insecure attachment has a negative correlation with self-compassion (Moreira et al., 2015; Pepping et al., 2015; Raque-Bogdan et al., 2011). To explain this relationship, self-care representations of internalizing soothing qualities results from sensitive careful and available attachment which helps the individual to cope with stress-inducing situations with a compassionate attitude toward their 'self' and self-care (Moreira et al., 2015). The initial stable experience of soothing increases self-soothing and self-compassion. However, the experience of rejection and punishment by parents may lead to a self-blame in times of distress or difficulty, which is considered the opposite of self-compassion (Hackmann, 2011). According to neuroscience research, it is believed that parents' behavior is essential for the development of the nervous system which regulates the individual's capacity for self-soothing and self-compassion. Hence, the impact of attachment theory is related to the effect of early relationships with caregivers has on the development of styles related to 'self' or others (Hackmann, 2011). The compassionate or non-compassionate view on an individual toward himself or herself is, in fact, a reflection of his or her primary caregivers' view.

Our correlational analyses among the components of the three-dimensional model of personality self-regulation and psychopathological variables showed that integrative self-knowledge, mindfulness, self-control, and self-compassion, had moderate to high negative significant correlation with depression, anxiety, and stress. These findings are consistent with those of previous research (e.g., Ghorbani et al., 2012; Ghorbani et al.,

2014; Ju & Lee, 2015; Li et al., 2015). On the one hand, self-knowledge is considered as a self-regulation process promoting the wellbeing of 'self' (Ghorbani et al., 2003). On the other hand, individuals with high self-knowledge have high understanding of themselves and their abilities, and in the face of problems, they are able to solve their problems by integrating their past and present experiences and circumstances. Further, people with high level of mindfulness have non-judgmental and nonreactive awareness of their problems and this probably causes them not to ruminate about their problems. As a result, they have a high rate of stable mental health.

Self-control acts as a coping skill for anxiety (Hamama, Ronen, & Feigin, 2000) and psychological distress. Indeed, the ability to cope, manage and moderate thoughts, emotions, and behaviors in a right manner is likely to provide a ground for ignoring impaired cognitions and emotional dysregulation which are related to depression, anxiety, and stress. Self-control can contribute to creating an extensive range of positive outcomes in people's life. People with high self-control have positive behavioral outcomes in a variety of areas such as failure tolerance, ethical behaviors, and discipline (Bauer & Baumeister, 2011; Tangney et al., 2004). People with high self-compassion have sincere and receptive view of 'self' coupled with a conscious and speculative view which places emphasis on the current experience, place and time (Tanaka, Wekerle, Schmuck, Paglia-Boak, & MAP Research Team, 2011). Moreover, they understand and accept their incompetency, failures, and painful life events (Neff & Germer, 2013), and have a tendency to relieve their pain and suffering (Barnard & Curry, 2011). Applying all these methods and strategies to coping with problems and difficulties of life probably results in less vulnerability to psychopathology and higher rates of mental health.

The results of our mediation model showed that of the components of the three-dimensional model of personality self-regulation, integrative self-knowledge, self-control, and self-compassion were relative mediators in the relationship between insecure attachment and symptoms of depression. In fact, according to the findings of this study, insecure attachment would lead to depression by producing deficiencies in the level of self-knowledge, self-control, and self-compassion. In the meantime, according to the findings of this study, the role of self-compassion and integrative self-knowledge, respectively, is more than that of self-control, suggesting that more attention should be paid to these two components. Other results of our mediation model indicated that of the components of the three-dimensional model of personality self-regulation, integrative self-knowledge, mindfulness, and self-compassion relatively functioned as mediators in the relationship between insecure attachment and symptoms of anxiety.

Therefore, as indicated by the results of our study, insecure attachment negatively affects self-knowledge, mindfulness, and self-compassion and subsequently leads to an increase in the level of depression. We also found that integrative self-knowledge and mindfulness had more prominent roles than self-compassion. Therefore, in psychotherapy and counseling, attention to these variables in people with insecure attachment is of high importance. Results of the last mediation model showed that of the components of the three-dimensional model of personality self-regulation, integrative self-knowledge, self-control, and self-compassion were the relative mediators between insecure attachment and symptoms of stress with self-compassion having a greater role than the other variables. Thus, insecure attachment functions as a vulnerability variable in that, by disrupting self-knowledge, mindfulness, and self-compassion, it makes people vulnerable to stress. Therefore, training skills related to self-knowledge, mindfulness, and self-compassion specifically for individual with stress problems and insecure attachment style can reduce their mental pressure.

Another result of this study was that of the components of the three-dimensional model of personality self-regulation, it was only mindfulness and self-compassion that could moderate the relationship between insecure attachment and depression. In other words, suffering from insecure attachment, which is accompanied by low mindfulness and self-compassion, increases the levels of depression. In other words, an individual with insecure attachment who has higher mindfulness and self-compassion experiences has a lower level of depression compared to an individual with insecure attachment who has lower levels of mindfulness and self-compassion. As a result, in psychotherapy and counseling, mindfulness and self-compassion can be therapeutic targets for people with insecure attachment who also suffer from depression.

It can be claimed that depression is a mood disorder and related to negative emotions. Mindfulness (English, 2012; Snyder et al., 2012) and self-compassion (Diedrich, Grant, Hofmann, Hiller, & Berking, 2014; Vettese et al., 2011) are also both considered to be regulation emotion strategies. In fact, mindfulness and self-compassion act as self-regulation of emotion. However, self-control is more related to preventing or ignoring certain behaviors (Tangney et al., 2004) and it is kind of self-regulation of behavior, not emotion. That is why mindfulness and self-compassion can moderate the relationship between insecure attachment and depression, but not self-control. In addition, based on correlational coefficients, the rate of relationships between insecure attachment and mindfulness and self-compassion were -0.48 and -0.47, respectively. However, the rate of the relationship between insecure attachment and self-control was -0.38, which was low, compared to those. This may affect the relationships between insecure attachment and mindfulness and self-compassion and moderate its effects on depression. And it may explain why self-control could not moderate the relationship between insecure attachment and mindfulness and self-compassion.

Therapeutic Implications

This study showed that the components of the three-dimensional model of personality self-regulation (integrative self-knowledge, mindfulness, and self-control and self-compassion) are relevant for understanding and treating mental disorders. Since numerous theoretical and empirical foundations have ignored the effect of insecure attachment on the development of mental disorders (e.g., depression, anxiety, and stress), discovering malleable variables that are derived from attachment is very important in clinical practices. Further, discovering positive mediators (structures related to positive psychology) may require a lower resistance in therapeutic interventions and set more feasible goals in their attempt to change the orientation of one's attachment. Attention to these structures can be useful for clinicians to shorten treatment time (Raque-Bogdan et al., 2011) and to make the treatment more effective. Thus, according to the findings of this study, mediation models of the components of the three-dimensional model of personality self-regulation were identified as relative mediators in the relationship between insecure attachment and the development of mental disorders.

Using the findings of this study, psychotherapists and counselors should deal with self-control and specifically self-compassion in insecurely attached individuals who suffer from depression. Further, they should try to enhance the level of self-compassion and specifically integrative self-knowledge and mindfulness in insecure people who suffer from anxiety, and deal with self-knowledge, mindfulness, and self-compassion in insecure people who have high levels of mental pressure. Furthermore, according to the results of analyses related to moderators, therapists and counselors can reduce depression in insecure patients who suffer from depression using self-compassion- and mindfulness-based interventions.

It is likely that the Third-Wave cognitive behavioral therapies which emphasize acceptance, mindfulness, faulting, dialectic, values, spirituality, and relationship (Hayes, 2004) can be used to increase the level of the components of the three-dimensional model of personality self-regulation.

The third-wave cognitive behavioral therapies include mindfulness-based meditation and stress reduction plan, cognitive therapy, dialectical behavior therapy, acceptance and commitment therapy, mindful self-compassion, compassion-focused therapy, compassionate mind training, compassionate image, and loving-kindness meditation, which stress mindfulness and self-compassion as their basic pillars. They also include psychotherapies such as affect phobia treatment (Schanche, Stiles, McCullough, Svartberg, & Nielsen, 2011) and intensive short-term dynamic psychotherapy which lead to increased self-knowledge and self-control, and also mindfulness of the patient. Besides, attachment-based therapies and interventions such as mentalization-based treatment (Lorenzini & Fonagy, 2013), transference-focused psychotherapy (Levy et al., 2006; Lorenzini, & Fonagy, 2013), and schema-focused therapy (Lorenzini & Fonagy, 2013), with some mainly emphasizing patients' attachment and others considering patients' attachment as one of their therapeutic principles, can be helpful for clinical work on patient's insecure attachment.

Limitations and Conclusion

This study has several limitations that should be considered in interpreting the results. First, according to the research design and correlational nature of the study, our findings may not have causal implications. Second, the population under investigation was healthy normal rather than clinical, thus limiting the generalization of the results to clinical populations. Third, the participants in this study were selected using a student population rather than a general population with a certain age, economic status, and cultural background which makes the generalizability of the results restricted. Accordingly, it is recommended that future studies replicate this study using different populations. Despite these limitations, the results of the mediation models showed that although insecure attachment directly functions as vulnerability in relation to psychopathology, this relationship can partly be explained by the components of the three-dimensional model of self-regulation.

Further, based on the three-dimensional model of self-regulation, the correlation between insecure attachment and different mental disorders (stress, depression, and anxiety) cannot be explained by a single similar variable. Moreover, by further providing evidence on the role of insecure attachment in the discovery of self, mindfulness, self-control, and self-compassion as mediators in the relationship between insecure attachment and psychopathology, this study contributed to the existing literature on psychology, counseling, and psychotherapy. This study also made an important contribution by introducing and developing the three-dimensional model of self-regulation as the foundation of successful self-regulation which is based on self-knowledge, self-control, and self-compassion.

Disclosure Statement

The authors declare that they have no conflict of interest.

References

Alizadeh-Navaei, R., & Hosseini, S. H. (2014). Mental health status of Iranian students until 2011: A systematic review. *Clinical Excellence*, *2*(1), 1–10. Retrieved from http://ce.mazums.ac.ir/article-1-75-en.html

Asghari, M. S., & Besharat, M. A. (2011). The relation of perceived parenting with integrative self-knowledge. *Procedia-Social and Behavioral Sciences*, *30*, 226–230. doi:10.1016/j.sbspro.2011.10.045

Bandura, A. (1991). Social cognitive theory of self-regulation. *Organizational Behavior and Human Decision Processes*, *50*(2), 248–287. doi:10.1016/0749-5978(91)90022-L

Barnard, L. K., & Curry, J. F. (2011). Self-compassion: Conceptualizations, correlates, & interventions. *Review of General Psychology*, *15*(4), 289–303. doi:10.1037/a0025754

Baron, R. M., & Kenny, D. A. (1986). The moderator–mediator variable distinction in social psychological research: Conceptual, strategic, and statistical considerations. *Journal of Personality and Social Psychology*, *51*(6), 1173–1182. doi:10.1037/0022-3514.51.6.1173

Bauer, I. M., & Baumeister, R. F. (2011). Self-regulatory strength. In K. D. Vohs and R. F. Baumeister (Eds.). *Handbook of self-regulation: Research, theory, and applications* (2nd ed., pp. 64–82). New York & London: Guilford Press.

Baumeister, R. F., & Heatherton, T. F. (1996). Self-regulation failure: An overview. *Psychological Inquiry*, *7*(1), 1–15. doi:10.1207/s15327965pli0701_1

Baumeister, R. F., Gailliot, M., DeWall, C. N., & Oaten, M. (2006). Self-regulation and personality: How interventions increase regulatory success, and how depletion moderates the effects of trait on behavior. *Journal of Personality*, *74*(6), 1773–1802. doi:10.1111/j.1467-6494.2006.00428.x

Blatt, S. J., & Levy, K. N. (2003). Attachment theory, psychoanalysis, personality development, and psychopathology. *Psychoanalytic Inquiry*, *23*(1), 102–150. doi:10.1080/07351692309349028

Bowlby, J. (1973). *Attachment and loss, II: Separation, anxiety and anger*. New York, NY: Basic Books.

Brown, K. W., & Ryan, R. M. (2003). The benefits of being present: Mindfulness and its role in psychological well-being. *Journal of Personality and Social Psychology*, *84*(4), 822–848. doi:10.1037/0022-3514.84.4.822

Caldwell, J. G., & Shaver, P. R. (2013). Mediators of the link between adult attachment and mindfulness. *Interpersona: An International Journal on Personal Relationships*, *7*, 299–310. doi:10.1007/s12671-015-0390-y

Caldwell, J. G., & Shaver, P. R. (2015). Promoting attachment-related mindfulness and compassion: A wait-list-controlled study of women who were mistreated during childhood. *Mindfulness*. *Mindfulness*, *6*(3), 624–636. doi:10.1007/s12671-014-0298-y

Cicognani, E., Pirini, C., Keyes, C., Joshanloo, M., Rostami, R., & Nosratabadi, M. (2008). Social participation, sense of community and social well being: A study on American, Italian and Iranian university students. *Social Indicators Research*, *89*(1), 97–112. doi:10.1007/s11205-007-9222-3

Collins, N. L. (1996). Working models of attachment: Implications for explanation, emotion, and behavior. *Journal of Personality and Social Psychology*, *71*(4), 810–832. doi:10.1037//0022-3514.71.4.810

Collins, N. L., & Read, S. J. (1990). Adult attachment, working models, and relationship quality in dating couples. *Journal of Personality and Social Psychology*, *58*(4), 644–663. doi:10.1037/0022-3514.58.4.644

Dadkhah, B., Mohammadi, M., & Mozaffari, N. (2006). Mental health status of the students in Ardabil University of medical sciences, 2004. *Journal of Ardabil University of Medical Sciences*, *6*(1), 31–36. Retrieved from http://jarums.arums.ac.ir/article-1-475-en.html

de Acedo Lizarraga, M. L. S., Ugarte, M. D., Cardelle-Elawar, M., Iriarte, M. D., & de Acedo Baquedano, M. T. S. (2003). Enhancement of self-regulation, assertiveness, and empathy. *Learning and Instruction*, *13*(4), 423–439. doi:10.1016/S0959-4752(02)00026-9

Dejman, M. (2010). *Cultural explanatory model of depression among Iranian women in three ethnic groups (Fars, Kurds and Turks) (doctoral dissertation)*. Department of Clinical Neuroscience, Karolinska Institutet, Stockholm, Sweden.

Delker, B. C., Noll, L. K., Kim, H. K., & Fisher, P. A. (2014). Maternal abuse history and self-regulation difficulties in preadolescence. *Child Abuse & Neglect*, *38*(12), 2033–2043. doi:10.1016/j.chiabu.2014.10.014

Dibajnia, P., & Bakhtiari, M. (2002). Mental health status of the students in the faculty of Rehabilitation, Shahid Beheshti University, 2002. *Journal of Ardabil University of Medical Sciences*, *2*(2), 27–32. Retrieved from http://jarums.arums.ac.ir/article-1-561-en.html

Diedrich, A., Grant, M., Hofmann, S. G., Hiller, W., & Berking, M. (2014). Self-compassion as an emotion regulation strategy in major depressive disorder. *Behaviour Research and Therapy*, *58*, 43–51. doi:10.1016/j.brat.2014.05.006

Diehl, M., Semegon, A. B., & Schwarzer, R. (2006). Assessing attention control in goal pursuit: A component of dispositional self-regulation. *Journal of Personality Assessment*, *86*(3), 306–317. doi:10.1207/s15327752jpa8603_06

DiTommaso, E., Brannen, C., & Burgess, M. (2005). The universality of relationship characteristics: A cross-cultural comparison of different types of attachment and loneliness in Canadian and visiting Chinese students. *Social Behavior and Personality: An International Journal*, *33*(1), 57–68. doi:10.2224/sbp.2005.33.1.57

Drake, K., Belsky, J., & Fearon, R. M. (2014). From early attachment to engagement with learning in school: The role of self-regulation and persistence. *Developmental Psychology, 50*(5), 1350–1361. doi:10.1037/a0032779

Dyrbye, L. N., Thomas, M. R., & Shanafelt, T. D. (2006). Systematic review of depression, anxiety, and other indicators of psychological distress among US and Canadian medical students. *Academic Medicine, 81*(4), 354–373. doi:10.1097/00001888-200604000-00009

Ebrahimnejad, H. (2002). Religion and medicine in Iran: From relationship to dissociation. *History of Science, 40*(1), 91–112. doi:10.1177/007327530204000104

Eisenberg, D., Gollust, S. E., Golberstein, E., & Hefner, J. L. (2007). Prevalence and correlates of depression, anxiety, and suicidality among university students. *American Journal of Orthopsychiatry, 77*(4), 534–542. doi:10.1037/0002-9432.77.4.534

Eisenberg, D., Hunt, J., & Speer, N. (2013). Mental health in American colleges and universities: Variation across student subgroups and across campuses. *The Journal of Nervous and Mental Disease, 201*(1), 60–67. doi:10.1097/NMD.0b013e31827ab077

English, L. (2012). *Investigating childhood emotional maltreatment, adult attachment, and mindfulness as predictors of internalizing symptoms and emotional processing* (Doctoral dissertation). University of Guelph, Canada.

Facundes, V. L. D., & Ludermir, A. B. (2005). Common mental disorders among health care students. *Revista Brasileira De Psiquiatria, 27*(3), 194–200. doi:10.1590/S1516-44462005000300007

Farahani, M. K., & Nouri, R. (2016). Concepts of health and disease in individualistic and collectivistic cultures: A cross-cultural study. *Journal of Research in Psychological Health, 9*(4), 1–16. doi:10.18869/acadpub.rph.9.4.1

Fishbach, A., & Converse, B. A. (2011). Identifying and battling temptation. In K. D. Vohs and R. F. Baumeister (Eds.). *Handbook of self-regulation: Research, theory and applications* (2nd ed., pp. 244–260). New York & London: Guilford Press.

Fonagy, P. (2000). Attachment and borderline personality disorder. *Journal of the American Psychoanalytic Association, 48*(4), 1129–1146. doi:10.1177/00030651000480040701

Fonagy, P., & Target, M. (2002). Early intervention and the development of self-regulation. *Psychoanalytic Inquiry, 22*(3), 307–335. doi:10.1080/07351692209348990

Friedman, M. D. (2010). *Adult attachment and self-construal: A cross-cultural analysis (Doctoral dissertation).* Texas A & M University, College Station, TX.

Ghorbani, N., Watson, P. J., & Hargis, M. B. (2008). Integrative self-knowledge scale: Correlations and incremental validity of a cross-cultural measure developed in Iran and the United States. *The Journal of Psychology, 142*(4), 395–412. doi:10.3200/JRPL.142.4.395-412

Ghorbani, N., Watson, P. J., & Weathington, B. L. (2009). Mindfulness in Iran and the United States: Cross-cultural structural complexity and parallel relationships with psychological adjustment. *Current Psychology, 28*(4), 211–224. doi:10.1007/s12144-009-9060-3

Ghorbani, N., Watson, P. J., Bing, M. N., Davison, H. K., & LeBreton, D. (2003). Two facets of self-knowledge: cross-cultural development of measures in Iran and the United States. *Genetic, Social, and General Psychology Monographs, 129*, 238–268. Retrieved from https://www.ncbi.nlm.nih.gov/pubmed/15134127

Ghorbani, N., Watson, P. J., Chen, Z., & Norballa, F. (2012). Self-compassion in Iranian Muslims: Relationships with integrative self-knowledge, mental health, and religious orientation. *International Journal for the Psychology of Religion, 22*(2), 106–118. doi:10.1080/10508619.2011.638601

Ghorbani, N., Watson, P. J., Farhadi, M., & Chen, Z. (2014). A multi-process model of self-regulation: Influences of mindfulness, integrative self-knowledge and self-control in Iran. *International Journal of Psychology, 49*(2), 115–122. doi:10.1002/ijop.12033

Gibbs, J. J., Giever, D., & Martin, J. S. (1998). Parental management and self-control: An empirical test of Gottfredson and Hirschi's general theory. *Journal of Research in Crime and Delinquency, 35*(1), 40–70. doi:10.1177/0022427898035001002

Gilmour, H. (2014). Positive mental health and mental illness. *Health Reports, 25*(9), 3–9. Retrieved from https://www.ncbi.nlm.nih.gov/pubmed/25229895

Gollust, S. E., Eisenberg, D., & Golberstein, E. (2008). Prevalence and correlates of self-injury among university students. *Journal of American College Health*, *56*(5), 491–498. doi:10.3200/JACH.56.5.491-498

Gottfredson, M., & Hirschi, T. (1990). *A general theory of crime*. Stanford: Stanford University Press.

Hackmann, C., J. (2011). *Investigation of a developmental account of self-compassion: The recall of parental behaviour during childhood and the potential roles of attachment and mindfulness* (Doctoral dissertation). University of East Anglia, Norwich, England.

Haghshenas, M., Noorbala, A. A., Akabary, S. A., Laeein, V. N., Sahlei, M., & Tayyebi, Z. (2016). The study of relationship between spiritual intelligence and modes of students' attachment. *Medical Ethics Journal*, *5*(14), 18–167. Retrieved from http://journals.sbmu.ac.ir/en-me/article/view/12858

Hamama, R., Ronen, T., & Feigin, R. (2000). Self-control, anxiety, and loneliness in siblings of children with cancer. *Social Work in Health Care*, *31*(1), 63–83. doi:10.1300/J010v31n01_05

Hayes, S. C. (2004). Acceptance and commitment therapy, relational frame theory, and the third wave of behavioral and cognitive therapies. *Behavior Therapy*, *35*(4), 639–665. doi:10.1016/S0005-7894(04)80013-3

Heydari, A., Teymoori, A., & Nasiri, H. (2015). The effect of parent and peer attachment on suicidality: The mediation effect of self-control and anomie. *Community Mental Health Journal*, *51*(3), 359–364. doi:10.1007/s10597-014-9809-5

Ibánez, M. I., Ruipérez, M. A., Moya, J., Marqués, M. J & Ortet, G. (2005). A short version of the self-regulation inventory (SRI-S). *Personality and Individual Differences*, *39*(6), 1055–1059.0 doi:10.1016/j.paid.2005.02.029

Ibrahim, A. K., Kelly, S. J., Adams, C. E., & Glazebrook, C. (2013). A systematic review of studies of depression prevalence in university students. *Journal of Psychiatric Research*, *47*(3), 391–400. doi:10.1016/j.jpsychires.2012.11.015

Jones, K. C., Welton, S. R., Oliver, T. C., & Thoburn, J. W. (2011). Mindfulness, spousal attachment, and marital satisfaction: A mediated model. *The Family Journal: Counseling and Therapy for Couples and Families*, *19*(4), 357–361. doi:10.1177/1066480711417234

Joshanloo, M., Wissing, M. P., Khumalo, I. P., & Lamers, S. M. (2013). Measurement invariance of the Mental Health Continuum-Short Form (MHC-SF) across three cultural groups. *Personality and Individual Differences*, *55*(7), 755–759. doi:10.1016/j.paid.2013.06.002

Ju, S., J., & Lee, W., K. (2015). Mindfulness, non-attachment, and emotional well-being in Korean adults. *Advanced Science and Technology Letters*, *87*, 68–72. doi:10.14257/astl.2015.87.15

Kelly, A. C., Zuroff, D. C., Foa, C. L., & Gilbert, P. (2010). Who benefits from training in self-compassionate self-regulation? A study of smoking reduction. *Journal of Social and Clinical Psychology*, *29*(7), 727–755. doi:10.1521/jscp.2010.29.7.727

Keyes, C. L. (2005). Mental illness and/or mental health? Investigating axioms of the complete state model of health. *Journal of Consulting and Clinical Psychology*, *73*(3), 539–548. doi:10.1037/0022-006X.73.3.539

Khosravi, S., Sadeghi, M., & Yabande, Y. (2014). Psychometric properties of self-compassion scale (SCS). *Journal Management System*, *4*(13), 47–59. Retrieved from http://jpmm.miau.ac.ir/article_339_en.html

Kord, B., & Pashasharifi, H. (2014). Psychometric characteristics self-compassion scale among students. *Educational Measurement*, *4*(16), 76–92. Retrieved from http://jem.atu.ac.ir/article_310_en.html

Levy, K. N., Meehan, K. B., Kelly, K. M., Reynoso, J. S., Weber, M., Clarkin, J. F., & Kernberg, O. F. (2006). Change in attachment patterns and reflective function in a randomized control trial of transference-focused psychotherapy for borderline personality disorder. *Journal of Consulting and Clinical Psychology*, *74*(6), 1027–1040. doi:10.1037/0022-006X.74.6.1027

Li, J. B., Delvecchio, E., Lis, A., Nie, Y. G., & Di Riso, D. (2015). Parental attachment, self-control, and depressive symptoms in Chinese and Italian adolescents: Test of a mediation model. *Journal of Adolescence*, *43*, 159–170. doi:10.1016/j.adolescence.2015.06.006

Loess, P., & Waltz, J. (2014). *Borderline personality disorder, emotion regulation, and self-compassion. Graduate Student Research Conference. Paper 20.* Retrieved from http://scholarworks. umt.edu/gsrc/2014/posters/20.

Lorenzini, N., & Fonagy, P. (2013). Attachment and personality disorders: A short review. *FOCUS, 11*(2), 155–166. doi:10.1176/appi.focus.11.2.155

Lovibond, S. H., & Lovibond, P. F. (1995). *Manual for the depression anxiety stress scale.* Sydney: The Psychology Foundation of Australia In.

Luszczynska, A., Diehl, M., Gutiérrez-Doña, B., Kuusinen, P., & Schwarzer, R. (2004). Measuring one component of dispositional self-regulation: Attention control in goal pursuit. *Personality and Individual Differences, 37*(3), 555–566. doi:10.1016/j.paid.2003.09.026

MarshPow, A. (2014). *Coping with catastrophe: emotion regulation, adult attachment security, and mindfulness as predictors of posttraumatic stress among mental health disaster responders* (Doctoral dissertation). University of North Carolina, Chapel Hill, North Carolina.

Martin, D. M. (2009). *Mindfulness and Attachment Security as Predictors of Sucess in Therapy* (Doctoral dissertation). University of Kansas, Lawrence, KS.

Mirabzadeh, A., Eftekhari, M. B., Falahat, K., Sajjadi, H., Vameghi, M., & Harouni, G. G. (2018). Positive Mental Health from the perspective of Iranian society: A qualitative study. *F1000Research, 7*, 103–115. doi:10.12688/f1000research.13394.1

Mokhtari, M., Dehghan, S. F., Asghari, M., Ghasembaklo, U., Mohamadyari, G., Azadmanesh, S. A., & Akbari, E. (2013). Epidemiology of mental health problems in female students: A questionnaire survey. *Journal of Epidemiology and Global Health, 3*(2), 83–88. doi:10.1016/j.jegh.2013.02.005

Moon, Y. S., & Han, S. J. (2009). Impact of parent-adolescent attachment and self-control on problem behavior in middle school students. *The Journal of Korean Academic Society of Nursing Education, 15*(2), 302–310. doi:10.5977/JKASNE.2009.15.2.302

Moreira, H., Gouveia, M. J., Carona, C., Silva, N., & Canavarro, M. C. (2015). Maternal attachment and children's quality of life: The mediating role of self-compassion and parenting stress. *Journal of Child and Family Studies, 24*(8), 2313–2332. doi:10.1007/s10826-014-0036-z

Morf, C. C., & Koole, S. L. (2012). The self. In M. Hewstone, W. Stroebe and K. Jonas (Eds.). *An Introduction to Social Psychology* (5th ed.). London: John Wiley & Sons.

Nakash-Eisikovits, O., Dutra, L., & Westen, D. (2002). Relationship between attachment patterns and personality pathology in adolescents. *Journal of the American Academy of Child & Adolescent Psychiatry, 41*(9), 1111–1123. doi:10.1097/00004583-200209000-00012

Neff, K. (2003). The development and validation of a scale to measure self-compassion. *Self and Identity, 2*(3), 223–250. doi:10.1080/15298860309027

Neff, K. D., & Germer, C. K. (2013). A pilot study and randomized controlled trial of the mindful self-compassion program. *Journal of Clinical Psychology, 69*(1), 28–44. doi:10.1002/jclp.21923

Noorbala, A. A., Yazdi, S. A. B., Faghihzadeh, S., Kamali, K., Faghihzadeh, E., Hajebi, A., …., Asadi, A. (2017). Trends of mental health status in Iranian population aged 15 and above between 1999 and 2015. *Archives of Iranian Medicine, 20*(11), 2–6.

Nosratabadi, M., Joshanloo, M., Mohammadi, F., & Shahmohammadi, K. (2010). Are Iranian students flourishing? *Journal of Iranian Psychologists, 7*(25), 83–94. Retrieved from http://jip.azad.ac.ir/article_512305_en.html

Pakdaman, S. (2001). *Examining the relationship between attachment and community-minded teenager* (Doctoral dissertation). University of Tehran, Tehran, Iran.

Papies, E. K., & Aarts, H. (2011). Nonconscious self-regulation or the automatic pilot of human behavior. In D. V. Kathleen & F. B. Roy (Eds.) *Handbook of self-regulation: Research, theory, and applications* (2nd ed., pp. 125–142). New York & London: Guilford Press.

Pepping, C. A., Davis, P. J., & O'Donovan, A. (2013). Individual differences in attachment and dispositional mindfulness: The mediating role of emotion regulation. *Personality and Individual Differences, 54*(3), 453–456. doi:10.1016/j.paid.2012.10.006

Pepping, C. A., Davis, P. J., O'Donovan, A., & Pal, J. (2015). Individual differences in self-compassion: The role of attachment and experiences of parenting in childhood. *Self and Identity, 14*(1), 104–117. doi:10.1080/15298868.2014.955050

Pepping, C. A., O'Donovan, A., & Davis, P. J. (2014). The differential relationship between mindfulness and attachment in experienced and inexperienced meditators. *Mindfulness*, 5(4), 392–399. doi:10.1007/s12671-012-0193-3

Pepping, C. A., O'Donovan, A., Zimmer-Gembeck, M. J., & Hanisch, M. (2015). Individual differences in attachment and eating pathology: The mediating role of mindfulness. *Personality and Individual Differences*, 75, 24–29. doi:10.1016/j.paid.2014.10.040

Pidgeon, A., & Grainger, A. (2013). Mindfulness as a factor in the relationship between insecure attachment style, neurotic personality and disordered eating behavior. *Open Journal of Medical Psychology*, 02(04), 25–33. doi:10.4236/ojmp.2013.24B005

Pipp, S., Easterbrooks, M., & Brown, S. R. (1993). Attachment status and complexity of infants' self-and other-knowledge when tested with mother and father. *Social Development*, 2(1), 1–14. doi:10.1111/j.1467-9507.1993.tb00001.x

Pipp, S., Easterbrooks, M., & Harmon, R. J. (1992). The relation between attachment and knowledge of self and mother in one-to three-year-old infants. *Child Development*, 63(3), 738–750. doi:10.1111/j.1467-8624.1992.tb01658.x

Preacher, K. J., & Hayes, A. F. (2008). Asymptotic and resampling strategies for assessing and comparing indirect effects in multiple mediator models. *Behavior Research Methods*, 40(3), 879–891. doi:10.3758/BRM.40.3.879

Rachlin, H. (1974). Self-control. *Behaviorism*, 2, 94–107. Retrieved from https://www.jstor.org/stable/27758811

Raes, F., Pommier, E., Neff, K. D., & Van Gucht, D. (2011). Construction and factorial validation of a short form of the Self-Compassion Scale. *Clinical Psychology & Psychotherapy*, 18(3), 250–255. doi:10.1002/cpp.702

Rahmati, M., Rahmani, S., Akbarzadeh, B. A., Fathollahzadeh, F., & Gharibnavaz, P. (2015). Investigation of relationship between quality of sleep and mental health of rehabilitation sciences students of Shahid Beheshti University of Medical Sciences. *Scientific Journal of Rehabilitation Medicine*, 4(3), 55–147. Retrieved from http://medrehab.sbmu.ac.ir/article_1100159_1016.html

Raque-Bogdan, T. L., Ericson, S. K., Jackson, J., Martin, H. M., & Bryan, N. A. (2011). Attachment and mental and physical health: Self-compassion and mattering as mediators. *Journal of Counseling Psychology*, 58(2), 272–278. doi:10.1037/a0023041

Rothbaum, F., Weisz, J., Pott, M., Miyake, K., & Morelli, G. (2000). Attachment and culture: Security in the United States and Japan. *American Psychologist*, 55(10), 1093–1104. doi:10.1037/0003-066X.55.10.1093

Sahebi, A., Asghari, M. J., & Salari, R. S. (2005). Validation of depression anxiety and stress scale (DASS-21) for an Iranian population. *Iranian Psychologists*, 4, 299–313. Retrieved from http://jip.azad.ac.ir/article_512443.html

Schanche, E., Stiles, T. C., McCullough, L., Svartberg, M., & Nielsen, G. H. (2011). The relationship between activating affects, inhibitory affects, and self-compassion in patients with Cluster C personality disorders. *Psychotherapy*, 48(3), 293–303. doi:10.1037/a0022012

Schmitt, D. P., Alcalay, L., Allensworth, M., Allik, J., Ault, L., Austers, I., … ZupanÈiÈ, A. (2004). Patterns and universals of adult romantic attachment across 62 cultural regions: Are models Of Self and of Other Pancultural Constructs? *Journal of Cross-Cultural Psychology*, 35(4), 367–402. doi:10.1177/0022022104266105

Schore, J. R., & Schore, A. N. (2008). Modern attachment theory: The central role of affect regulation in development and treatment. *Clinical Social Work Journal*, 36(1), 9–20. doi:10.1007/s10615-007-0111-7

Shahmohammadi, K., Ghorbani, N., & Besharat, M. A. (2007). The role of self-knowledge in stress, defensive styles, and physical health. *Journal of Developmental Psychology*, 3(10), 145–156. Retrieved from http://jip.azad.ac.ir/article_512505_en.html

Shaver, P. R., Lavy, S., Saron, C. D., & Mikulincer, M. (2007). Social foundations of the capacity for mindfulness: An attachment perspective. *Psychological Inquiry*, 18(4), 264–271. doi:10.1080/10478400701598389

Snyder, R., Shapiro, S., & Treleaven, D. (2012). Attachment theory and mindfulness. *Journal of Child and Family Studies, 21*(5), 709–717. doi:10.1007/s10826-011-9522-8

Sroufe, L. A., Duggal, S., Weinfield, N., & Carlson, E. (2000). Relationships, development, and psychopathology. A. J. Sameroff, M. Lewis, and S. M. Miller (Eds). *Handbook of developmental psychopathology* (2nd ed., pp. 75–91). New York, NY: Kluwer Academic/Plenum Publishers.

Tanaka, M., Wekerle, C., Schmuck, M. L., Paglia-Boak, A., & Research Team, M. A. P. (2011). The linkages among childhood maltreatment, adolescent mental health, and self-compassion in child welfare adolescents. *Child Abuse & Neglect, 35*(10), 887–898. doi:10.1016/j.chiabu.2011.07.003

Tangney, J. P., Baumeister, R. F., & Boone, A. L. (2004). High self-control predicts good adjustment, less pathology, better grades, and interpersonal success. *Journal of Personality, 72*(2), 271–322. doi:10.1111/j.0022-3506.2004.00263.x

Terry, M. L., & Leary, M. R. (2011). Self-compassion, self-regulation, and health. *Self and Identity, 10*(3), 352–362. doi:10.1080/15298868.2011.558404

Vaingankar, J. A., Subramaiam, M., Lim, Y. W., Sherbourne, C., Luo, N., Ryan, G., … Chong, S. A. (2012). From well-being to positive mental health: Conceptualization and qualitative development of an instrument in Singapore. *Quality of Life Research, 21*(10), 1785–1794. doi:10.1007/s11136-011-0105-3

Valikhani, A., & Goodarzi, M. A. (2017). Contingencies of self-worth and psychological distress in Iranian patients seeking cosmetic surgery: Integrative self-knowledge as mediator. *Aesthetic Plastic Surgery, 1,* 9. doi:10.1007/s00266-017-0853-8

Valikhani, A., Goodarzi, M. A., & Hashemi, R. (2017). Psychometric properties of dispositional self-regulation scale in Iranian population and predicting inhibitory/initiatory self-control on the basis of it. *Current Psychology, 1,* 11. doi:10.1007/s12144-017-9574-z

Valikhani, A., Sarafraz, M. R., & Moghimi, P. (2018). Examining the role of attachment styles and self-control in suicide ideation and death anxiety for patients receiving chemotherapy in Iran. *Psycho-Oncology, 27*(3), 1057–1060. doi:10.1002/pon.4466

van Ijzendoorn, M. H., & Sagi, A. (1999). *Cross-cultural patterns of attachment: Universal and contextual dimensions.* In J. Cassidy & P.R. Shaver (Eds.) *Handbook of attachment: Theory, research, and clinical applications* (pp. 713–734). New York, NY: The Guilford Press.

Vettese, L. C., Dyer, C. E., Li, W. L., & Wekerle, C. (2011). Does self-compassion mitigate the association between childhood maltreatment and later emotion regulation difficulties? A preliminary investigation. *International Journal of Mental Health and Addiction, 9*(5), 480–491. doi:10.1007/s11469-011-9340-7

Vohs K. D., & Baumeister, R. F. (Eds.). (2011). *Handbook of self-regulation: Research, theory, and applications.* New York & London: Guilford Press.

Vondra, J. I., Shaw, D. S., Swearingen, L., Cohen, M., & Owens, E. B. (2001). Attachment stability and emotional and behavioral regulation from infancy to preschool age. *Development and Psychopathology, 13*(1), 13–33. Retrieved from https://www.ncbi.nlm.nih.gov/pubmed/11346048

Walsh, J. J., Balint, M. G., Smolira Sj, D. R., Fredericksen, L. K., & Madsen, S. (2009). Predicting individual differences in mindfulness: The role of trait anxiety, attachment anxiety and attentional control. *Personality and Individual Differences, 46*(2), 94–99. doi:10.1016/j.paid.2008.09.008

Warren, R. (2015). Emotion regulation in borderline personality disorder: The role of self-criticism, shame, and self-compassion. *Personality and Mental Health, 9*(1), 84–86. doi:10.1002/pmh.1290

Westen, D., Nakash, O., Thomas, C., & Bradley, R. (2006). Clinical assessment of attachment patterns and personality disorder in adolescents and adults. *Journal of Consulting and Clinical Psychology, 74*(6), 1065–1085. doi:10.1037/0022-006X.74.6.1065

Whitebread, D., & Basilio, M. (2012). The emergence and early development of self-regulation in young children. *Profesorado, 16,* 15–33. Retrieved from http://www.ugr.es/local/recfpro/rev161ART2en.pdf

Self-Criticism, Neediness, and Distress in the Prediction of Suicide Ideation: Results from Cross-Sectional and Longitudinal Studies

Rui C. Campos, Ronald R. Holden, Cristina Baleizão, Berta Caçador, and Ana Sofia Fragata

ABSTRACT
The aim of the present study was to test whether the maladaptive personality traits of self-criticism and neediness predict suicide ideation when controlling for general distress. Further, potential interactive effects on suicide ideation of the two traits and distress were also evaluated. Two studies with nonclinical samples were conducted. The first investigation was cross-sectional and involved a final sample of 202 community adults while the second study was longitudinal with a final sample of 207 college students. Results of Study 1 demonstrated that self-criticism, but not neediness, associated with suicide ideation and, in doing so, also interacted with distress. Neediness also tended to interact with self-criticism in the prediction of suicide ideation. Results from Study 2 were similar and confirmed the Study 1 results. Changes in self-criticism, but not changes in neediness, predicted changes in suicide ideation after statistically controlling for changes in distress. Changes in the interaction between self-criticism and distress predicted changes in suicide ideation and changes in the interaction between self-criticism and neediness tended to predict changes in suicide ideation. Results are discussed with regard to their implications for psychological intervention.

Identifying variables associated with suicide risk and suicide ideation and articulating how these variables interact with each other and how they express themselves as risk factors can allow for an increased understanding of a problem as complex and multifactorial as suicide (Hawton & van Heeringen, 2009; Overholser, Braden, & Dieter, 2012; Pompili et al., 2012). Importantly, suicide ideation, itself, is a highly relevant indicator of suicide risk with suicide ideation being strongly related to suicide attempts and death by suicide (Brown, Beck, Steer, & Grisham, 2000; Prieto & Tavares, 2005; Wetzel et al., 2011).

General psychopathology and distress are factors that contribute to suicide risk and suicide ideation (e.g., Lund, Nadorff, & Seader, 2016; Overholser et al., 2012). However, although the presence of a mental illness increases the risk for suicide, not all individuals who experience distress or psychopathology, or who have even received a psychiatric diagnosis are at risk for suicide or experience suicide ideation. As such, it becomes important to investigate other variables that potentiate the relationship between distress or general psychopathology and suicide ideation (Overholser et al., 2012; Pompili, Lester, Leenaars, Tatarelli, & Girardi, 2008). Thus, although distress or general psychopathology of themselves may be important (Bertolote & Fleischmann, 2002; Jacobs et al., 2010), they are insufficient to understand and explain a high percentage of the variance in suicide ideation.

Based on Blatt's (2008) model, we hypothesised that the dysfunctional personality traits of neediness and self-criticism may be moderators of the relationship between distress and suicide ideation. According to this model, optimal personality development and adaptation implies an integration of two central developmental tasks: establishing mutually satisfactory and evolved relationships; and constructing a coherent, differentiated, and integrated sense of self. However, the extensive and distorted emphasis given by self-critical and needy individuals, respectively, to the developmental processes of self-definition and relatedness are linked to dysfunctional forms of adaptation and to poor mental health (e.g., Besser & Priel, 2005, 2011; Blatt, 2008; Blatt & Zuroff, 1992). Self-criticism refers to a personality dimension comprising maladaptive traits that combine having high personal standards with high self-criticism, perfectionism, and a tendency toward feelings of unworthiness, guilt failure, and to engage in a harsh self-scrutiny. Neediness includes a preoccupation with abandonment, rejection, separation, and helplessness, as well as feelings of being unloved. These individuals fear loss and tend to seek help and support from others, especially when they are confronted with stressful situations or feeling lonely (Blatt, 2008). Individuals with maladaptive personality characteristics or dysfunctional personality functioning manage in a deficient way with distress and traumatic events (e.g., Besser & Priel, 2010). It follows that they may be able to cope better or worse depending on the rigidity and adaptability of these characteristics. Avoidance strategies, for example, may generate or potentiate the effects of distress, although other forms of coping will not necessarily have this effect (e.g., Dunkley, Blankstein, Halsall, Williams, & Winkworth, 2000).

Ineffective coping strategies may explain, for example, why perfectionism generates a vulnerability to distress (Dunkley & Blankstein, 2000) and possibly even to suicide ideation. Perfectionism that is intrinsically linked to self-criticism, albeit distinct, can explain the relation of the latter to suicide risk, because this perfectionism results in the occurrence of internal experiences of self-punishment based in self-evaluations of the individual that are performed in an unrealistic manner (e.g., Morrison & O'Connor, 2008; see also Falgares et al., 2017; Flett, Hewitt, & Heisel, 2014). Perfectionism also results in experiences of guilt and deeper feelings of devaluation attributable to an excessive concern about not having an ideal or a perfect self (Flett, Hewitt, Blankstein, & Gray, 1998). Individuals with more introjective personality traits (i.e., self-critical traits) may, in fact, be more likely to present with suicide intent than would anaclitic (i.e., dependent) individuals (with high levels of neediness) (Fazaa & Page, 2003, 2009; Sobrinho, Campos, & Holden, 2016). Fazaa and Page (2003), for example, also found that suicide attempts among self-critical (introjective) college students were often in response to intrapsychic distress.

However, anaclitic or dependent personality traits can also increase a vulnerability to cope poorly with negative experiences (e.g., Besser & Priel, 2005, 2010; Blatt, 1990, 2008). Some studies (e.g., Loas & Defélice, 2012) have also shown that dependency is a stable personality trait in individuals who have attempted suicide. Anaclitic traits, in addition to introjective traits, may be a risk factor (Klomek et al., 2008), although with less importance than introjective traits (Fazaa & Page, 2003, 2009). Dependent individuals because of their great need for reassurance from others may, in some cases, elicit rejection from others, especially when they present with poor social abilities (Bornstein, 1996). This rejection and withdrawal of interpersonal support may then increase future risk for suicidal behavior (Stellrecht & Rudd, 2006).

Previous research has shown that distress (e.g., Campos, Besser, & Blatt, 2012) and depression (Campos, Besser, & Blatt, 2013; Sobrinho et al., 2016) were mediating variables in the association of introjective personality traits with suicide risk. The effect of neediness on suicide risk was either only indirect (Campos et al., 2012) or just marginal (Sobrinho et al., 2016). In the Campos, Besser, Abreu, Parreira, and Blatt (2014) study, however, distress fully mediated the relationship between dependency and suicide risk in a sample of Portuguese adolescents. But, to our knowledge, no investigation has tested the interaction between the dysfunctional personality traits proposed by Blatt and distress in the prediction of suicide ideation. Of note, an extensive body of literature, including cross-sectional (e.g., Campos, Besser, & Blatt, 2010), longitudinal (e.g., Yao, Fang, Zhu, & Zuroff, 2009), and experimental (e.g., Besser, Guez, & Priel, 2008) studies, has examined and confirmed the vulnerability role of maladaptive personality traits, particularly self-criticism, for depression (Blatt, 2004), neuroticism and distress (Bagby & Rector, 1998), and anxiety (e.g., Mongrain & Zuroff, 1995; Overholser & Freiheit, 1994). Each of these can ultimately contribute to suicide risk via a meditational effect (e.g., Campos et al., 2012). Nevertheless, testing the moderating effects of personality traits on distress in its relationship to suicide risk and suicide ideation is still clearly a research task that is called for.

Dysfunctional personality traits may, in fact, augment difficulties in coping and recovering from acute distress states such as depression. For example, Shahar, Gallagher, Blatt, Kuperminc, and Leadbeater (2004) demonstrated that patients' perfectionism had an adverse effect on treating depression and that this effect may be due in part to having a less positive sustained social network. Also in researching perfectionism, Hewitt, Flett, and Weber (1994) reported that stress interacted with each of self-oriented and socially prescribed perfectionism in the prediction of suicide ideation among university undergraduates. The importance of individual differences in moderating the association between stress and suicide ideation also extends beyond dysfunctional traits. For example, emotional intelligence has been found to moderate (reducing) the relationship between stress and suicide ideation among a sample of depressed adolescent inpatients (Abdollahi, Carlbring, Khanbani, & Ghahfarokhi, 2016).

Aim of the Study

In the present investigation, we test the hypothesis that dysfunctional personality traits, in addition to their previously documented direct effect on distress, may also enhance or potentiate (i.e., moderate) the effect of distress on suicide risk, as assessed by an important clinical indicator—suicide ideation. In this research, two studies are presented: a cross-sectional investigation and a longitudinal study; both testing the impact of the same variables on suicide ideation.

In the first study, the participant sample was comprised of community adults. It was hypothesised that self-criticism and neediness as proposed in Blatt's model (1990, 2004,

2008) would potentiate the effect of distress on suicide ideation and also that both traits would interact with each other in the prediction of suicide ideation.

In the second study, a nonclinical sample composed of young adult university students participated. Data were collected at two time points, with an interval of approximately 5 months. Analyses examined the impact on changes in suicide ideation of changes in distress, changes in the dysfunctional personality traits of self-criticism and neediness, changes in the interaction between these dysfunctional traits, and changes in the interaction between distress and the dysfunctional personality traits. It was hypothesised that changes in the interaction between distress and the dysfunctional personality traits and changes in the interaction between the two dysfunctional personality traits would predict changes in suicide ideation.

In the present research, current suicide ideation was studied, unlike previous studies in Portugal that have investigated life-long suicide risk and personality. Further, distress in general was assessed, not just depression or other specific distress dimensions such as anxiety. Our rationale for this was that dysfunctional personality traits are linked to a wide range of psychopathologies (Blatt, 2004, 2008), such as bipolar depression (Rosenfarb, Becker, Khan, & Mintz, 1998), social anxiety (Kopala–Sibley, Zuroff, Russell, & Moskowitz, 2014) and borderline personality disorder (Levy, Edell, & McGlashan, 2007), and not only to depression.

Study 1

Participants and Procedures

Initially, 270 community individuals were contacted and, of these, 242 agreed to participate in the study. However, 40 protocols were subsequently removed because of either excessive missing responses or invalid response styles. This resulted in a final sample of 202 participants, including 115 (56.9%) women and 87 (43.1%) men.

Participants' ages ranged from 18 to 65 years ($M = 41.36$, $SD = 12.11$). Their number of years of education was between 6 and 19 years ($M = 12.45$, $SD = 3.13$). In addition, 26 (12.9%) of the participants were unemployed and 111 (55.0%) were married or living together. According to data available in the National Institute of Statistics (2011), the Portuguese population is composed of 52.2% women; the average age is 41.8 years, with a mean of 7.9 years of schooling and an unemployment rate of 13.2%. Therefore, the sample that participated in the present study was similar to the general population except that the level of schooling was higher.

Potential participants were approached by trained research assistants in public places (including small shops, cafes, supermarkets, offices, and a university) and invited to take part in an investigation related to suicide risk. Some individuals participated immediately; others later participated at home after scheduling a convenient date and time with a research assistant. Individuals, who agreed to participate, signed an informed consent form that indicated the confidentiality of their research data and, then, the individuals completed the research protocol. Participants were not compensated for responding to the research questionnaires. The order of presentation of the questionnaires was random and the questionnaires were administered individually by the research assistants. Informed consent provided telephone numbers for any individuals who wished to talk with a mental health professional. The study was approved by the research ethics committee of the university.

Measures

SocioDemographic Questionnaire This questionnaire collected information regarding demographic variables, including age, gender, marital status, nationality, schooling, and employment status.

Depressive Experiences Questionnaire (DEQ; Blatt, D'Afflitti, & Quinlan, 1976, 1979) This questionnaire assesses two types of depressive experiences or, more generally, two personality dimensions or traits (Blatt, 2008; Blatt & Zuroff, 1992; Blatt et al., 1976). It consists of 66 items answered on seven-point Likert ratings, in which 1 corresponds to "totally disagree" and 7 to "totally agree." A 4 is considered as the midpoint. The Depressive Experiences Questionnaire yields scores on factors derived through principal components analysis based on the responses of American college students (Blatt et al., 1976, 1979). Factor I labelled as "dependency" has two subfactors, neediness and connectedness, based on subsequent research (Blatt, Zohar, Quinlan, Zuroff, & Mongrain, 1995; Rude & Burnham, 1995). The items with the greatest component weights on this first subfactor relate to interpersonal relationships, addressing issues such as concern about being abandoned or rejected and feeling lonely, and helpless (e.g., "Without support from others who are close to me, I would be helpless"). Factor II, named "self-criticism," encompasses items that express concern about feeling an inner emptiness, hopelessness, guilt, insecurity, dissatisfaction, and feelings of not meeting expectations and goals (e.g., "I often found that I don't live up to my own standards or ideals"). Despite these two main factors being consistent with the two dimensions of depression and personality described by Blatt (e.g., Blatt & Blass, 1990; Blatt & Luyten, 2009; Luyten & Blatt, 2013), factor analysis has revealed the existence of a third factor, referred to as "efficacy" (Blatt et al., 1976). It includes items relating to trust in one's own abilities and resources, ability to take on responsibilities, feelings of independence, pride, satisfaction, and inner strength [e.g., "I have many inner resources (abilities, strengths)"]. With regard to internal consistency reliability, Cronbach's alpha values for scores on DEQ scales were adequate both in the original study (Blatt, D'Afflitti, & Quinlan, 1979) and in the replication study (Zuroff, Quinlan, & Blatt, 1990). In the present study, we used the factor scales of neediness, the maladaptive component of dependency, and self-criticism because we were interested only in maladaptive personality traits. The DEQ has been translated into various languages in several countries and its validity in these other versions has been established in numerous studies (see Falgares et al., 2017). In the Portuguese version (Campos, 2009, 2016) of the DEQ, previous data have been obtained for samples of 1545 community adults and 488 university students. With regard to Cronbach's alpha, in the community sample, values were .79 for self-criticism and .64 for neediness. For university students, Cronbach's alphas were .78 and .68 for the self-criticism and neediness scales, respectively. In the current study, the Cronbach's alpha values for the self-criticism and neediness scales were .78 and .63, respectively.

Brief Symptom Inventory (BSI; Derogatis, 1993) The BSI is a self-report inventory consisting of 53 items assessing the degree to which each symptom has affected the respondent in the week prior to the evaluation. Higher values represent a greater level of distress. The BSI allows for the evaluation of psychopathological symptoms in terms of nine dimensions—somatization, obsessions-compulsions, interpersonal sensitivity, depression, anxiety, hostility, phobic anxiety, paranoid ideation, and psychoticism. Responses are on Likert ratings, ranging from 0 to "never" to 4 "very many times." Examples of items are: "Feeling alone," "Feeling sad." The BSI can generate three global indexes that evaluate general distress: The Global Severity Index (GSI), the Positive Symptoms Total (PST), and the Positive Symptom Distress Index (PSDI). The PSDI provides a measure of the severity or intensity of the presented symptoms. The test manual reports that when a sample of American psychiatric patients completed the BSI, the internal consistency assessed by Cronbach's alpha ranged from .71 to .85 and, and test-retest reliability for a 2-week interval ranged from .68 to .91 for the different symptom scales. Psychometric studies with the Portuguese version of the inventory (Canavarro, 1999, 2007) have revealed that it presents adequate levels of scale score internal consistency, with Cronbach's alpha values varying between .62 and .80 for the nine dimensions of psychopathological symptomatology. In the current study, the overall level of distress in terms of symptom intensity was indexed with the PSDI. In calculating the internal consistency reliability for total scale scores, a Cronbach's alpha of .97 was obtained.

Suicidal Ideation Questionnaire (SIQ; Reynolds, 1988)

The SIQ is a self-report questionnaire that measures the frequency and severity of suicidal thoughts in the month prior to assessment. Applicable to adolescents and adults, the instrument consists of 30 items, each directed to a specific form of suicide ideation. Example items include: "I thought about killing myself," "I thought killing myself would solve my problems," "I thought about people dying." The items are based on clinical interviews with adolescents and adults who had depressive symptoms, some of whom had also had a prior suicide attempt. Numerous studies have supported the validity of SIQ scales scores (Reynolds, 1988) demonstrating substantial correlations with other relevant psychological variables such as self-esteem, anxiety, and depression. Item responses are as Likert ratings, ranging from 0 "never thought of it" to 6 "almost every day." Higher scores indicate a greater severity of suicide ideation. Possible scores can vary between 0 and 180 points. According to the author, a score equal to or greater than 41 points may be indicative of potential suicide risk (Reynolds, 1988). In adapting the SIQ to the Portuguese language, scale score Cronbach's alpha coefficient was .96 (Ferreira & Castela, 1999). In the present study, the Cronbach's alpha value was .97.

Data Analytic Strategy

Initially, correlations between sociodemographic variables (i.e., gender, age, schooling, unemployment, marital status) and suicide ideation were tested. If a sociodemographic variables correlated significantly with suicide ideation, it was to be considered as a variable to be statistically controlled for in the subsequent hierarchical multiple linear regression analysis. Correlations among other variables in the study were also computed.

To test the contribution of distress (intensity of presented symptoms) and personality, as well as their interactions to suicide ideation, the multivariate statistical technique of hierarchical multiple linear regression analysis was employed. Suicide ideation was entered as the outcome variable. In the first step, distress was entered. The personality variables of self-criticism and neediness were entered in the second step. In the third step, the interaction term between the two personality variables was entered (see Aiken & West, 1991). In the fourth step, the two interaction terms between each of the personality variables and distress were entered. Finally, in the fifth step, the three-way interaction term between the two personality variables and distress was entered. In order to avoid issues related to nonnormality and heterocedasticity, bootstrapping (using 1000 samples to construct 95% bias-corrected confidence intervals) was used to test the significance levels of the estimated parameters (e.g., Yung & Bentler, 1996). The variables were standardized before obtaining the interaction terms and the calculation of the model parameters.

Results

Preliminary Analysis

Correlations between sociodemographic variables and suicide ideation were calculated. Because, there were no significant correlations between any of the demographic variables and suicide ideation, the former were not further considered in the regression analysis. The correlation values between the psychological variables under study were also calculated and are presented in Table 1.

Hierarchical Multiple Linear Regression Analysis

Results of the hierarchical multiple linear regression analysis are summarized in Table 2. With the exception of Step 5, each step of analysis resulted in a significant increase in accounting for variance in suicide ideation. In Step 1, distress was related significantly to suicide ideation. In Step 2, self-criticism, but not neediness, enhanced significantly the prediction of suicide ideation. In Step 3, the interaction of self-criticism × neediness accounted for further unique variance in ideation if we consider the confidence interval obtained for B, but not according to a t-test using the standard error obtained through bootstrapping. This interaction is represented in Figure 1A. In Step 4, there is a significant interaction between self-criticism and distress in predicting suicide ideation. This interaction is represented in Figure 1B. Finally, in Step 5, the three-way interaction term did not make a significant contribution to the prediction of suicide ideation.

As a supplementary analysis, a similar regression model was tested where neediness (and not self-criticism) was the only personality variable tested. This was undertaken in order to assess whether neediness provided a contribution to suicide ideation prediction that was being obfuscated by the presence of self-criticism. In that analysis, neediness tended toward providing an additional contribution ($B = 2.31$, $SE = 1.34$, $p <$ .10, 95% CI [.31–4.80]) beyond distress ($B = 7.94$, $SE = 2.51$, $p < .05$, 95% CI [4.08–12.83]) in predicting suicide ideation, with the interaction of neediness and distress ($B = 4.05$, $SE = 1.74$, $p < .05$, 95% CI [1.38–7.82]) also explaining unique suicide ideation variance. In this supplementary regression analysis, each of the three steps enhanced significantly the prediction of suicide ideation variance.

Table 1. Descriptive Statistics and Bivariate Correlations for Study 1 Psychological Variables ($N = 202$).

Variables	1	2	3	M	SD
1. Self-criticism	——			−0.86	0.97
2. Neediness	.48[*]	——		−0.39	0.81
3. Distress	.49[*]	.34[*]	——	1.35	0.43
4. Suicide Ideation	.40[*]	.28[*]	.47[*]	8.22	17.34

Note: [*]$p < .001$ (two-tailed).

Table 2. Hierarchical Multiple Regression Analysis for Suicide Ideation (Study 1; $N = 202$).

Predictors	R^2	ΔR^2	B	$SE\ B$	t/F	95% CI of B LL	95% CI of B UL	Overall F	df
Step 1	.22	.22			56.33***			56.33***	1, 200
Distress			7.94	2.25	3.53*	4.24	12.21		
Step 2	.26	.04			4.46**			23.26***	2, 198
Self-criticism			3.40	.92	3.70**	1.96	5.07		
Neediness			1.11	1.20	.93	−.96	3.37		
Step 3	.29	.03			7.24**			19.80***	3, 197
Self-criticism × Neediness			2.88	1.89	1.52	.09	6.73		
Step 4	.37	.08			13.46***			19.34***	5, 195
Self-criticism × Distress			4.27	1.98	2.16*	1.18	8.42		
Neediness × Distress			1.54	1.14	1.35	−.58	3.69		
Step 5	.38	.01			2.82			17.15***	6, 194
Self-criticism × Neediness × Distress			1.53	1.72	.89	−.78	5.57		

Note: ΔR^2 = increase in R^2; t = value associated with B; F = F ratio associated with increase in R^2.
*$p < .05$.
**$p < .01$.
***$p < .001$ (two-tailed).

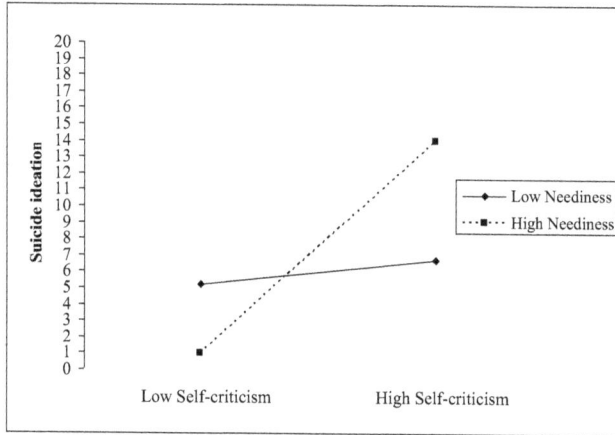

(A)

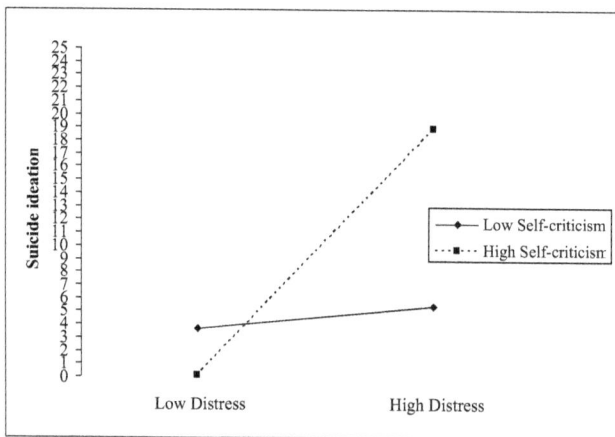

(B)

Figure 1. (A) Interaction between self-criticism and neediness (Study 1; $N = 202$). (B) Interaction between distress and self-criticism (Study 1; $N = 202$). Note: Both figures report mean values.

Study 2

Participants and Procedures

Data were collected at two time points, with a 5-month interval between them (mean interval of 22 weeks). At Time 1, 347 college students were contacted, 6 of whom declined to participate. Of the remaining 341, 31 protocols were eliminated because of nonidentification (not providing up to three or four initials of their full name that permitted anonymity but still allowed for pairing with their Time 2 protocols) or, in a very few cases, by the presence of excessive missing data. The final sample at Time 1 was thus composed of 310 individuals, of whom 118 were men (38.1%) and 192 (61.9%) were women. Participants' ages varied between 18 and 29 years ($M = 20.10$, $SD = 2.17$).

One hundred and two students did not participate at Time 2 and data for one participant were removed due to an excessive number of missing items. As such, the final sample for Study 2 was composed of 207 participants. The group of 103 that did not participate did not differ significantly from the final sample of 207 participants with respect to either gender, χ^2 (1, $N = 310$) $= 0.89$, ns, or age, $t(308) = 1.88$, ns, nor in any of the psychological study variables, self-criticism, $t(308) = 0.45$, ns, neediness, $t(308) = 0.91$, ns, distress, $t(308) = 0.57$, ns, or suicide ideation, $t(308) = 0.64$, ns. This final sample consisted of 75 (36.2%) male and 132 (63.8%) female students. Ages ranged between 18 and 29 years ($M = 19.90$, $SD = 1.85$). Participants were between the first and fifth year of university ($M = 2.27$, $SD = 0.93$).

During class time, potential participants were invited by the authors to take part in an investigation of personality, life events, distress, and suicide ideation. Individuals who agreed to participate signed an informed consent form where the confidentiality of the responses was assured and, subsequently, they completed the research protocol. Students were then asked to respond again to the same research protocol 5 months later. This time period was chosen as a matter of convenience by the researchers. Participants were not compensated for their participation. The order of presentation of the questionnaires was random. Informed consent provided telephone numbers for participants who wished to talk with a mental health professional. The study was approved by the research ethics committee of the university.

Measures

SocioDemographic Questionnaire The sociodemographic questionnaire collected information regarding age, gender, course year and topic, employment status, and course satisfaction.

Depressive Experiences Questionnaire The same measure was used as in Study 1. In this second study, for the final sample, the Cronbach's alpha reliabilities for the neediness scale scores were .69 and .74 at Time 1 and Time 2, respectively. For the self-criticism scale scores, alpha reliabilities were .77 and .80 for Time 1 and Time 2, respectively.

Brief Symptom Inventory The same measure was used as in Study 1. Cronbach's alpha reliability was .97 at each of Time 1 and Time 2.

Suicide Ideation Questionnaire The same measure was used as in Study 1. In Study 2, Cronbach's alpha reliability was .97 at Time 1 and .93 at Time 2.

Data Analytic Strategy Possible associations between sociodemographic variables and suicide ideation were tested. The sociodemographic variables considered were gender, age (whether or not older than 25 years), whether or not the student was a student-worker, year of the course and degree of satisfaction with the course. Correlations among the psychological variables, distress, personality (self-criticism and neediness), and suicide ideation were calculated for each time point.

To evaluate how changes in distress and personality (i.e., self-criticism and neediness) and their interactions predicted changes in suicide ideation over 5 months, the multivariate statistical technique of hierarchical multiple linear regression analysis was again used. Suicide ideation at Time 2 was entered as the outcome variable. In Step 1, suicide ideation at Time 1 was entered. In this covarying out of Time 1 suicide ideation, the residual variance that remained represented change in suicide ideation over 5 months. Distress assessed both at Time 1 and at Time 2 was entered in Step 2 to control for this general covariate. The personality variables of self-criticism and neediness variables assessed each of Time 1 and Time 2 were entered in Step 3. In Step 4, the interaction terms (see Aiken & West, 1991) between the two personality variables at each of Time 1 and Time 2 were entered. In the fifth step, the interaction terms between each of the personality variables and distress at each of Times 1 and 2 were entered. Finally, in a sixth step, two three-way interaction terms of the two personality variables and distress at each of Times 1 and 2 were entered.

To avoid issues associated with data nonnormality and heterocedasticity, bootstrapping (with 1000 samples to construct 95% bias-corrected confidence intervals) was used to test the significance levels of the estimated parameters. The variables were standardized before obtaining the interaction terms and the calculation of the model parameters.

Results

Preliminary Analysis

The correlations between the sociodemographic variables and the suicide ideation variable assessed at Time 2 were calculated and none was significant and, consequently, they were not included in the subsequent regression analysis. Correlations for the psychological variables (distress, self-criticism, neediness, and suicide ideation) at each of Time 1 and Time 2 are displayed in Table 3.

Hierarchical Multiple Linear Regression Analysis

Results of the hierarchical multiple linear regression analysis are summarized in Table 4. In Step 1, suicide ideation assessed at Time 1 was related to suicide ideation assessed at Time 2. In Step 2, distress intensity assessed at Time 2 was related to changes in suicide ideation when distress assessed at Time 1 was introduced as a covariate, meaning that changes in distress related to changes in suicide ideation over 5 months. In Step 3, self-criticism evaluated at Time 2 was related to the suicide ideation assessed at Time 2, when self-criticism evaluated at Time 1 was introduced as a covariate, meaning that changes in self-criticism predicted 5-month changes in suicide ideation beyond the prediction associated with changes in distress. In Step 4, changes in the interaction between self-criticism and neediness significantly predicted 5-month changes in suicide ideation over and beyond what was predicted by changes in main effects for the personality variables and by distress. That is, an

Table 3. Descriptive Statistics and Bivariate Correlations for Study 2 Variables ($N = 207$).

Variables	1	2	3	4	5	6	7	M	SD
1. Distress T1	——							1.52	0.48
2. Distress T2	.63**	——						1.53	0.45
3. Self-criticism T1	.51**	.36**	——					−0.42	0.89
4. Self-criticism T2	.43**	.48**	.76**	——				−0.43	0.91
5. Neediness T1	.26**	.23**	.35**	.34**	——			−0.10	0.82
6. Neediness T2	.18*	.24**	.30**	.46**	.76**	——		−0.12	0.84
7. Suicide ideation T1	.57**	.40**	.53**	.37**	.32**	.21*	——	9.81	18.83
8. Suicide ideation T2	.37**	.40**	.37**	.45**	.31**	.28**	.52**	8.81	11.62

Note: T1 = Time 1; T2 = Time 2 (5 months later).
*$p < .01$.
**$p < .001$ (two-tailed).

increase in suicide ideation covaried with an increase in the interaction between the two personality variables. It should be noted, however, that this effect only attained significance when considering confidence intervals for *B*, but not for the t-test that used bootstrapping to calculate the standard error associated with the parameter. A graphic representation of this interaction effect is shown in Figure 2A. In Step 5, changes in the interaction between self-criticism and distress were related to changes in suicide ideation over 5 months. This interaction is represented in Figure 2B. None of the three-way interactions of Step 6 was related to the dependent variable so, for simplification, the results for that regression step were not included in Table 4.

When a supplementary analysis, analogous to that of Study 1 where the only personality variable of neediness was considered, was performed, neither neediness, its changes, nor its interactions predicted changes in suicidal ideation.

Table 4. Hierarchical Multiple Regression Analysis for Changes in Suicide Ideation (Study 2; $N = 207$).

Predictors	R^2	ΔR^2	B	SE B	t/F	95% CI of B LL	95% CI of B UL	Overall F	df
Step 1	.27	.27			74.47***			74.47***	1, 205
Suicide ideation T1			6.65	2.75	2.42**	2.74	14.58		
Step 2	.31	.04			6.91***			30.86***	3, 203
Distress T1			−.52	1.03	.50	−2.51	1.34		
Distress T2			2.96	1.11	2.67*	.83	4.86		
Step 3	.38	.07			5.25***			17.39***	7, 199
Self-criticism T1			−2.12	1.20	1.77	−5.11	.35		
Self-criticism T2			4.17	1.49	2.80**	1.61	6.47		
Neediness T1			1.42	1.16	1.22	−.65	3.36		
Neediness T2			−.38	1.27	.29	−2.86	2.29		
Step 4	.42	.04			6.33**			15.61***	9, 197
Self-criticism × Neediness T1			−2.74	1.49	1.84	−5.95	.92		
Self-criticism T2 × Neediness T2			2.11	1.21	1.74	.08	3.78		
Step 5	.49	.07			6.46***			13.97***	13, 193
Self-criticism × Distress T1			−4.08	1.90	2.14*	−7.30	1.49		
Self-criticism T2 × Distress T2			2.66	.99	2.68**	.80	4.40		
Neediness × Distress T1			.84	1.34	0.63	−1.75	2.72		
Neediness T2 × Distress T2			−1.29	1.04	1.24	−3.40	1.18		

Note: T1 = Time 1; T2 = Time 2, ΔR^2 = increase in R^2; t = value associated with B; F = F ratio associated with increase in R^2.
*$p < .05$.
**$p < .01$.
***$p < .001$ (two-tailed).

Discussion

We tested whether the maladaptive personality traits of self-criticism and neediness predicted suicide ideation beyond the predictive ability of distress and whether these two personality factors interacted with each other or with distress in the prediction of suicide ideation. Results of Study 1, a cross-sectional study with a community adult sample, demonstrated that self-criticism, but not neediness, associated with suicide ideation and interacted with distress in this association. Neediness also tended to interact with self-criticism in the prediction of suicide ideation. When considered alone as a trait, neediness also predicted suicide ideation and interacted with distress in the prediction of suicide ideation. Results from Study 2 with a college sample indicated that changes in self-criticism, but not changes in neediness, predicted changes in suicide ideation. Changes in the interaction between self-criticism and distress enhanced this prediction of changes in suicide ideation and changes in the interaction between self-criticism and neediness tended to further enhance the prediction of changes in suicide ideation. Results from the longitudinal study are in accordance with results from our cross-sectional study and support the importance of self-criticism as a suicide ideation variable.

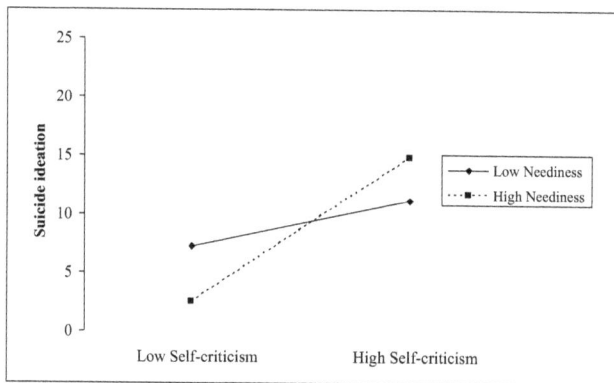

(A)

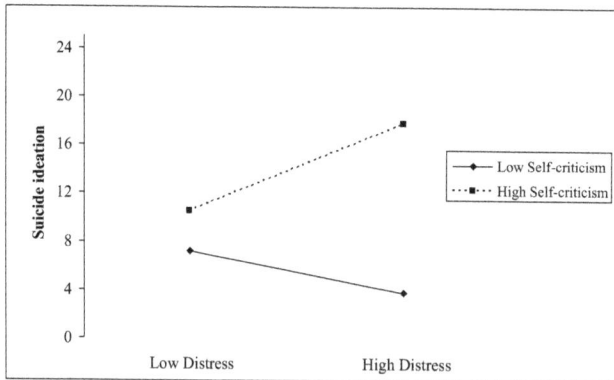

(B)

Figure 2. (A) Interaction between self-criticism and neediness (Study 2; $N = 207$). (B) Interaction between distress and self-criticism (Study 2; $N = 207$). Note: Both figures report mean values.

The current analyses confirm the major importance of self-criticism for suicide ideation. According to the present results, neediness has clearly a secondary role relative to self-criticism (see Sobrinho et al., 2016). Recently, Falgares et al. (2017) failed to obtain a relationship between the dependency factor of the DEQ and suicidal behaviors in a nonclinical sample. However, neediness did potentiate the effect of self-criticism in its relation with suicide ideation. In clinical samples, individuals presenting both types of traits have been described as presenting a more severe form of pathology than individuals that manifest only one configuration of psychopathology, either anaclitic (i.e., focused on relationships) or introjective (i.e., focused on autonomy and self-definition) (Blatt, Quinlan, Chevron, McDonald, & Zuroff, 1982; Shahar, Blatt, & Ford, 2003). Purely anaclitic or purely introjective patients may likely be able to construct a relatively focal form of adaptation which allows them to function at a more adjusted level (Shahar et al., 2003). Another possibility is that there is a synergistic effect between the two types of traits. As in normal development, when considering psychopathology, relatedness, and self-definition can also operate synergistically. For example, when dependent individuals have the perception of failing at a given goal, they feel worthless but they may also fear being rejected by others because of having failed. Alternatively, self-critical individuals may at times experience interpersonal rejection or abandonment but, reactively, turn those feelings into a threat to their self-esteem and a proof of their worthlessness (Shahar et al., 2004). According to our current results, individuals with both types of traits may be at greater risk for experiencing suicide ideation.

Based on present findings, self-criticism also interacts with distress in the prediction of suicide ideation. Self-critically vulnerable individuals are characterized by feelings of unworthiness, indignity, failure, and guilt and they tend to engage in a harsh self-scrutiny. They often strive for excessive achievement and perfection, are very demanding of themselves, and often achieve greatly but with little lasting satisfaction (Blatt, 1995, 2004). Their focus on issues of self-worth and failure can be particularly insidious and these individuals may be vulnerable to serious suicide attempts under high distress (Blatt, 1995, 2008; Fazaa & Page, 2003; Flett et al., 2014). Self-critical "individuals may be at risk for suicide when they experience high levels of psychological distress .... [because it] makes it difficult for them to seek and accept support from others" (Campos et al., 2014, pp. 130–131).

In each of our cross-sectional and longitudinal studies, under high levels of self-criticism, distress predicted suicide ideation. Interestingly, under low levels of self-criticism in our cross-sectional study, the relation between distress and suicide ideation was nonsignificant but, in the longitudinal study and under low levels of self-criticism, high distress presented a negative relation with suicide ideation. We speculate that, under high levels of distress, individuals with low self-criticism may actually use that distress to adapt, accessing greater resilience and coping abilities that promote adjusting to life and, consequently, not desiring death.

Theoretically, it is logical to consider self-criticism as an important modifier of the link between distress and suicide ideation (see Luyten & Blatt, 2016). However, demonstrating this as a causal inference is always challenging. Causal inferences require that a cause and its effect covary (in both association by presence and association by change), that a cause precedes an effect, and that other causal explanations be ruled out (Kenny, 1979). In the present research, we evaluated whether self-criticism and neediness were associated as main effects or interactions with suicide ideation and whether this association continued when another suicide-relevant variable of distress was controlled

statistically. In addition, using a two-wave study, we more extensively tested concomitant variation by evaluating whether changes in self-criticism and neediness (Time 2
controlling for Time 1) and changes in the effect (Time 2 suicide ideation controlling
for Time 1 suicide ideation) covaried longitudinally and independently of changes in
distress (Time 2 distress controlling for Time 1 distress). We also tested whether self-
criticism and neediness interacted with distress.

Here, we have demonstrated that self-criticism and neediness covaried with suicide
ideation (Tables 1 and 3), that changes in self-criticism as a main effect and as a moderator
covaried with changes in suicide ideation (Table 4), and that these influences for self-criticism on suicide ideation continued when an alternative causal explanation based on distress
was statistically controlled. We also verified that self-criticism interacted with distress in the
prediction of suicide ideation. As such, although not established experimentally, the results
offer compelling support for the role of self-criticism as a causal agent for suicide ideation
and, potentially, for other forms of suicidal behavior.

Limitations and Conclusions

The present study has potential limitations. The first limitation is that, in testing for the
contribution of self-criticism and neediness and interactions beyond the contribution of distress, nonclinical low risk samples were used. In future research, it would be informative to
compare present results with those obtained for clinical samples: suicide at-risk samples and
samples of patients manifesting personality disorders focused on issues of relatedness or on
self-definition such as dependent and narcissistic personality disorders, respectively. Further,
our longitudinal findings were based on two time-points and would be strengthened by
including more than two waves of data collection. A third limitation is that the elapsed time
between the two points of data collection in the longitudinal study was a relatively small
interval of 5 months. Fourth, data collection was self-report, an issue that may be particularly
relevant in assessing suicide ideation. However, countering this, it can be argued that some
suicide ideators tend to conceal their negative feelings from others (Flett & Hewitt, 2013)
and may be more likely to self-report suicidal ideation by the means of a confidential questionnaire than to report it to an interviewer. Fifth, the Neediness scale that we used provided
scores with limited reliability. Future studies should look to establish the generalizability of
present findings in samples of high-risk individuals with previous suicide attempts, in longitudinal designs with more and longer time intervals between assessments, and with methods
other than self-report such as clinical interviews. Finally, because large samples are needed
to detect two-way and three-way interactions, the current sample may not have been
adequately powered for the analyses.

Based on our results, self-critical, distressed individuals who concomitantly present needy
traits may be at risk for experiencing suicide ideation. In assessing potentially suicide at risk
individuals prior to any psychological intervention, evaluations should go beyond assessing
current levels of distress and should also focus on maladaptive personality traits (especially
self-critical personality traits) that can actually increase risk under high levels of distress.
Psychotherapy for suicide at-risk individuals should "go deeply" and not only be concerned
with reducing psychopathological symptoms. Issues of failure, guilt, and worthlessness associated with a self-critical personality must be addressed and adaptive coping strategies must
be implemented. Future research could explore interventions that focus on experimentally

treating self-criticism. Given recent research emphasizing both the static and dynamic nature of self-criticism (Zuroff, Sadikaj, Kelly, & Leybman, 2016) and findings that cognitive-behavioral therapy interacts with self-criticism in alleviating depression (Kelly, Zuroff, & Shapira, 2009), a randomized control trial for addressing the self-criticism—suicide ideation link becomes a promising avenue to pursue.

Acknowledgments

The authors would like to thank all research participants in this study and all the research assistants that helped in the collection of data of study one.

Funding

This study was partially supported by Centro de Investigação em Educação e Psicologia—CIEP-UE with founds from Fundação para a Ciência e Tecnologia—Ref. "UID/CED/04312/2016."

References

Addollani, A., Carlbring, P., Khanbani, M., & Ghahfarokhi, S. A. (2016). Emotional intelligence moderates perceived stress and suicidal ideation among depressed adolescent inpatients. *Personality and Individual Differences, 102*, 223–228. doi.10.1016/j.paid.2016.07.015.

Aiken, S., & West, G. (1991). *Multiple regression: Testing and interpreting interactions.* Newbury Park, CA: Sage Publications.

Bagby, R. M., & Rector, N. A. (1998). Self-criticism, dependency and the five factor model of personality in depression: Assessing construct overlap. *Personality and Individual Differences, 24*, 895–897 doi:10.1016/s0191-8869(97)00238-9.

Bertolote, J., & Fleishman, A. (2002). A global perspective in the epidemiology of suicide. *Suicidology, 7*, 6–8. doi:10.5617/suicidologi.2330

Besser, A., Guez, J., & Priel, B. (2008). The associations between self-criticism and dependency and incidental learning of interpersonal and achievement words. *Personality and Individual Differences, 44*, 1696–1710. doi:10.1016/j.paid.2008.01.017.

Besser, A., & Priel, B. (2003). A multisource approach to self-critical vulnerability to depression: The moderating role of attachment. *Journal of Personality, 71*, 515–555. doi:10.1111/1467-6494.7 104002.

Besser, A., & Priel, B. (2010). Personality vulnerability, low social support, and maladaptive cognitive emotion regulation under ongoing exposure to terrorist attacks. *Journal of Social and Clinical Psychology, 29*, 166–201. doi:10.1521/jscp.2010.29.2.166.

Besser, A., & Priel, B. (2011). Dependency, self-criticism and negative affective responses following imaginary rejection and failure threats: Meaning-making processes as moderators or mediators. *Psychiatry, 74*, 31–39. doi:10.1521/psyc.2011.74.1.31.

Blatt, S. J. (1990). Interpersonal relatedness and self-definition: Two primary configurations and their implications for psychopathology and psychotherapy. In J. L. Singer (Ed.), *Repression and dissociation: Implications for personality theory, psychopathology, and health* (pp. 299–335). Chicago: University of Chicago Press.

Blatt, S. J. (1995). The destructiveness of perfectionism: Implications for the treatment of depression. *American Psychologist, 53*, 103–120. doi:10.1037//0003-066x.50.12.1003

Blatt, S. J. (2004). *Experiences of depression: Theoretical, clinical, and research perspectives.* Washington, DC: American Psychological Association.

Blatt, S. J. (2008). *Polarities of experience: Relatedness and self-definition in personality development, psychopathology, and the therapeutic process.* Washington, DC: American Psychological Association Press.

Blatt, S. J., & Blass, R. B. (1990). Attachment and separateness: A dialectic model of the products and processes of development throughout the life cycle. *Psychoanalytic Study of the Child, 45*, 107–127. doi:10.1080/00797308.1990.11823513.

Blatt, S., D'Afflitti, J., & Quinlan, D. (1976). Experiences of depression in normal young adults. *Journal of Abnormal Psychology, 85*, 383–389. doi:10.1037/0021-843X.85.4.383.

Blatt, S., D'Afflitti, J., & Quinlan, D. (1979). *Depressive Experiences Questionnaire.* Unpublished manual, New Haven, CT: Yale University

Blatt, S., & Luyten, P. (2009). A structural–developmental psychodynamic approach to psychopathology: Two polarities of experience across the life span. *Development and Psychopathology, 21*, 793–814. doi:10.1017/s0954579409000431.

Blatt, S. J., Quinlan, D. M., Chevron, E. S., McDonald, C., & Zuroff, D. (1982). Dependency and self-criticism: Psychological dimensions of depression. *Journal of Consulting and Clinical Psychology, 50*, 113–124. doi:10.1037//0022-006x.50.1.113.

Blatt, S. J., Zohar, A. H., Quinlan, D. M., Zuroff, D. C., & Mongrain, M. (1995). Subscales within the dependency factor of the Depressive Experiences Questionnaire. *Journal of Personality Assessment, 64*, 319–339. doi:10.1207/s15327752jpa6701_4.

Blatt, S. J., & Zuroff, D. C. (1992). Interpersonal relatedness and self-definition: Two prototypes for depression. *Clinical Psychology Review, 12*, 527–562. doi:10.1016/0272-7358(92)90070-o.

Bornstein, R. F. (1996). Beyond orality: Toward an object-relations/interactionist reconceptualization of the etiology and dynamics of dependency. *Psychoanalytic Psychology, 13*, 177–203. doi:10.1037/0736-9735.13.2.177.

Brown, G. K., Beck, A. T., Steer, R. A., & Grisham, J. R. (2000). Risk factors for suicide in psychiatric outpatients: A 20-year prospective study. *Journal of Consulting and Clinical Psychology, 68*, 371–377. doi:10.1037//0022-006x.68.3.371.

Campos, R. C. (2016). *Questionário de Experiência Depressivas: Manual Técnico—Edição Atualizada e Revista.* Évora, Portugal: Centro de Investigação em Educação e Psicologia—Universidade de Évora (CIEP-UE)

Campos, R. C., Besser, A., & Blatt, S. J. (2010). The mediating role of self-criticism and dependency in the association between perceptions of maternal caring and depressive symptoms. *Depression and Anxiety, 27*, 1149–1157. doi:10.1002/da.20763.

Campos, R., Besser, A., & Blatt, S. (2012). Distress mediates the association between personality predispositions and suicidality: A preliminary study in a Portuguese community sample. *Archives of Suicide Research, 16*, 44–58. doi:10.1080/13811118.2012.640583.

Campos, R. C. (2009). *Questionário de Experiências Depressivas: Manual.* Évora: Departamento de Psicologia, Escola de Ciências Sociais, Universidade de Évora.

Campos, R. C., Besser, A., & Blatt, S. J. (2013). Recollections of parental rejection, self-criticism and depression in suicidality. *Archives of Suicide Research, 17,* 58–74. doi:10.1080/13811118.2013.748416.

Campos, R. C., Besser, A., Abreu, H., Parreira, T., & Blatt, S. J. (2014). Personality vulnerabilities in adolescent suicidality: The mediating role of psychological distress. *Bulletin of the Meninger Clinic, 78,* 115–139. doi:10.1521/bumc.2014.78.2.115.

Canavarro, M. C. (1999). Inventário de Sintomas Psicopatológicos: BSI. In M. R. Simões, M. Gonçalves, & L. S. Almeida (Eds.), *Testes e provas psicológicas em Portugal* (vol. *II,* pp. 87–109). Braga: SHO/APPORT.

Canavarro, M. (2007). Inventário de Sintomas Psicopatológicos (BSI): Uma revisão crítica dos estudos realizados em Portugal. In M. R. Simões, C. Machado, M. Gonçalves, & L. Almeida (Eds.), *Avaliação psicológica: Instrumentos validados para a população Portuguesa* (pp. 305–331). Coimbra: Quarteto Editora.

Derogatis, L. (1993). *BSI: Administration, scoring, and procedures for the Brief Symptom Inventory* (3rd ed.). Minneapolis, MN: National Computer Systems.

Dunkley, D. M., & Blankstein, K. R. (2000). Self-critical perfectionism, coping, hassles, and current distress: A structural equation modeling approach. *Cognitive Therapy and Research, 24,* 713–730. doi:10.1023/A:1005543529245.

Dunkley, D. M., Blankstein, K. R., Halsall, J., Williams, M., & Winkworth, G. (2000). The relation between perfectionism and distress: Hassles, coping, and perceived social support as mediators and moderators. *Journal of Counseling Psychology, 47,* 437–453. doi:10.1037//0022-0167.47.4.437.

Falgares, G., De Santis, S., Gullo, S., Kopala-Sibley, D. C., Scrima, F., & Livi, S. (2018). Psychometric aspects of the Depressive Experiences Questionnaire: Implications for clinical assessment and research. *Journal of Personality Assessment, 100*(2), 207–218. First published online. doi:10.1080/00223891.2017.1282493

Falgares, G., Marchetti, D., De Santis, S., Carrozzino, D., Kopala-Sibley, D. C., Fulcheri, M., & Verrocchio, M. C. (2017). Attachment styles and suicide-related behaviors in adolescence: The mediating role of self-criticism and dependency. *Frontiers in Psychiatry, 8,* 36. Published online. doi:10.3389/fpsyt.2017.00036.

Fazaa, N., & Page, S. (2003). Dependency and self-criticism as predictors of suicidal behavior. *Suicide and Life-Threatening Behavior, 33,* 172–185. doi:10.1521/suli.33.2.172.22777.

Fazaa, N., & Page, S. (2009). Personality style and impulsivity as determinants of suicidal subgroups. *Archives of Suicide Research, 13,* 31–45. doi:10.1080/13811110802572122.

Ferreira, J., & Castela, M. (1999). Questionário de Ideação Suicida (QIS). In M. Simões, M. Gonçalves, & L. Almeida (Eds.), *Testes e provas psicológicas em Portugal* (pp. 123–130). Braga: Sistemas Humanos e Organizacionais, Lda. [Suicide Ideation Questionnaire (SIQ)]

Flett, G. L., & Hewitt, P. L. (2013). Disguised distress in children and adolescents "flying under the radar": Why psychological problems are underestimated and how schools must respond. *Canadian Journal of School Psychology, 28,* 12–27. doi:10.1177/0829573512468845.

Flett, G. L., Hewitt, P. L., Blankstein, K. R., & Gray, L. (1998). Psychological distress and the frequency of perfectionistic thinking. *Journal of Personality and Social Psychology, 75,* 13–63. doi:10.1037//0022-3514.75.5.1363.

Flett, G. L., Hewitt, P. L., & Heisel, M. J. (2014). The destructiveness of perfectionism revisited: Implications for the assessment of suicide risk and the prevention of suicide. *Review of General Psychology, 18,* 156–172. doi:10.1037/gpr0000011.

Hawton, K., & van Heeringen, K. (2009). Suicide. *The Lancet, 373,* 1372–1381. doi:10.1016/s0140-6736(09)60372-x.

Hewitt, P. L., Flett, G. L., & Weber, C. (1994). Dimensions of perfectionism and suicide ideation. *Cognitive Theory and Research, 18,* 439–460. doi:10.1007/bf02357753.

Jacobs, D., Baldessarini, R., Conwell, Y., Fawcett, J., Horton, L., Meltzer, H., ... Simon, R. I. (2010). *Practice guidelines for the assessment and treatment of patients with suicidal behaviors.* Washington, DC: American Psychiatric Association.

Kelly, A. C., Zuroff, D. C., & Shapira, L. B. (2009). Soothing oneself and resisting self-attacks: The treatment of two intrapersonal deficits in depression vulnerability. *Cognitive Therapy and Research, 33*, 301–313. doi:10.1007/s10608-008-9202-1.

Kenny, D. A. (1979). *Correlation and causality.* New York: Wiley.

Klomek, A., Orbach, I., Sher, L., Sommerfeld, E., Diller, R., Apter, A., Shahar, G., & Zalsman, G. (2008). Quality of depression among suicidal inpatient youth. *Archives of Suicide Research, 12*, 133–140. doi:10.1037/e528192007-001.

Kopala–Sibley, D. C., Zuroff, D. C., Russell, J. J., & Moskowitz, D. S. (2014). Understanding heterogeneity in social anxiety disorder: Dependency and self–criticism moderate fear responses to interpersonal cues. *British Journal of Clinical Psychology, 53*, 141–156. doi:10.1111/bjc.12032.

Levy, K. N., Edell, W. S., & McGlashan, T. H. (2007). Depressive experiences in inpatients with borderline personality disorder. *Psychiatric Quarterly, 78*, 129–143. doi:10.1007/s11126-006-9033-8.

Loas, G., & Défélice, E. (2012). Absolute and relative short-term stability of interpersonal dependency in suicide attempters. *Journal of Nervous & Mental Disease, 200*, 904–907. doi:10.1097/nmd.0b013e31826ba141.

Lund, E., Nadorff, M., & Seader, K. (2016). Relationship between suicidality and disability when accounting for depressive symptomology. *Rehabilitation Counseling Bulletin, 59*, 185–188. doi:10.1177/0034355215586388.

Luyten, P., & Blatt, S. J. (2013). Interpersonal relatedness and self-definition in normal and disrupted personality development. *American Psychologist, 68*, 172–183. doi:10.1037/a0032243.

Luyten, P., & Blatt, S. J. (2016). A hierarchical multiple-level approach to the assessment of interpersonal relatedness and self-definition: Implications for research, clinical practice, and DSM planning. *Journal of Personality Assessment, 98*, 5–13. doi:10.1080/00223891.2015.1091773.

Mongrain, M., & Zuroff, D. C. (1995). Motivational and affective correlates of dependency and self-criticism. *Personality and Individual Differences, 18*, 347–354. doi:10.1016/0191-8869(94)00139-j.

Morrison, R., & O'Connor, R. C. (2008). A systematic review of the relationship between rumination and suicidality. *Suicide and Life-Threatening Behavior, 38*, 523–538. doi:10.1521/suli.2008.38.5.523.

National Institute of Statistics. (2011). *Censos 2011: Resultados Definitivos.* Lisboa: Instituto Nacional de Estatística.

Overholser, J., Braden, A., & Dieter, L. (2012). Understanding suicide risk: Identification of high-risk groups during high-risk times. *Journal of Clinical Psychology, 68*, 334–348. doi:10.1002/jclp.20859.

Overholser, J. C., & Freiheit, S. R. (1994). Assessment of interpersonal dependency using the Millon Clinical Multiaxial Inventory-II (MCMI-II) and the Depressive Experiences Questionnaire. *Personality and Individual Differences, 17*, 71–78. doi:10.1016/0191-8869(94)90263-1.

Pompili, M., Forte, A., Palermo, M., Stefani, H., Lamis, A., Serafini, G., ... Girardi, P. (2012). Suicide risk in multiple sclerosis: A systematic review of current literature. *Journal of Psychosomatic Research, 73*, 411–417. doi:10.1016/j.jpsychores.2012.09.011.

Pompili, M., Lester, D., Leenaars, A., Tatarelli, R., & Girardi, P. (2008). Psychache and suicide: A preliminary investigation. *Suicide and Life-Threatening Behavior, 38*, 116–121. doi:10.1521/suli.2008.38.1.116.

Prieto, D., & Tavares, M. (2005). Fatores de risco para suicídio e tentativa de suicídio: Incidência, eventos estressores e transtornos mentais. *Jornal Brasileiro de Psiquiatria, 54*, 146–154.

Reynolds, W. (1988). *Suicidal Ideation Questionnaire (SIQ): Professional manual.* Odessa, FL: Psychological Assessment Resources.

Rosenfarb, I. S., Becker, J., Khan, A., & Mintz, J. (1998). Dependency and self-criticism in bipolar and unipolar depressed women. *British Journal of Clinical Psychology, 37*, 409–414. doi:10.1111/j.2044-8260.1998.tb01398.x.

Rude, S., & Burnham, B. (1995). Connectedness and Neediness: Factors of the DEQ and SAS Dependency scales. *Cognitive Therapy and Research, 19*, 323–340. doi:10.1007/bf02230403.

Shahar, G., Blatt, S. J., & Ford, R. (2003). Mixed anaclitic-introjective psychopathology in treatment-resistant inpatients undergoing psychoanalytic psychotherapy. *Psychoanalytic Psychology, 20*, 84–102. doi:10.1037/0736-9735.20.1.84.

Shahar, G., Gallagher, E. F., Blatt, S. J., Kuperminc, G. P., & Leadbeater, B. J. (2004). An interactive-synergetic approach to the assessment of personality vulnerability to depression: Illustration using the adolescent version of the Depressive Experiences Questionnaire. *Journal of Clinical Psychology*, *60*, 605–625. doi:10.1002/jclp.10237.

Sobrinho, A. T., Campos, R. C., & Holden, R. R. (2016). Parental rejection, personality, and depression in the prediction of suicidality in a sample of nonclinical young adults. *Psychoanalytic Psychology*, *33*, 554–570. doi:10.1037/pap0000051.

Stellrecht, N. E., & Rudd, M. D. (2006). Responding to and treating negative interpersonal processes in suicidal depression. *Journal of Clinical Psychology*, *62*, 1129–1140. doi:10.1002/jclp.20298 .

Wetzel, H., Gehl, C., Dellefave-Castillo, L., Schiffman, J., Shannon, K., & Paulsen, J. (2011). Suicidal ideation in Huntington disease: The role of comorbidity. *Psychiatry Research*, *15*, 372–376. doi:10.1016/j.psychres.2011.05.006.

Yao, S., Fang, J., Zhu, X., & Zuroff, D. (2009). The Depressive Experience Questionnaire: Construct validation and prediction of depressive symptoms in a sample of Chinese undergraduates. *Depression and Anxiety*, *26*, 930–937. doi:10.1002/da.20465.

Yung, Y. F., & Bentler, P. M. (1996). Bootstrapping techniques in analysis of mean and covariance structures. In G. A.. Marcoulides & R. E. Schumacker (Eds.), *Advanced structural equation modeling techniques*. Hillsdale, NJ: Lawrence Erlbaum.

Zuroff, D. C., Quinlan, D. M., & Blatt, S. J. (1990). Psychometric properties of the Depressive Experiences Questionnaire in a college population. *Journal of Personality Assessment*, *55*, 65–72. doi:10.1207/s15327752jpa5501&2_7.

Zuroff, D. C., Sadikaj, G., Kelly, A. C., & Leybman, M. J. (2016). Conceptualizing and measuring self-criticism as both a personality trait and a personality state. *Journal of Personality Assessment*, *98*, 14–21. doi:10.1080/00223891.2015.1044604.

Obsessive-Compulsive and Depressive Symptoms: The Role of Depressive Cognitive Styles

Ashley M. Shaw (ID), Julia Y. Carbonella, Kimberly A. Arditte Hall (ID), and Kiara R. Timpano (ID)

ABSTRACT

Obsessive-compulsive disorder (OCD) commonly co-occurs with depression, resulting in heightened severity and poorer treatment response. Research on the associations between specific obsessive-compulsive symptoms (OCS) and depressive symptoms has utilized measures that have not fully considered the relationship across OCS dimensions. Little is known about which factors explain the overlap between OCS and depressive symptoms. OCS and depressive symptoms may be related via depressive cognitive styles, such as rumination or dampening (i.e., down-regulating positive emotions). We evaluated the associations of OCS dimensions with depressive symptoms and cognitive styles. We also examined the indirect effects of rumination and dampening in the relationship between OCS and depressive symptoms. Participants ($N = 250$) completed questionnaires online. Greater depressive symptoms, rumination, and dampening were associated with greater levels of all OCS dimensions. Path analysis was utilized to examine a model including the direct effect of depressive symptoms on overall OCS and two indirect effects (through rumination and dampening). There was a significant indirect effect of depressive cognitive styles on the relationship between OCS and depressive symptoms, through rumination and dampening. Replication in a clinical sample and experimental manipulations may bear important implications for targeting depressive cognitive styles in treatments for OCD and depression.

Obsessive-Compulsive Disorder (OCD) is a debilitating condition characterized by recurrent, intrusive thoughts (i.e., obsessions), and compulsive urges to perform rituals to neutralize these obsessions (American Psychiatric Association, 2013). Approximately two percent of the population meet diagnostic criteria (Benito & Storch, 2011), and an additional 8.7% experience subclinical obsessive compulsive symptoms (OCS; Adam, Meinlschmidt, Gloster, & Lieb, 2012; Angst et al., 2004). OCS are thematically heterogeneous, and factor analytic research has detected four primary symptom dimensions: (1) *responsibility for harm* (e.g., fears about being accountable for something bad happening, and checking rituals to prevent a feared outcome), (2) *contamination* (e.g., obsessions about germs and dirt, and washing or cleaning rituals), (3) *symmetry* (e.g., obsessions about things being symmetrical, and rituals involving ordering and arranging items), and *unacceptable thoughts* (e.g., repugnant thoughts with a sexual, aggressive, or religious content; Abramowitz et al., 2010; Mataix-Cols, Rosario-Campos, & Leckman, 2005; McKay et al., 2004). OCD is associated with financial and psychosocial impairment, and is severely distressing to the individual and their family (Lopez & Murray, 1998; Markarian et al., 2010). A hallmark feature of OCD is its remarkably high rates of comorbidity with other psychiatric disorders; in fact, merely eight percent of OCD patients present with OCD alone, in the absence of comorbidities (LaSalle et al., 2004).

Major depressive disorder (MDD) is the most common comorbidity with OCD (Black & Noyes, 1990; LaSalle et al., 2004; Ruscio, Stein, Chiu, & Kessler, 2010). Up to 70% of individuals with OCD also suffer from lifetime MDD (LaSalle et al., 2004; Nestadt et al., 2009; Nestadt et al., 2001; Ruscio et al., 2010) – in contrast with 13% of the general population with a lifetime diagnosis of MDD (Hasin, Goodwin, Stinson, & Grant, 2005). Approximately one-third of OCD patients suffer from current MDD (Perugi et al., 1997; Rasmussen & Eisen, 1992; Steketee, Eisen, Dyck, Warshaw, & Rasmussen, 1999), with the onset of OCD preceding that of MDD in the majority of cases (Black & Noyes, 1990). Moreover, greater depressive symptoms have been associated with increased OCS severity (Quarantini et al., 2011; Tükel, Polat, Özdemir, Aksüt, & Türksoy, 2002), even in individuals not experiencing a current major depressive episode (Ricciardi & McNally, 1995). This comorbidity has been linked with worse treatment outcomes with regards to cognitive-behavioral therapy and combined medication and therapy interventions (Maher et al., 2010; Overbeek, Schruers, Vermetten, & Griez, 2002; Steketee, Chambless, & Tran, 2001).

Rachman's (1997) cognitive model of obsessions provides a theoretical rationale for why patients with OCD may frequently experience depressive symptoms. This model specifies that when an individual experiences a shameful or repulsive obsession, it is often interpreted as an indication or reflection of one's own flawed morals or belief systems. This leads the person to interpret the thought as having personal and catastrophic significance. For example, an intrusive thought of stabbing a loved one could lead to the interpretation of "I am a terrible person and pose a threat to loved ones". Because those with OCD attribute these thoughts as bearing a negative meaning – whether by forecasting a future occurrence or indicating a shameful personal characteristic – they are apt to experience a range of negative emotions (e.g., guilt and/or anxiety), which perpetuate dysphoric mood over time. Individuals may try to suppress the obsession or develop compulsions to negate or prevent it from occurring. Inadvertently, this increased dysphoric mood and resulting compulsive behaviors have the effect of making individuals more likely to experience the obsessions, which over time, reinforces their negative self-views. As a result, these negative self-interpretations become deeply ingrained and increase in a vicious cycle, which may make individuals more susceptible to developing depressive symptoms.

Despite the striking overlap between OCS and depressive symptoms and the theoretical model outlined by Rachman (1997), relatively few studies have investigated how depressive symptoms are linked with specific OCS dimensions. The relationship between depressive symptoms and specific OCS is important to consider in light of the heterogeneous symptom structure of OCD. Preliminary evidence is somewhat varied; one study found that depressive symptoms bore a unique association with *unacceptable thoughts* in particular (e.g., aggressive, sexual, and religious obsessions), as well as with checking compulsions (Hasler et al.,

2005). In contrast, other research suggests that all four primary OCS dimensions (i.e., unacceptable thoughts, responsibility for harm, symmetry, and contamination) may be linked with depressive symptoms (Quarantini et al., 2011), and that levels of depressive symptoms may not differ among patients with different primary obsessions (Ricciardi & McNally, 1995). Notably, these investigations relied on measures that do not reflect recent findings on the nature and dimensional structure of obsessions and compulsions (for a discussion of this, see Abramowitz et al., 2010). Thus, research utilizing measures consistent with structural research and diagnostic criteria per the latest Diagnostic and Statistical Manual of Mental Disorders (DSM-5; American Psychiatric Association, 2013) is warranted to clarify which OCS dimensions have a unique relationship with depressive symptoms.

Potential mechanisms that may help explain the overlap between MDD and OCD are also in need of further exploration. Several studies have proposed that shared etiological factors, such as deficient reward processing and cognitive inflexibility, may predispose individuals to experience both OCD and depression (Overbeek et al., 2002; Quarantini et al., 2011; Tükel et al., 2002). Recent findings have also linked OCD to anhedonia, which may play an important role in the onset of depressive symptoms (Abramovitch, Pizzagalli, Reuman, & Wilhelm, 2014). Consideration of these theoretical links between OCD and depression brings into question the role of common depressive cognitive styles as a related factor that may underlie both disorders.

One of the most common depressive cognitive styles is *rumination*: the passive, repetitive, inward focus on one's experience of distress (Nolen-Hoeksema, 1991). Though most commonly studied as a risk factor for depression (Nolen-Hoeksema, Wisco, & Lyubomirsky, 2008), rumination has recently been conceptualized as a transdiagnostic emotion regulation strategy that also underlies anxiety disorders (Aldao & Nolen-Hoeksema, 2010). Across several studies, elevated rumination has been associated with OCS severity, even in individuals who do not endorse depressive symptoms (Dar & Iqbal, 2014; Exner, Martin, & Rief, 2009; Moradi, Fata, Ahmadi Abhari, & Abbasi, 2014; Wahl, Ertle, Bohne, Zurowski, & Kordon, 2011). Indeed, the frequency of ruminative thoughts in individuals with OCD is similar to that of obsessive thoughts and on par with levels of rumination in depressed patients (Wahl, Schönfeld, et al., 2011). It may be the case that ruminative thinking gives rise to depressed mood, which perpetuates recurrent depressive episodes in those with pre-existing OCD (Wahl, Schönfeld, et al., 2011). In terms of the relationship between rumination and specific dimensions of OCS, checking (Exner et al., 2009) and washing (Wahl, Schönfeld, et al., 2011) compulsions appear to have strong links to rumination.

Meanwhile, other depressive cognitive styles remain understudied in relation to OCS. *Dampening* is one such style, defined by a pessimistic manner of thinking that down-regulates positive emotions (Feldman, Joormann, & Johnson, 2008). Several explanations for dampening have been proposed; individuals may be pessimistic about their ability to maintain a positive mood (Heimpel, Wood, Marshall, & Brown, 2002; Smith & Petty, 1995) or do not feel deserving of experiencing positive affect due to low self-esteem (Parrott, 1993). Greater levels of dampening have been associated with greater depressive symptom severity (Feldman et al., 2008). One preliminary investigation found dampening to be linked with OCS, even after controlling for lifetime depressive symptoms (Eisner, Johnson, & Carver, 2009).

Additional investigations are needed to clarify the nature of depressive cognitive styles in the context of OCS. Within the extant literature, few studies have examined cognitive styles (a) other than rumination, or (b) in conjunction with rumination, in an effort to better understand the overlap between OCS and depressive symptoms. Moreover, the conclusions of extant studies are limited by the approach of considering individuals with OCD and individuals with depression as distinct groups; exploring OCS and depressive symptoms in conjunction using continuous symptom measures will help shed light on cognitive styles that may underlie the high comorbidity of these two conditions.

The current study aims to contribute to the small body of literature within this realm, by examining the relationship between OCS and depressive symptoms in a sample of participants from Amazon's Mechanical Turk (MTurk). MTurk is an online data collection platform, which allows researchers to administer surveys to a variety of registered users in an efficient and inexpensive manner. Increasingly, MTurk is being used to study psychological phenomena, as the samples have been found to be more representative and diverse than undergraduate samples and other online samples (Chandler & Shapiro, 2016). Additionally, online data collection allows participants to more comfortably report on psychological constructs than they would feel in person (Shapiro, Chandler, & Mueller, 2013). Moreover, MTurk workers have been found to be relatively honest and consistent when reporting on psychological constructs (Chandler & Shapiro, 2016). Several previous studies have utilized MTurk to study OCS (Fergus & Bardeen, 2014) and depression (Winer, Veilleux, & Ginger, 2014; Yang, Friedman-Wheeler, & Pronin, 2014). Although some studies have found that levels of depressive symptoms in MTurk samples are similar to (Shapiro et al., 2013), or lower than, typical community samples (Veilleux, Salomaa, Shaver, Zielinski, & Pollert, 2015), our group and others have found marked elevations in OCS, depression, and emotional regulation difficulties (Arditte, Çek, Shaw, & Timpano, 2015; Fergus & Bardeen, 2014). Based on these previous findings (Arditte et al., 2015; Fergus & Bardeen, 2014), we predicted that MTurk would allow us to examine OCS, depressive symptoms, and depressive cognitive styles in a sample with a full range of symptomatology, from nonclinical to clinically-significant symptoms.

Our first aim examined the associations between OCS dimensions and depressive symptoms. We predicted that depressive symptoms would be robustly associated with the *responsibility for harm* and *unacceptable thoughts* dimensions (controlling for *symmetry* and *contamination* symptoms, as well as co-occurring anxiety symptoms). We controlled for anxiety symptoms, given their frequent co-occurrence with and relevance for both MDD and OCD. Our second aim investigated the relationship between OCS and two depressive cognitive styles, dampening and rumination. We predicted that greater levels of overall OCS severity would be associated with greater levels of dampening and rumination (controlling for depressive and anxiety symptoms). In line with previous research (Exner et al., 2009; Wahl, Schönfeld, et al., 2011), we hypothesized that the *responsibility for harm* and *contamination* dimensions, in particular, would be associated with rumination. Given the scarcity of literature, we did not have a specific hypothesis about which OCS dimensions would be associated with dampening. For our third aim, we examined the indirect effects of overall OCS on depressive symptoms through depressive cognitive styles. We predicted that there would be significant indirect effects through dampening and rumination. For aim 3, to examine the most parsimonious model, we focused on overall OCS rather than specific symptom dimensions given that depressive symptoms have previously been tied to all symptom dimensions and since individuals with OCD often endorse several different symptom dimensions at once and/or across time. The direction of all predicted pathways was rooted in the theoretical understanding of the relationships between these constructs, as well as data to support the directionality of these effects (Black & Noyes, 1990; Nolen-Hoeksema et al., 2008; Rachman, 1997; Wahl, Schönfeld, et al., 2011). For example, we modeled OCS as a predictor of depressive symptoms, since OCD onsets before depression in the majority of cases (Black & Noyes, 1990).

Methods

Participants

Participants included 335 individuals recruited using Amazon's MTurk website. To ensure the highest quality data based on guidelines for collecting MTurk data, only MTurk workers who resided in the United States (US) and had completed 90% or more of their previous surveys in a satisfactory manner (as determined by the survey administrator) were eligible to participate (Chandler & Shapiro, 2016). We adhered to data cleaning procedures used in previous MTurk research (e.g., Behrend, Sharek, Meade, & Wiebe, 2011), by excluding participants from analyses who completed the survey in less than 60% of the projected survey completion time ($n = 85$). The final sample consisted of 250 participants.

It is estimated that MTurk has approximately 500,000 registered users, approximately 15,000 from the US. In terms of the characteristics of US MTurk workers, these samples are not fully representative of any particular population. Specifically, MTurk samples (1) are younger, more liberal, more educated, more likely to be unemployed, less religious, and less likely to be married, and (3) include more White/Caucasian and Asian Americans, but less Hispanics and African Americans than the general US population (Chandler & Shapiro, 2016).

Within our final sample ($N = 250$), 52.0% of participants were female and the mean age was 31.9 years old ($SD = 9.3$; Range $= 19$–67). The racial distribution was: 85.6% White/Caucasian, 5.6% Black/African American, 5.2% Asian, 1.2% American Indian/Alaska Native, 0.4% Native Hawaiian/Pacific Islander, and 2.0% "Other." Additionally, 7.6% of the sample was Hispanic or Latino. A small portion of our sample (17.2%) reported that they had previously received a psychiatric diagnosis, including depression ($n = 26$), OCD ($n = 2$), an anxiety disorder (e.g., agoraphobia, social anxiety disorder, panic disorder, generalized anxiety disorder; $n = 26$), attention deficit hyperactivity disorder ($n = 5$), bipolar disorder ($n = 4$), post-traumatic stress disorder ($n = 3$), anorexia nervosa ($n = 1$), and borderline personality disorder ($n = 1$).

Measures

Internal consistency of measures in our sample ranged from good to excellent (Table 1).

The Dimensional Obsessive-Compulsive Scale (DOCS; Abramowitz et al., 2010) is a 20-item questionnaire measuring OCS over the past month. Participants rate items on a scale from *0* to *4*. The DOCS measures four symptom dimensions supported by factor analysis: *responsibility for harm, contamination, symmetry*, and *unacceptable thoughts* (Abramowitz et al., 2010). For example, one of the *responsibility for harm* items asks, "To what extent has your daily routine (work, school, self-care, social life) been disrupted by thoughts about harm or disasters and excessive checking or asking for reassurance?" In line with DSM-5

Table 1. Descriptive statistics and internal consistency values for all variables in our sample.

Variable	N	M	SD	Range	α	Skew	Kurtosis
DOCS tot	250	12.60	11.16	0–53	.93	1.12	1.04
DOCS harm	250	3.32	3.65	0–19	.91	1.18	1.15
DOCS contam	250	2.97	3.61	0–17	.90	1.55	2.16
DOCS symm	250	2.58	3.22	0–13	.91	1.20	0.61
DOCS unaccept	250	3.73	4.10	0–20	.93	1.42	2.20
DASS dep	222	12.21	11.14	0–42	.93	0.69	−0.61
DASS anx	222	8.23	9.00	0–38	.87	1.13	0.41
Dampening	203	15.40	5.05	8–27	.86	0.41	−0.83
Rumination	250	47.24	14.72	22–85	.95	0.17	−0.85

Note. DOCS = Dimensional Obsessive-Compulsive Scale; DOCS tot = DOCS total score; DOCS harm = DOCS responsibility for harm subscale; DOCS contam = DOCS contamination subscale; DOCS symm = DOCS symmetry subscale; DOCS unaccept = DOCS unacceptable thoughts subscale; DASS dep = Depression, Anxiety, Stress Scales depression subscale; DASS anx = Depression, Anxiety, Stress Scales anxiety subscale.

criteria, the DOCS assesses obsessions together with compulsions, rather than separately. As an illustration, one of the *contamination* items asks, "About how much time have you spent each day thinking about contamination and engaging in washing or cleaning behaviors because of contamination?" The DOCS total and subscale scores have previously demonstrated strong internal consistency, good test-retest reliability, and good convergent and discriminant validity across individuals with OCD and nonclinical samples (Abramowitz et al., 2010).

The Depression, Anxiety, Stress Scales (DASS-21; Henry & Crawford, 2005) is a self-report measure of depression, anxiety, and stress. The current study only utilized the *depression* and *anxiety* subscales. The extent to which participants have experienced symptoms over the past week is rated on a scale from *0 (did not apply to me at all)* to *3 (applied to me very much)*. Sample items include: "I felt I was close to panic" (*anxiety*) and "I felt down-hearted and blue" (*depression*). The DASS-21 has previously exhibited strong internal consistency (Henry & Crawford, 2005).

The Responses to Positive Affect Scale (RPA; Feldman et al., 2008) includes a dampening subscale, which measures the habitual use of strategies to reduce positive affect. The subscale consists of eight items. Participants rate the extent to which they generally do each item when they feel happy on a scale from *1 (Almost never)* to *4 (Almost always)*. Sample items include: "Think about things that could go wrong" and "Remind yourself these feelings won't last." The dampening subscale has demonstrated acceptable internal consistency in previous studies (Feldman et al., 2008).

The Ruminative Responses Scale (RRS; Conway, Csank, Holm, & Blake, 2000) measures rumination in response to dysphoric affect, including focus on the self, symptoms, and possible causes and consequences of depressed mood. Each of the 22 items is rated from *1 (Almost Never)* to *4 (Almost Always)*. Illustrative items include: "Think about how sad you feel" and "Analyze recent events to try to understand why you are depressed." Although the RRS can be sub-divided into the brooding and pondering subscales (Treynor, Gonzalez, & Nolen-Hoeksema, 2003), we elected to use the full RRS to make findings comparable to previous studies on OCS and rumination (Dar & Iqbal, 2014; Exner et al., 2009; Moradi et al., 2014; Wahl, Ertle, et al., 2011). The RRS has demonstrated good internal consistency previously (Conway et al., 2000).

Procedure

Procedures were approved by the University's institutional review board. Participants were assured in writing of our procedures for maintaining confidentiality and written informed consent was collected from participants online before starting the survey. Participants were also informed that they could contact investigators to answer any specific questions regarding the information provided in the online consent form and survey. The email addresses and phone numbers of the study investigators were provided for this purpose. No inquiries regarding the meaning of survey questions were received. The questionnaire battery took approximately 30 minutes, and participants were compensated $6.00 for participation.

Study procedures have also been reported in an earlier report on a subset ($N = 228$) of the current sample (Arditte, Shaw, & Timpano, 2016). While there is some overlap in the variables examined, the current investigation and the previous report do not overlap, and each reflects an independent and separate set of aims and hypotheses. We expanded on this previous investigation by (1) examining how depressive symptoms, rumination, and post-event processing specifically relate to the four different OC symptom dimensions and (2) exploring rumination and dampening as mediators of the relationship between OCS and depressive symptoms.

Data Analytic Plan

For Aim 1, zero-order correlations were used to examine the associations between OCS (total and subscale scores) and depressive symptoms. Next, we conducted a multiple regression analysis, with anxiety symptoms entered in Step 1, and all four DOCS dimensions entered in Step 2 of the equation, to predict depressive symptoms.

For Aim 2, zero-order correlations were used to examine the associations between OCS and depressive cognitive styles (rumination and dampening). To test the robustness of these associations, we conducted partial correlations, controlling for depressive and anxiety symptoms.

For Aim 3, path analysis was conducted using Mplus statistical software (version 7; Muthen & Muthen, 1998) to examine the indirect effect of depressive cognitive styles in the relationship between OCS and depressive symptoms. Path analysis was selected as the statistical approach for this aim because it allowed us to estimate the indirect effects of both depressive cognitive styles (rumination and dampening) simultaneously. We used maximum likelihood estimation with robust standard errors, which provides accurate standard errors even when data are non-normal and when there are missing data (Muthen & Muthen, 1998).

Results

Preliminary Analyses

The descriptive statistics for all variables are included in Table 1. Mean scores across measures did not significantly differ based on gender, race, or ethnicity (all p's $> .05$). Participant's mean DOCS scores were similar to mean scores obtained from previous nonclinical samples (Abramowitz et al., 2010), although 16% of our sample scored above the clinical cut-off of 21. DASS depression scores in our sample were higher than other nonclinical samples (Osman et al., 2012), and fell into the mild depression range. RRS scores were also higher than typical nonclinical samples, and were actually more similar to mean scores for individuals with MDD (Zetsche, D'Avanzato, & Joormann, 2012). In contrast, RPA-dampening scores were similar to mean scores in undergraduates (Feldman et al., 2008).

We carefully examined data for violations of the assumptions of normality. All variables were normally distributed according to skewness and kurtosis (i.e., skewness $< |2|$ and kurtosis $< |7|$; Table 1) (Kline, 2011). However, we also conducted the Kolmogorov-Smirnov and the Shapiro-Wilk tests of normality, and found that the distributions of each variable listed in Table 1 were significantly ($p < .05$) different from a normal distribution. Due to non-normal data, we corroborated significance values of zero-order and partial correlations for Aims 1 and 2 with bootstrapping, which does not assume normally-distributed data (Mooney & Duval, 1993). Per bootstrapping procedures, we examined the bias corrected and accelerated (BCa) 95% confidence intervals (CIs) for all correlations (Field, 2013). Significant positive associations can be corroborated when the 95% CI only includes positive values (i.e., does not includes zero), whereas non-significant associations can be corroborated when the 95% CI includes zero (Field, 2013).

Aim 1: Associations Between OCS and Depressive Symptoms

We found that greater depressive symptoms were associated with greater levels of overall OCS and all four symptom dimensions (Table 2). These significant correlations were corroborated via bootstrapping. Controlling for anxiety symptoms and the other symptom dimensions, unacceptable thoughts was the only OCS dimension which significantly predicted depressive symptoms, $\beta = .29, b = .81, t\,(216) = 4.05, p < .001$, BCa 95% CI $= .29–1.36$.

Aim 2: Associations Between OCS and Depressive Cognitive Styles

As predicted, greater rumination and dampening were associated with greater overall OCS and all four symptom dimensions (Table 2). These significant zero-order correlations were corroborated via bootstrapping.

Table 2. Inter-correlations (and bias corrected and accelerated 95% confidence intervals) for all variables (N = 203–250).

Variable	2	3	4	5	6	7	8	9
1. DOCS tot	.80 (.74–.85)	.79 (.71–.85)	.75 (.66–.82)	.76 (.69–.83)	.49 (.36–.61)	.62 (.53–.70)	.53 (.44–.62)	.52 (.39–.65)
2. DOCS harm	1	.54 (.43–.64)	.47 (.34–.59)	.49 (.37–.61)	.39 (.25–.52)	.52 (.39–.63)	.46 (.34–.56)	.45 (.33–.57)
3. DOCS contam		1	.52 (.39–.63)	.43 (.26–.58)	.29 (.16–.42)	.38 (.24–.51)	.34 (.24–.46)	.37 (.24–.50)
4. DOCS symm			1	.39 (.22–.54)	.28 (.13–.43)	.38 (.23–.53)	.34 (.22–.47)	.33 (.19–.47)
5. DOCS unaccept				1	.55* (.44–.66)	.62 (.51–.70)	.50 (.39–.60)	.46 (.32–.60)
6. DASS dep					1	.53 (.42–.63)	.68 (.60–.76)	.56 (.47–.66)
7. DASS anx						1	.62 (.53–.70)	.55 (.44–.64)
8. Rumination							1	.62 (.53–.70)
9. Dampening								1

Note. DOCS = Dimensional Obsessive-Compulsive Scale; DOCS tot = DOCS total score; DOCS harm = DOCS responsibility for harm subscale; DOCS contam = DOCS contamination subscale; DOCS symm = DOCS symmetry subscale; DOCS unaccept = DOCS unacceptable thoughts subscale; DASS dep = Depression, Anxiety, Stress Scales depression subscale; DASS anx = Depression, Anxiety, Stress Scales anxiety subscale.
All *p's* < .001.

Controlling for depressive and anxiety symptoms, greater levels of rumination remained significantly associated with responsibility for harm ($r = .14$, $p < .05$, BCa 95% CI $= .02–.27$). However, the significant associations between rumination and overall OCS ($r = .12$, $p = .07$, BCa 95% CI $= −.01–.27$), contamination ($r = .11$, $p = .12$, BCa 95% CI $= −.01–.24$), symmetry ($r = .11$, $p = .11$, BCa 95% CI $= −.02–.24$), and unacceptable thoughts ($r = −.02$, $p = .82$, BCa 95% CI $= −.18–.15$) disappeared, controlling for depressive and anxiety symptoms.

Controlling for depressive and anxiety symptoms, greater levels of dampening remained significantly associated with overall OCS ($r = .20$, $p < .01$, BCa 95% CI $= .04–.38$), responsibility for harm ($r = .19$, $p < .01$, BCa 95% CI $= .05–.33$), and contamination ($r = .18$, $p < .05$, BCa 95% CI $= .02–.35$). However, dampening was no longer associated with symmetry ($r = .13$, $p = .07$, BCa 95% CI $= −.01–.25$) or unacceptable thoughts ($r = .06$, $p = .39$, BCa 95% CI $= −.12–.24$), after controlling for depressive and anxiety symptoms.

Aim 3: Indirect Effect of Depressive Cognitive Styles in the Relationship Between OCS and Depressive Symptoms

The model included the direct effect of overall OCS on depressive symptoms and two indirect effects (through rumination and dampening). Figure 1 includes standardized factor loadings, unstandardized path coefficients, and standard errors for the direct effects. The model explained 53.00% of the variance in depressive symptoms, 26.80% of the variance in dampening, and 28.30% of the variance in rumination. Controlling for rumination and dampening, greater levels of overall OCS significantly predicted greater depressive symptoms. The combination of the two indirect paths partially mediated the relationship between OCS and depressive symptoms ($\beta = .37$, b $= .37$, SE $= .05$, $p < .001$, 95% CI $= .28–.46$), specifically through rumination ($\beta = .28$, b $= .28$, SE $= .05$, $p < .001$, 95% CI $= .19–.35$) and dampening ($\beta = .09$, b $= .09$, SE $= .04$, $p = .01$, 95% CI $= .02–.15$).

Discussion

This is the first comprehensive examination of the relations between OCS, depressive symptoms, and cognitive styles. When examining zero-order correlations, we found that overall OCS and all four symptom dimensions were associated with depressive symptoms. We clarified previous mixed findings on whether depressive symptoms are linked to all OCS

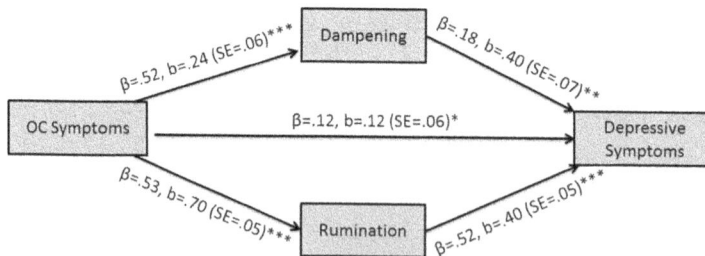

Figure 1. Standardized factor loadings (β), unstandardized path coefficients (b), and standard errors (SE) for the structural model of depressive cognitive styles mediating the association between OCS and depressive symptoms. *Note.* $^*p < .05$, $^{**}p < .01$, $^{***}p < .001$

(Quarantini et al., 2011; Ricciardi & McNally, 1995) or specific OCS (e.g., unacceptable thoughts and responsibility for harm) (Hasler et al., 2005). Specifically, we found that unacceptable thoughts had the largest unique variance with depressive symptoms (of all four OCS dimensions), when taking into account anxiety symptoms and other OCS dimensions. In addition, we found that greater levels of overall OCS and all four symptom dimensions were associated with greater rumination and dampening. This is in line with previous findings (Dar & Iqbal, 2014; Eisner et al., 2009; Exner et al., 2009; Moradi et al., 2014; Wahl, Schönfeld, et al., 2011). Controlling for depressive and anxiety symptoms, responsibility for harm was associated with rumination and dampening, and contamination was correlated with dampening. Depressive cognitive styles exhibited a significant indirect effect in the relationship between overall OCS and depressive symptoms. If replicated in a clinical sample, these findings may suggest the importance of targeting depressive cognitive styles to simultaneously reduce OCS and depressive symptoms.

In line with one previous study (Quarantini et al., 2011), all four OCS dimensions were associated with depressive symptoms. Yet, when controlling for anxiety symptoms and the other symptom dimensions, only unacceptable thoughts was associated with depressive symptoms. Perhaps, OCS that are considered most ego-dystonic (i.e., unacceptable thoughts) are more likely to lead to depressive symptoms because they are tied most closely to negative self-interpretations and deep-seated core beliefs. Additionally, unacceptable obsessive thoughts are considered a form of repetitive negative thinking with similar qualities to rumination and dampening, though there are also some important differences. For example, although patients may have positive beliefs about forms of repetitive negative thinking, such as worry, unacceptable thoughts in OCD are viewed as completely unwanted and intrusive. Overall, individuals prone to repetitive negative thinking may be at greater risk for both OCD and MDD. Interestingly, we did not find the predicted robust relationship between responsibility for harm and depressive symptoms (Hasler et al., 2005). This may be because Hasler et al. (2005) found a unique relationship between checking compulsions (rather than responsibility for harm more broadly) and depressive symptoms. Our findings for Aim 2 suggest that responsibility for harm may be more closely tied to depressive cognitive styles than current depressive symptoms.

When controlling for depressive and anxiety symptoms, we found support for unique relationships between specific OCS and depressive cognitive styles. Specifically, we found that responsibility for harm was robustly associated with rumination, which replicates previous findings (Exner et al., 2009). Although we used the full RRS scale to be more parsimonious and in line with past research, future studies should more closely examine the relationship between OCS, rumination, and depressive symptoms by exploring the brooding subscale, which is unconfounded with depression content (Treynor et al., 2003). If findings replicate with the brooding subscale, this would provide even stronger evidence that responsibility for harm is linked with ruminative thinking processes. In contrast to Wahl, Schönfeld, et al. (2011), we did not find a robust relationship between washing and rumination. This may be because the authors examined obsessions and compulsions separately, rather than considering the overarching contamination dimension. Another previous study found that repetitive negative thinking, a broad transdiagnostic construct thought to encompass rumination, was not associated with overall OCS (Reese, Pollert, & Veilleux, 2016), although a different measure of OCS was utilized. Our study highlights the importance of clarifying the relationship of rumination with each separate symptom dimension, in addition to overall OCS, given that OCD is a heterogeneous disorder.

The current study was the first to consider how dampening related to specific OCS. We found that both greater responsibility for harm and contamination were significantly associated with greater levels of dampening, after controlling for depression and anxiety. It is interesting to contemplate why responsibility for harm and contamination might be most linked to dampening. Since these two symptom dimensions involve completing overt compulsions (checking and washing, respectively), it is possible that individuals with these symptoms do not feel deserving of positive affect if they have not satisfactorily completed their rituals. Alternatively, individuals with checking and washing compulsions may feel that positive affect would distract them from completing compulsions, and thus may seek to dampen positive emotional experiences. Future research in clinical samples should examine such hypotheses.

We expanded on past literature by examining the indirect effect of depressive cognitive styles in the relationship between OCS and depressive symptoms. As predicted, we found a significant indirect effect of depressive cognitive styles in the relationship between OCS and depressive symptoms, with specific pathways through rumination and dampening. Although future longitudinal work is necessary to determine the temporal order of the constructs in this model, patients with OCD may develop depressive cognitive styles in an attempt to understand or cope with their distressing symptoms, and these styles may put them at risk for developing depression (Wahl, Schönfeld, et al., 2011). Overall, repetitive negative thinking may serve as an important transdiagnostic factor for affective disorders that plays a role in explaining comorbidity and is relevant for treatment (Arditte et al., 2016).

The results of the current study should be interpreted in light of its limitations. Symptoms in our sample ranged from nonclinical to clinically-meaningful levels of OCD and depressive symptoms, including a portion of participants who had received a psychiatric diagnosis of depression, anxiety, or OCD. Our sample also exhibited elevated levels of rumination compared to other nonclinical samples. Nevertheless, it should be noted that participants represented an online convenience sample. As discussed previously, MTurk is not fully representative of the general population, particularly in terms of the racial demographics (i.e., more White/Caucasian and Asian Americans, but less Hispanics and African Americans) (Chandler & Shapiro, 2016). In particular, given that MTurk participants are less likely to be employed than the general population and have higher rates of social anxiety (Chandler & Shapiro, 2016), the results may be limited to individuals who spend time earning money through online activities. Overall, by restricting our sample to 250 MTurk workers, this somewhat limits the generalizability of our findings. The results of the current study should be replicated in a large clinical sample, prior to drawing conclusions about patients with OCD and MDD. Replicating these findings in a clinical sample would aid in drawing conclusions about patients with OCD and MDD as well as treatment implications. Also, due to our cross-sectional and self-report design, the causal relations examined in Aim 3 cannot be confirmed. Though the direction of predicted pathways tested in this investigation was rooted in our theoetical and empicial understanding of these constructs, OCS, depressive symptoms, and depressive cognitive styles may be related by complex feedback loops. More advanced methods, such as longitudinal investigations, ecological momentary assessment, or experimental investigations, should be utilized to confirm the causal nature of investigated relationships.

To conclude, this study clarified and expanded upon past literature on the relations between distinct OCS dimensions, depressive symptoms, and depressive cognitive styles. Specifically, unacceptable thoughts were uniquely associated with depressive symptoms. Responsibility for harm was uniquely related to rumination and dampening, and contamination was associated with dampening. Depressive cognitive styles exhibited an indirect effect in the relationship between overall OCS and depressive symptoms, suggesting that rumination and dampening may play a role in spurring and/or maintaining depressive symptoms in those with OCD. Importantly, rumination and dampening are considered transdiagnostic processes that can be targeted in cognitive behavioral interventions, and thus could be important to incorporate when treating patients with OCD. For example, therapists could emphasize using problem-solving or mindfulness strategies when patients engage in ruminative thinking and address cognitive errors such as discounting the positive to target dampening.

ORCID

Ashley M. Shaw http://orcid.org/0000-0003-2625-372X
Kimberly A. Arditte Hall http://orcid.org/0000-0002-3095-1099
Kiara R. Timpano http://orcid.org/0000-0002-0665-8722

References

Abramovitch, A., Pizzagalli, D. A., Reuman, L., & Wilhelm, S. (2014). Anhedonia in obsessive-compulsive disorder: Beyond comorbid depression. *Psychiatry Research, 216*(2), 223–229. doi: 10.1016/j.psychres.2014.02.002

Abramowitz, J. S., Deacon, B. J., Olatunji, B. O., Wheaton, M. G., Berman, N. C., Losardo, D., … Adams, T. (2010). Assessment of obsessive-compulsive symptom dimensions: Development and evaluation of the dimensional obsessive-compulsive scale. *Psychological Assessment, 22*(1), 180–198. doi: 10.1037/a0018260

Adam, Y., Meinlschmidt, G., Gloster, A. T., & Lieb, R. (2012). Obsessive–compulsive disorder in the community: 12-month prevalence, comorbidity and impairment. *Social Psychiatry and Psychiatric Epidemiology, 47*(3), 339–349. doi: 10.1007/s00127-010-0337-5

Aldao, A., & Nolen-Hoeksema, S. (2010). Specificity of cognitive emotion regulation strategies: A transdiagnostic examination. *Behaviour Research and Therapy, 48*(10), 974–983. doi: 10.1016/j.brat.2010.06.002

American Psychiatric Association. (2013). *Diagnostic and statistical manual of mental disorders* (Fifth ed.). Arlington, VA: American Psychiatric Publishing.

Angst, J., Gamma, A., Endrass, J., Goodwin, R., Ajdacic, V., Eich, D., & Rössler, W. (2004). Obsessive-compulsive severity spectrum in the community: Prevalence, comorbidity, and course. *European Archives of Psychiatry and Clinical Neuroscience, 254*(3), 156–164. doi: 10.1007/s00406-004-0459-4

Arditte, K. A., Çek, D., Shaw, A. M., & Timpano, K. R. (2015). The importance of assessing clinical phenomena in Mechanical Turk research. *Psychological Assessment, 28*, 684–691. doi: 10.1037/pas0000217

Arditte, K. A., Shaw, A. M., & Timpano, K. R. (2016). Repetitive negative thinking: A transdiagnostic correlate of affective disorders. *Journal of Social and Clinical Psychology, 35*, 181–201. doi: 10.1521/jscp.2016.35.3.181

Behrend, T. S., Sharek, D. J., Meade, A. W., & Wiebe, E. N. (2011). The viability of crowdsourcing for survey research. *Behavior Research Methods, 43*(3), 800–813. doi: 10.3758/s13428-011-0081-0

Benito, K., & Storch, E. A. (2011). Assessment of obsessive-compulsive disorder: Review and future directions. *Expert Review of Neurotherapeutics, 11*(2), 287–298. doi: 10.1586/ern.10.195

Black, D. W., & Noyes, R. (1990). Comorbidity and obsessive-compulsive disorder. *Comorbidity of Mood and Anxiety Disorders.* Washington, DC: American Psychiatric Press, Inc, 305–316.

Chandler, J., & Shapiro, D. (2016). Conducting clinical research using crowdsourced convenience samples. *Annual Review of Clinical Psychology, 12*, 53–81. doi: 10.1146/annurev-clinpsy-021815-093623

Conway, M., Csank, P. A. R., Holm, S. L., & Blake, C. K. (2000). On assessing individual differences in rumination on sadness. *Journal of Personality Assessment, 75*(3), 404–425. doi: 10.1207/s15327752jpa7503_04

Dar, K. A., & Iqbal, N. (2014). Worry and rumination in generalized anxiety disorder and obsessive compulsive disorder. *The Journal of Psychology, 149*(8), 866–880. doi: 10.1080/00223980.2014.986430

Eisner, L. R., Johnson, S. L., & Carver, C. S. (2009). Positive affect regulation in anxiety disorders. *Journal of Anxiety Disorders, 23*(5), 645–649. doi: 10.1016/j.janxdis.2009.02.001

Exner, C., Martin, V., & Rief, W. (2009). Self-focused ruminations and memory deficits in obsessive-compulsive disorder. *Cognitive Therapy and Research, 33*(2), 163–174. doi: 10.1007/s10608-009-9266-6

Feldman, G. C., Joormann, J., & Johnson, S. L. (2008). Responses to positive affect: A self-report measure of rumination and dampening. *Cognitive Therapy and Research, 32*(4), 507–525. doi: 10.1007/s10608-006-9083-0

Fergus, T. A., & Bardeen, J. R. (2014). Emotion regulation and obsessive-compulsive symptoms: A further examination of associations. *Journal of Obsessive-Compulsive Related Disorders, 3*, 243–248. doi: 10.1016/j.jocrd.2014.06.001

Field, A. (2013). *Discovering statistics using IBM SPSS Statistics* (4th ed.). London, UK: Sage Publications.

Hasin, D. S., Goodwin, R. D., Stinson, F. S., & Grant, B. F. (2005). Epidemiology of major depressive disorder: Results from the national epidemiologic survey on alcoholism and related conditions. *Archives of General Psychiatry, 62*(10), 1097–1106. doi: 10.1001/archpsyc.62.10.1097

Hasler, G., LaSalle-Ricci, V Holland, Ronquillo, J. G., Crawley, S. A., Cochran, L. W., Kazuba, D., … Murphy, D. L. (2005). Obsessive–compulsive disorder symptom dimensions show specific relationships to psychiatric comorbidity. *Psychiatry Research, 135*(2), 121–132. doi: 10.1016/j.psychres.2005.03.003

Heimpel, S. A., Wood, J. V., Marshall, M. A., & Brown, J. D. (2002). Do people with low self-esteem really want to feel better? Self-esteem differences in motivation to repair negative moods. *Journal of Personality and Social Psychology, 82*(1), 128–147. doi: 10.1037/0022-3514.82.1.128

Henry, J. D., & Crawford, J. R. (2005). The short-form version of the Depression Anxiety Stress Scales (DASS-21): Construct validity and normative data in a large non-clinical sample. *British Journal of Clinical Psychology, 44*(2), 227–239. doi: 10.1348/014466505x29657

Kline, R. B. (2011). Data preparation. In R. B. Kline (Ed.), *Principles and practice of structural equation modeling* (3rd ed., pp. 63–64). New York, NY: The Guilford Press.

LaSalle, V Holland, Cromer, K. R., Nelson, K. N., Kazuba, D., Justement, L., & Murphy, D. L. (2004). Diagnostic interview assessed neuropsychiatric disorder comorbidity in 334 individuals with obsessive–compulsive disorder. *Depression and Anxiety, 19*(3), 163–173. doi: 10.1002/da.20009

Lopez, A. D., & Murray, C. C. (1998). The global burden of disease, 1990–2020. *Nature Medicine, 4* (11), 1241–1243. doi: 10.1038/3218

Maher, M. J., Huppert, J. D., Chen, H., Duan, N., Foa, E. B., Liebowitz, M. R., & Simpson, H. B. (2010). Moderators and predictors of response to cognitive-behavioral therapy augmentation of pharmacotherapy in obsessive–compulsive disorder. *Psychological Medicine, 40*(12), 2013–2023. doi: 10.1017/S0033291710000620

Markarian, Y., Larson, M. J., Aldea, M. A., Baldwin, S. A., Good, D., Berkeljon, A., … McKay, D. (2010). Multiple pathways to functional impairment in obsessive-compulsive disorder. *Clinical Psychology Review, 30*(1), 78–88. doi: 10.1016/j.cpr.2009.09.005

Mataix-Cols, D., Rosario-Campos, M. C., & Leckman, J. F. (2005). A multidimensional model of obsessive-compulsive disorder. *American Journal of Psychiatry, 162*(2), 228–238. doi: 10.1176/appi.ajp.162.2.228

McKay, D., Abramowitz, J. S., Calamari, J. E., Kyrios, M., Radomsky, A., Sookman, D., … Wilhelm, S. (2004). A critical evaluation of obsessive–compulsive disorder subtypes: Symptoms versus mechanisms. *Clinical Psychology Review, 24*(3), 283–313. doi: 10.1016/j.cpr.2004.04.003

Mooney, C. Z., & Duval, R. D. (1993). *Bootstrapping: A nonparametric approach to statistical inference.* Newbury Park, CA: Sage Publications.

Moradi, M., Fata, L., Ahmadi Abhari, A., & Abbasi, I. (2014). Comparing attentional control and intrusive thoughts in obsessive-compulsive disorder, generalized anxiety disorder and non clinical population. *Iranian Journal of Psychiatry, 9*(2), 69–75.

Muthen, L. K., & Muthen, B. O. (1998). *Mplus user's guide.* Los Angeles, CA: Muthen & Muthen.

Nestadt, G., Di, C. Z., Riddle, M. A., Grados, M. A., Greenberg, B. D., Fyer, A. J., … Rasmussen, S. A. (2009). Obsessive–compulsive disorder: Subclassification based on co-morbidity. *Psychological Medicine, 39*(9), 1491–1501. doi: 10.1017/S0033291708004753

Nestadt, G., Samuels, J., Riddle, M. A., Liang, K.-Y., Bienvenu, O. J., Hoehn-Saric, R., … Cullen, B. (2001). The relationship between obsessive–compulsive disorder and anxiety and affective disorders: Results from the Johns Hopkins OCD Family Study. *Psychological Medicine, 31*(3), 481–487. doi: 10.1017/S0033291701003579

Nolen-Hoeksema, S. (1991). Responses to depression and their effects on the duration of depressive episodes. *Journal of Abnormal Psychology, 100*(4), 569–582. doi: 10.1037/0021-843X.100.4.569

Nolen-Hoeksema, S., Wisco, B. E., & Lyubomirsky, S. (2008). Rethinking rumination. *Perspectives on Psychological Science, 3*(5), 400–424. doi: 10.1111/j.1745-6924.2008.00088.x

Osman, A., Wong, J. L., Bagge, C. L., Freedenthal, S., Gutierrez, P. M., & Lozano, G. (2012). The depression anxiety stress scales-21 (DASS-21): Further examination of dimensions, scale reliability, and correlates. *Journal of Clinical Psychology, 68*(12), 1322–1338. doi: 10.1002/jclp.21908

Overbeek, T., Schruers, K., Vermetten, E., & Griez, E. (2002). Comorbidity of obsessive-compulsive disorder and depression: Prevalence, symptom severity, and treatment effect. *The Journal of Clinical Psychiatry, 63*(12), 1106–1112.

Parrott, W Gerrod (1993). Beyond hedonism: Motives for inhibiting good moods and for maintaining bad moods. In D. M. Wegner & J. W. Pennebaker (Eds.), *Handbook of mental control* (pp. 278–305). Englewood Cliffs, NJ: Prentice-Hall.

Perugi, G., Akiskal, H. S., Pfanner, C., Presta, S., Gemignani, A., Milanfranchi, A., … Cassano, G. B. (1997). The clinical impact of bipolar and unipolar affective comorbidity on obsessive–compulsive disorder. *Journal of Affective Disorders, 46*(1), 15–23. doi: 10.1016/S0165-0327(97)00075-X

Quarantini, L. C., Torres, A. R., Sampaio, A. S., Fossaluza, V., de Mathis, M. A., Do Rosário, M. C., … Petribu, K. (2011). Comorbid major depression in obsessive-compulsive disorder patients. *Comprehensive Psychiatry, 52*(4), 386–393. doi: 10.1016/j.comppsych.2010.09.006

Rachman, S. (1997). A cognitive theory of obsessions. *Behaviour Research and Therapy, 35*(9), 793–802. doi: 10.1016/S0005-7967(97)00040-5

Rasmussen, S. A., & Eisen, J. L. (1992). The epidemiology and clinical features of obsessive compulsive disorder. *Psychiatric Clinics of North America, 15*(4), 743–758.

Reese, E. D., Pollert, G. A., & Veilleux, J. C. (2016). Self-regulatory predictors of eating disorder symptoms: Understanding the contributions of action control and willpower beliefs. *Eat Behav, 20*, 64–69. doi: 10.1016/j.eatbeh.2015.11.005

Ricciardi, J. N., & McNally, R. J. (1995). Depressed mood is related to obsessions, but not to compulsions, in obsessive-compulsive disorder. *Journal of Anxiety Disorders, 9*(3), 249–256. doi: 10.1016/0887-6185(95)00006-A

Ruscio, A. M., Stein, D. J., Chiu, W. T., & Kessler, R. C. (2010). The epidemiology of obsessive-compulsive disorder in the National Comorbidity Survey Replication. *Molecular Psychiatry, 15*(1), 53–63. doi: 10.1038/mp.2008.94

Shapiro, D. N., Chandler, J., & Mueller, P. A. (2013). Using Mechanical Turk to study clinical populations. *Clinical Psychological Science, 1*, 213–220. doi: 10.1177/2167702612469015

Smith, S. M., & Petty, R. E. (1995). Personality moderators of mood congruency effects on cognition: The role of self-esteem and negative mood regulation. *Journal of Personality and Social Psychology, 68*(6), 1092–1107. doi: 10.1037/0022-3514.68.6.1092

Steketee, G., Chambless, D. L., & Tran, G. Q. (2001). Effects of axis I and II comorbidity on behavior therapy outcome for obsessive-compulsive disorder and agoraphobia. *Comprehensive Psychiatry, 42*(1), 76–86. doi: 10.1053/comp.2001.19746

Steketee, G., Eisen, J., Dyck, I., Warshaw, M., & Rasmussen, S. (1999). Predictors of course in obsessive compulsive disorder. *Psychiatry Research, 89*(3), 229–238. doi: 10.1016/S0165-1781(99)00104-3

Treynor, W., Gonzalez, R., & Nolen-Hoeksema, S. (2003). Rumination reconsidered: A psychometric analysis. *Cognitive Therapy and Research, 27*(3), 247–259. doi: 10.1023/a:1023910315561

Tükel, R., Polat, A., Özdemir, Ö., Aksüt, D., & Türksoy, N. (2002). Comorbid conditions in obsessive-compulsive disorder. *Comprehensive Psychiatry, 43*(3), 204–209. doi: 10.1053/comp.2002.32355

Veilleux, J. C., Salomaa, A. C., Shaver, J. A., Zielinski, M. J., & Pollert, G. A. (2015). Multidimensional assessment of beliefs about emotion: Development and validation of the emotion and regulation beliefs scale. *Assessment, 22*(1), 86–100. doi: 10.1177/1073191114534883

Wahl, K., Ertle, A., Bohne, A., Zurowski, B., & Kordon, A. (2011). Relations between a ruminative thinking style and obsessive–compulsive symptoms in non-clinical samples. *Anxiety, Stress & Coping: An International Journal, 24*(2), 217–225. doi: 10.1080/10615806.2010.482985

Wahl, K., Schönfeld, S., Hissbach, J., Küsel, S., Zurowski, B., Moritz, S., … Kordon, A. (2011). Differences and similarities between obsessive and ruminative thoughts in obsessive-compulsive and depressed patients: A comparative study. *Journal of Behavior Therapy and Experimental Psychiatry, 42*(4), 454–461. doi: 10.1016/j.jbtep.2011.03.002

Winer, E. S., Veilleux, J. C., & Ginger, E. J. (2014). Development and validation of the specific loss of interest and pleasure scale (SLIPS). *Journal of Affective Disorders, 152*, 193–201. doi: 10.1016/j.jad.2013.09.010

Yang, K. T., Friedman-Wheeler, D. G., & Pronin, E. (2014). Thought acceleration boosts positive mood among individuals with minimal to moderate depressive symptoms. *Cognitive Therapy and Research, 38*(3), 261–269. doi: 10.1007/s10608-014-9597-9

Zetsche, U., D'Avanzato, C., & Joormann, J. (2012). Depression and rumination: Relation to components of inhibition. *Cognition and Emotion, 26*(4), 758–767. doi: 10.1080/02699931.2011.613919

Faces of Shame: Implications for Self-Esteem, Emotion Regulation, Aggression, and Well-Being

Patrizia Velotti, Carlo Garofalo (iD), Federica Bottazzi, and Vincenzo Caretti

ABSTRACT
There is an increasing interest in psychological research on shame experiences and their associations with other aspects of psychological functioning and well-being, as well as with possible maladaptive outcomes. In an attempt to confirm and extend previous knowledge on this topic, we investigated the nomological network of shame experiences in a large community sample ($N = 380$; 66.1% females), adopting a multidimensional conceptualization of shame. Females reported higher levels of shame (in particular, bodily and behavioral shame), guilt, psychological distress, emotional reappraisal, and hostility. Males had higher levels of self-esteem, emotional suppression, and physical aggression. Shame feelings were associated with low self-esteem, hostility, and psychological distress in a consistent way across gender. Associations between characterological shame and emotional suppression, as well as between bodily shame and anger occurred only among females. Moreover, characterological and bodily shame added to the prediction of low self-esteem, hostility, and psychological distress above and beyond the influence of trait shame. Finally, among females, emotional suppression mediated the influence of characterological shame on hostility and psychological distress. These findings extend current knowledge on the nomological net surrounding shame experiences in everyday life, supporting the added value of a multidimensional conceptualization of shame feelings.

Shame is commonly defined as an intense negative emotion characterized by the perception of a global devaluation of the self (Tangney & Dearing, 2002). Shame feelings are often triggered by social events in which a drop of personal status or feelings of rejection are perceived. Of note, rather than representing a unidimensional construct, shame could actually refer to different aspects of the self, such as behaviors or body characteristics, as well to the broader identity (Andrews, Qian, & Valentine, 2002; Hejdenberg & Andrews, 2011). Specifically, a multidimensional conceptualization of shame has been proposed (Andrews et al., 2002) to identify: (a) experiences of characterological shame (i.e., regarding personal habits, manner with others, the kind of person one is, and personal skills); (b) experiences of behavioral shame (i.e., referred to doing something wrong, saying something stupid, and failing in competitive contexts); and (c) bodily shame (i.e., referred to being ashamed of one's physical appearance). There is substantial evidence linking shame with psychopathology in general, and internalizing symptoms in particular (Andrews et al., 2002; Velotti, Elison, & Garofalo, 2014). Yet, associations between specific experiences of shame and other psychological mechanisms have sparsely been investigated. In the current study, we sought to provide a fine-grained analysis of the nomological network surrounding shame feelings, adopting a multidimensional conceptualization of shame experiences. The concept of nomological network refers to a group of constructs that are theoretically or empirically expected to show consistent linkages, and as such nomological network analysis is used to measure construct validity (Cronbach & Meehl, 1955). Specifically, we aimed at confirming associations between shame feelings and psychopathological distress (Andrews et al., 2002). Furthermore, we sought to expand current knowledge broadening the scope of the nomological network of shame. To this end, we first reviewed prior literature to identify possible correlates of shame experiences.

Shame and Self-Esteem

Frequent experiences of shame may eventually crystallize into trait-like shame proneness. Trait shame, in turn, involves a particularly painful, and often incapacitating, negative feeling involving a sense of inferiority, hopelessness, and helplessness, as well as a desire to hide personal flaws (Andrews et al., 2002). Accordingly, it has been proposed that experiences of shame are tightly linked with fluctuation in self-esteem, and it is plausible that frequent experiences of shame could be conceptually related to chronically low levels of self-esteem (Elison, Garofalo, & Velotti, 2014). Furthermore, low levels of self-esteem could increase the individual vulnerability to experience negative emotional states, including shame. Accordingly, although the directionality of their association is not clear, several studies have reported a substantial relation between low self-esteem and negative emotions, such as guilt and shame (Garofalo, 2015; Marshall, Marshall, Serran, & O'Brien, 2009). Of note, both self-esteem and negative emotions have been linked to increased aggressive tendencies, yet few studies have empirically tested associations between shame and aggression.

Shame and Aggression

The link between shame and aggression was proposed by several scholars, and some went so far as to say that all forms of violence are anticipated by feelings of shame and humiliation (Gilligan, 1996). From this perspective, early experiences of rejection and abuse might lead to shame-proneness in adulthood. In turn, individuals with high levels of shame-proneness may believe that resorting to aggression and violence is the only possible way to get rid of their shame feelings. From an evolutionary perspective, the experience of shame early in the development may be later replaced by a condition of chronic anger, adopted as a means to keep others away so that shame feelings cannot be detected or triggered (Farmer & Andrews, 2009). Alternatively, the perception of self-devaluation – which is implicit in shame experiences – may represent the first step of a chain that connects shame and aggression (Elison et al., 2014). Specifically, the sequence could begin with a devaluation of the self that causes shame; in turn, shame feelings can lead to the experience of substantial anger and to the expression of aggressive behavior towards the source of the initial devaluation (Elison et al., 2014; Velotti et al., 2014). In line with this assumption, in a recent study shame experiences were associated with trait anger, and this relation was accounted for by the role of angry reactions to criticisms (Hejdenberg & Andrews, 2011). Specifically, behavioral shame was linked to both proneness toward angry reactions and trait anger, whereas characterological and bodily shame were only related to angry reactions to criticisms (Hejdenberg & Andrews, 2011). In this chain, maladaptive emotion regulation may play a mediating role (Garofalo, Holden, Zeigler-Hill, & Velotti, 2016; Roberton, Daffern & Bucks, 2012). Yet, this possibility has not been empirically tested so far.

Shame and Emotion Regulation

Shame is considered among the emotions that are more difficult to regulate (Elison et al., 2014). Of note, the way people regulate emotions has important consequences for their well-being (Gross & John, 2003). Cognitive reappraisal and expressive suppression have been identified among the emotion regulation strategies that people use more often (Gross & John, 2003; Gross & Levenson, 1993). Cognitive reappraisal entails thinking about an upsetting situation from a different angle in order to alter its meaning and modulate its emotional impact. Expressive suppression involves an attempt to inhibit or reduce the outward expression of an ongoing emotional experience (i.e., not showing the emotion that one is feeling). In general, reappraisal and suppression are inversely related to a wide range of outcomes in the domains of subjective well-being, affectivity, and social relationships. Specifically, reappraisal is typically associated with better, and suppression with poorer, outcomes (Gross & John, 2003). A recent experimental study has shown that trait shame was linked with emotional suppression (Lanteigne, Flynn, Eastabrook, & Hollenstein, 2014). This is important, because adopting maladaptive emotion regulation strategies for shame may ultimately lead to both internalizing (e.g., psychological distress) and externalizing (e.g., aggression) psychopathological symptoms (Elison, Pulos, & Lennon, 2006; Velotti et al., 2014). Therefore, it is possible that shame is associated with maladaptive emotion regulation, which in turn may explain the associations that shame has with psychopathological symptoms and aggression.

Overview of the Current Study

In the present study we sought to: (1) confirm and extend prior research on the nomological network of shame, investigating its associations with measures of psychological distress; self-esteem, aggression, and emotion regulation; and (2) examine the possible mediating role of maladaptive emotion regulation (i.e., emotional suppression) in the association between trait shame and external correlates (i.e., self-esteem, aggression and general psychopathology). Since gender differences in shame experiences (Andrews et al., 2002), emotion regulation (John & Gross, 2003), aggression (Fossati, Maffei, Acquarini, & Di Ceglie, 2003), and psychopathological distress (Prunas, Sarno, Preti, Madeddu, & Perugini, 2012) have consistenly been reported, we also examined gender differences in mean levels and patterns of associations.

Method

Participants and Procedures

The total sample comprised 380 adult participants (66.1% women, $N = 251$) recruited from the community. Participants were recruited by psychology graduate students with a snowball sampling technique: they started recruiting 5 participants from their acquaintances and asked them to recruit participants among their social networks. Men ($M_{age} = 31.00$, $SD = 11.42$, range 19–63) were slightly but significantly older than women ($M_{age} = 28.50$, $SD = 9.88$, range 18–58), $t(225.85) = 2.11$, $p = .04$. All participants were Italian. The majority of participants were university students ($N = 225$, 59.2%), whereas 6.3% ($N = 24$) were unemployed, 23.9% ($N = 91$) were employees, 9.5% ($N = 36$) were self-employed, and 1.1% ($N = 4$) were retired. Most participants ($N = 313$, 82.4%) reported to be (or to had been in the past) in a significant intimate relationship lasted at least 6 months. Finally, 64 participants (16.8%) did not have children, whereas 316 of them (83.2%) had at least one kid. All participants voluntarily and anonymously took part in the study and provided written informed consent. Participants were administered the questionnaires described below and returned them in a sealed envelope to ensure confidentiality. The local Institutional Review Board formally approved all procedures.

Measures

All measures were self-report Likert-type questionnaires. Participants were administered the Italian versions of the following measures. The translated items of all measures were obtained by the authors of the corresponding published Italian adaptations (see references below).

Experience of Shame Scale (ESS; Andrews et al., 2002)

The ESS is a 25-item questionnaire designed to capture the experience of shame across three components: characterological shame (sample item: 'Have you felt ashamed of any of your personal habits?'; $\alpha = .85$), behavioral shame (sample item: 'Do you feel ashamed when you do something wrong?'; $\alpha = .85$), and bodily shame (sample item: 'Have you felt ashamed of your body or any part of it?'; $\alpha = .87$). The sum of these three components provides an overall index of shame feelings ($\alpha = .91$). In the present study, the Italian version of the ESS was used (Caretti, Craparo, & Schimmenti, 2010), which substantially replicated the psychometric properties of the original version.

Differential Emotions Scale-IV (DES-IV; Izard et al., 1993)

The DES-IV consists of 36 items aimed at capturing the frequency of the experience of specific positive and negative emotions in the daily life. For the purpose of this study, only the six items assessing shame (e.g., 'Feel embarrassed when anybody sees you make a mistake'; $\alpha = .63$) and guilt (e.g., 'Feel regret, sorry about something you did'; $\alpha = .68$) of the Italian adaptation of the DES-IV (Zavattini et al., 2015) were administered.

Rosenberg Self-Esteem Scale (RSES; Rosenberg, 1965)

The 10-item RSES was used to assess the general level of self-esteem (e.g., 'On the whole, I am satisfied with myself'). The Italian version of the RSES has shown sound psychometric properties (Prezza, Trombaccia, & Armento, 1997). Cronbach's alpha was .88 in the present study.

Symptom Checklist-90-Revised (SCL-90-R; Derogatis, 1994)

The SCL-90-R is a 90-item inventory designed to measure general psychopathological distress suffered in the past month. The SCL-90-R estimates a global index of psychopathology (Global Severity Index, GSI), by averaging all item scores (e.g., 'To what extent do you feel/have you felt blue in the last month?'), rated on a Likert scale ($\alpha = .97$). The Italian adaptation of the SCL-R-90 was used in this study (Prunas et al., 2012).

Emotion Regulation Questionnaire (ERQ; Gross & John, 2003)

The 10-item ERQ was administered to assess individual differences in two emotion regulation strategies: cognitive reappraisal (e.g., 'I control my emotions by changing the way I think about the situation I'm in'; $\alpha = .87$) and expressive suppression (e.g., 'I keep my emotions to myself'; $\alpha = .79$). For the purpose of this study, we used the Italian version of the ERQ (Balzarotti, John, & Gross, 2010), which has shown adequate psychometric properties.

Aggression Questionnaire (AQ; Buss & Perry, 1992)

The AQ is a 29-item instrument composed by four subscales: physical aggression (e.g., 'Once in a while I can't control the urge to strike another person'; $\alpha = .83$); verbal aggression (e.g., 'I can't help getting into arguments when people disagree with me'; $\alpha = .76$); anger ('I sometimes feel like a powder keg ready to explode'; $\alpha = 80$); and hostility (e.g., 'When people are especially nice, I wonder what they want'; $\alpha = .81$). The AQ total score represent an index of trait aggression ($\alpha = 90$). The Italian version of the AQ has shown good reliability and validity (Fossati et al., 2003), and has been used in the present study.

Data Analytic Strategy

Descriptive statistics were computed for all study variables. Gender differences and associations with socio-demographic variables of interest were evaluated with one-way between-groups univariate or multivariate analyses of covariance (i.e., ANCOVA or MANCOVA, respectively). Pillai's Trace was used as the most robust test statistic, and Partial Eta squared ($\eta^2_{partial}$) was chosen as an estimate of the effect size of the univariate F tests. Pearson product-moment correlation coefficients among all measures were calculated. The homogeneity of correlation coefficients across gender was tested using the appropriate z statistic (Cohen, Cohen, West, & Aiken, 2003). To test whether the ESS scales explained additional variance in previously significant correlates, above and beyond the effect of DES-IV-assessed shame, hierarchical multiple regression analyses were conducted. The Variance Inflation Factor (VIF) was adopted to assess collinearity. Finally, to test the hypothesized indirect effect of shame on both aggression and psychopathological distress through the mediation of maladaptive emotion regulation, hierarchical regression and bootstrap analyses were conducted using the PROCESS Macro for SPSS (Hayes, 2013). All analyses were carried out holding constant the effect of age.

Results

Descriptive Analyses and Gender Differences

Descriptive statistics and gender differences are presented in Table 1.

Table 1. Means, Standard Deviations (*SD*), and Gender Comparisons (Controlling for Age) for All Study Variables (*N* = 380).

	Male participants (*N* = 129) Mean (*SD*)	Female participants (*N* = 251) Mean (*SD*)	Whole sample (*N* = 380) Mean (*SD*)	*F*	df	η^2 partial
ESS total score	46.89(11.79)	**52.96**(12.48)	50.89(12.57)	17.15***	1, 375	.04
ESS characterological	21.63(6.09)	22.73(6.49)	22.36(6.37)	1.37	1, 375	.00
ESS behavioral	18.70(5.15)	**20.65**(5.41	19.99(5.40)	9.79**	1, 375	.03
ESS bodily	6.57(2.53)	**9.54**(3.45)	8.53(3.46)	69.34***	1, 375	.16
DES-IV shame	5.24(1.71)	**6.03**(2.11)	5.75(2.01)	9.85**	1, 342	.03
DES-IV guilt	6.24(1.75)	**6.79**(1.97)	6.59(1.91)	4.45*	1, 342	.01
Self-esteem	**32.00**(4.75)	30.50(5.49)	31.01(5.29)	6.62*	1, 377	.02
SCL-90-R GSI	.54(.38)	**.76**(.53)	.69(.49)	15.55***	1, 377	.04
ERQ reappraisal	4.71(1.02)	**4.97**(1.05)	4.88(1.05)	4.93*	1, 377	.13
ERQ suppression	**3.70**(1.19)	3.18(1.24)	3.36(1.25)	12.98***	1, 377	.03
AQ total score	63.57(16.51)	62.18(15.75)	62.65(16.00)	1.14	1, 377	.00
AQ physical aggression	**17.42**(6.50)	14.13(5.34)	15.25(5.96)	29.26***	1, 377	.07
AQ verbal aggression	14.37(3.74)	13.67(4.24)	13.91(4.09)	2.59	1, 377	.01
AQ anger	15.47(5.24)	16.09(5.30)	15.88(5.28)	0.82	1, 377	.00
AQ hostility	16.33(5.02)	**18.29**(5.73)	17.63(5.57)	8.44**	1, 377	.02

Note. ESS = Experience of Shame Scale; DES-IV = Differential Emotions Scale-IV; SCL-90-R = Symptom Checklist-90-Revised; ERQ = Emotion Regulation Questionnaire; AQ = Aggression Questionnaire. Bolded mean values are significantly greater than the corresponding value in the opposite gender.
*$p < .05$. **$p < .01$. ***$p < .001$.

Females reported an overall greater level of ESS-assessed shame than males, and lower levels of self-esteem. Also, MANCOVA results revealed that there was a statistically significant difference between male and female participants on the combined ESS scale scores, $F(3, 372) = 26.57$, $p < .001$, Pillai's Trace = .18, $\eta^2_{partial} = .18$. Specifically, females scored higher than males on behavioral and bodily shame. Females also reported significantly greater levels of DES-IV-assessed guilt and shame, multivariate $F(2, 340) = 5.12$, $p < .01$, Pillai's Trace = .03, $\eta^2_{partial} = .03$. A subsequent ANCOVA revealed a significant gender difference on the SCL-90-R GSI score. Furthermore, a significant multivariate effect of gender occurred on the combined ERQ scales, $F(2, 375) = 9.52$, $p < .001$, Pillai's Trace = .05, $\eta^2_{partial} = .05$; in particular, females reported higher levels of cognitive reappraisal, and lower levels of expressive suppression than males. Finally, a significant difference across gender occurred when the AQ subscales were entered as combined dependent variables, $F(4, 373) = 19.28$, $p < .001$, Pillai's Trace = .17, $\eta^2_{partial} = .17$, but not when males and females when compared on the AQ total score using an ANCOVA design. When the AQ subscales were considered separately, only two differences reached statistical significance, in opposite directions: males reported higher levels of physical aggression, but lower levels of hostility, than females.

Furthermore, we tested whether levels of shame differed between people with and without children, as well as between people who reported to be (or to had been in the past) in a long lasting romantic relationship and people who did not. Controlling for gender and age, participants with children reported significantly lower scores on the ESS total score, $F(1, 373) = 3.95$, $p > .05$, $\eta^2_{partial} = .01$. However, the multivariate main effect of the parental condition (i.e., children yes/no) on the combined ESS scale scores was only approaching significance, $F(3, 371) = 2.22$, $p = .08$, Pillai's Trace = .02, $\eta^2_{partial} = .02$. Specifically, although participants with children reported lower levels of shame on all three dimensions, these differences were significant for characterological shame, $F(1, 373) = 3.98$, $p < .05$, $\eta^2_{partial} = .01$, and behavioral shame, $F(1, 373) = 4.79$, $p < .05$, $\eta^2_{partial} = .01$. On the other hand, although there was not significant difference on the ESS total score, $F(2, 372) = 1.49$, $p > .05$, $\eta^2_{partial} = .01$, a significant multivariate effect between participants with and without a current or past intimate relationship occurred on the combined ESS scales, $F(6, 742) = 2.57$, $p < .05$, Pillai's Trace $= .04$, $\eta^2_{partial} = .02$. Specifically, controlling for gender and age, individuals who had never had a long lasting intimate relationship reported significantly greater scores of bodily shame, $F(2, 372) = 4.33$, $p < .05$, $\eta^2_{partial} = .02$. The analyses in this paragraph were exploratory in nature, to test for associations between the ESS and demographics. However, since an interesting pattern of results occurred, we opted for reporting and discussing them, to stimulate further research in this area.

ESS Nomological Network

Correlation analysis results are displayed in Table 2. Of note, the ESS scales were all strongly related to the ESS total score (controlling for age, partial rs were .89, .84. and .63 for the characterologial shame, behavioral shame, and bodily shame scales, respectively). Further, the ESS scales were significantly associated to each other (rs ranging between .33 and .60). All ESS scales were significantly and positively related to the DES-IV shame and guilt scales. Of note, homogeneity tests did not show significant differences in correlation coefficient values of any ESS scale with shame *versus* guilt scale from the DES-IV, min. $z = 0.24$, max $z = 1.53$, all $ps > .05$. Conversely, homogeneity tests across gender revealed that only 1 out 8 pairs of correlation coefficients (12.5%) significantly differed across gender, with the association between bodily shame and guilt being stronger among males ($z = 2.27$, $p < .05$). All the ESS scales were also significantly and negatively associated with levels of self-esteem. As for the associations between the ESS and the ERQ, no significant correlations were found with cognitive reappraisal. Among females only, a significant positive correlations emerged between emotional suppression and both characterological shame and the ESS total score. Among males, no significant associations occurred between the ESS and the AQ total score; on the other hand, the AQ total score was significantly and positively related to the ESS bodily shame scale and the ESS total score among females. Physical aggression was negatively related with characterological shame among males. Among females, the direction of the association was inverse, but nonsignificant. Of note, correlation coefficients between physical aggression and ESS total and characterological shame scores significantly differed across gender ($z = 2.12$ and 2.41, respectively, both $ps < .05$). Verbal aggression was only significantly related to characterological shame (negatively) among females. Among females, anger showed a positive association with bodily shame. Moreover, the ESS total and subscale scores were significantly and positively related to hostility across gender. Finally, significant positive correlations were found between all ESS scales and the GSI scale of the SCL-90-R. Overall, only 3 out of 44 comparisons between correlation coefficients (across gender) turned out to be significant (6.82%), suggesting that the patterns of correlations between the ESS scales and external correlates are largely invariant across gender (min. $z = 0.00$, max $z = 1.68$, all $ps > .05$).

Incremental Variance of ESS Dimensions on Relevant Outcomes

We then tested whether the ESS scales significantly explained a portion of additional variance in self-esteem, hostility, and psychopathological distress (as these were the variables

Table 2. Partial Correlations (Controlling for Age) of the ESS Total and Scale Scores with the DES-IV Guilt and Shame Scales, Self-Esteem Level, Emotion Regulation Strategies, and Aggression Dimensions, in Both Male ($N = 129$) and Female ($N = 251$) Participants (Total $N = 380$).

		DES-IV shame	DES-IV guilt	Self-esteem	ERQ reappraisal	ERQ suppression	AQ total	AQ physical aggression	AQ verbal aggression	AQ anger	AQ hostility	SCL-90-R GSI
ESS total	Males	.45***	.56***	-.42***	.01	.03	.04	-.16[a]	-.04	.02	.37***	.43***
	Females	.51***	.54***	-.51***	-.06	.19**	.16*	.07[a]	-.12	.07	.41***	.52***
ESS characterological	Males	.40***	.54***	-.46***	.02	.12	.01	-.21*[a]	-.03	-.01	.34***	.45***
	Females	.50***	.59***	-.54***	-.05	.22**	.12	.05[a]	-.15*	.05	.34***	.52***
ESS behavioral	Males	.39***	.40***	-.25***	.02	-.04	.06	-.09	-.01	.05	.31***	.26***
	Females	.38***	.36***	-.30***	-.01	.12	.09	.03	-.12	-.02	.33***	.33***
ESS bodily	Males	.33**	.49***[a]	-.35***	-.04	-.06	.04	-.06	-.10	.01	.29**	.36***
	Females	.30***	.28***[a]	-.37***	-.11	.09	.22***	.12	.03	.17**	.33***	.39***

Note. ESS = Experience of Shame Scale; DES-IV = Differential Emotions Scale-IV; ERQ = Emotion Regulation Questionnaire; AQ = Aggression Questionnaire; SCL-90-R = Symptom Checklist-90-Revised; GSI = Global Severity Index scale of the SCL-90-R.

[a]Significant difference in correlation coefficients between male and female participants.

*$p < .05.$ **$p < .01.$ ***$p < .001.$

Table 3. Hierarchical Multiple Regression Analyses Predicting Self-Esteem, Hostility, and Psychopathological Distress ($N = 380$).

	Self-esteem B	AQ Hostility β	GSI β
Step 1			
Age	.21***	−.20***	−.10
Gender	.13*	−.15**	−.20***
Adjusted R2change	.06***	.06***	.05***
Step 2			
DES-IV shame	−.38***	.60***	.54***
Adjusted R2change	.13***	.33***	.27***
Step 3			
ESS characterological shame	−.39***	−.02	.30***
ESS behavioral shame	−.09	.08	−.08
ESS bodily shame	−.17***	.15**	.18***
Adjusted R2change	.13***	.02**	.10***

Note. AQ = Aggression Questionnaire; GSI = Global Severity Index of the Symptom Checklist-90-Revised; DES-IV = Differential Emotions Scale-IV; ESS = Experience of Shame Scale. Gender was dummy-coded with 0 = females.

most strongly associated at the bivariate level with the ESS scales), above and beyond the influence of DES-IV-assessed shame (see Table 3). None of the VIF values suggested that collinearity among predictors could have biased regression results. Hierarchical multiple regression analyses revealed that, controlling for age and gender, the ESS scales significantly explained a portion of incremental variance in all of the outcomes considered. Specifically, after removing the shared variance among ESS scales, characteriological and bodily shame scales significantly and independently predicted self-esteem level (negatively) and global psychopathological distress (positively). Further, bodily shame uniquely and positively predicted hostility, over and above the influence of the shame scale of the DES-IV.

Does Emotional Suppression Account for an Indirect Relationship between Sshame and Maladaptive Outcomes?

Based on partial correlation results (see Table 2), the significance of statistical indirect effects was assessed only among female participants (i.e., because among males the association between shame and emotional suppression was not significant, ruling out the possibility of any indirect effect of the former through the latter). A summary of the indirect effect analyses conducted is presented in Table 4. A total of seven indirect effects were tested, four of which yielded significant results with small effect size. Specifically, emotion suppression mediated the effect of ESS total score and characterological shame on both hostility and psychopathological distress. The other indirect effects (involving self-esteem and overall trait aggression) did not reach statistical significance.

Discussion

The aim of the current study was to confirm and extend previous knowledge on the nomological net surrounding the multidimensional construct of shame, also testing for invariance across gender. Further, the possible mechanisms underlying the association between shame and maladaptive outcomes were investigated, examining the mediating role of maladaptive emotion regulation (i.e., emotional suppression).

Table 4. Summary of Bootstrapping Analyses Examining the Indirect Effect of Shame on Self-Esteem, Aggression, and Psychopathological Distress Through the Role of Emotional Suppression, Controlling for Age (Among Females Only; N = 251; 5,000 Bootstrap Samples).

Predictor Variable(PV)	Mediating variable(M)	Criterion Variable (CV)	Effect of PV on M (a)	Effect of M on CV, controlling for the PV (b)	Total effect (c)	Direct effect (c')	Indirect effect (bias corrected intervals) (a × b)	95% CI	abcs [95% bias corrected CI]
ESS total	Emotional suppression	Self-esteem	.02**	−.39	−.23***	−.22***	−.007	[−.021, .000]	
ESS total	Emotional suppression	AQ total	.02**	.68	.21**	.20*	.012	[−.015, .053]	
ESS characterological shame	Emotional suppression	AQ total	.04**	.75	.31*	.28	.028	[−.028, .111]	
ESS total score	Emotional suppression	AQ hostility	.02**	.87**	.20***	.18***	.016	[.005, .035]	.034 [.009, .075]
ESS characterological shame	Emotional suppression	AQ hostility	.04**	.90**	.32***	.28***	.034	[.012, .075]	.039 [.013, .084]
ESS total score	Emotional suppression	GSI	.02**	.10***	.02***	.02***	.002	[.001, .003]	.041 [.012, .081]
ESS characterological shame	Emotional suppression	GSI	.04**	.09***	.04***	.04***	.003	[.001, .007]	.042 [.015, .085]

Note. ESS = Experience of Shame Scale; AQ = Aggression Questionnaire; GSI = Global Severity Index scale of the Symptom Checklist-90-Revised; CI = Confidence Intervals. Unstandardized coefficients are reported. ab_{cs} = completely standardized indirect effect, measure of the effect size for significant indirect effects.
* $p < .05$. ** $p < .01$. *** $p < .001$.

In line with the expectations, women reported greater levels of shame (specifically: behavioral and bodily shame), and lower levels of self-esteem, than men. Women also reported greater levels of psychopathological distress, cognitive reappraisal, and hostility, whereas men had greater levels of emotional suppression and physical aggression. Taken together, these findings are in line with prior findings (Andrews et al., 2002; Fossati et al., 2003; John & Gross, 2003) on gender differences in emotional experience, emotion regulation styles, as well as in the expression of aggressive tendencies. Notably, levels of characterological and behavioral shame were higher among people who did not have kids, and levels of bodily shame were higher among people who never had a significant romantic relationship. The correlational nature of the study did not allow to speculate about causal effects, but the interesting link between intimate attachment relationships (with children and/or romantic partners) and shame feelings in different domains warrants future investigation.

The nomological network surrounding shame experiences was largely consistent across gender. Behavioral, characterological, and bodily shame feelings were all related with trait shame and trait guilt. Furthermore, shame feelings were associated with decreased self-esteem, and with higher levels of hostility and psychological distress. This is consistent with previous literature (Garofalo, 2015; Elison, 2005; Gilligan, 1996; Marshall et al., 2009) and suggests that the experience of shame does not come in isolation. Rather, feelings of shame are likely associated with a more general lack of confidence in the self as well as in the outside world. As such, it is not surprising that feelings of shame and lack of confidence in the self and the others can be accompanied by overall psychological distress. Some gender differences in the nomological net emerged, suggesting that the experience of shame might have more pronounced consequences in women. Indeed, characterological shame was related with emotional suppression, indicating that women who are more prone to experience feeling of shame about their own personality may tend to adopt maladaptive emotion regulation strategies (Nyström & Mikkelsen, 2013). This might be due to an attempt to protect themselves from the effects of such unbearable feelings (Elison et al., 2014), which would probably increase the experience of shame itself. Therefore, it appears that women who experience characterological shame are likely to suppress, rather than show, their own emotions. In line with this, higher levels of characterological shame were also associated with lower levels of verbal aggression. Further, bodily shame was associated with angry feelings, suggesting that the perception of flaws in their physical aspect could be a trigger for angry and aggressive outbursts especially in females (Hejdenberg & Andrews, 2011). Finally, physical aggression was negatively related to characterological shame in men, indicating a possible inhibiting effect of shame toward aggressive tendencies. This is consistent with the idea that shame feelings are not always bad, and that the experience of shame might have healthy and adaptive consequences (Farmer & Andrews, 2009). For example, feeling ashamed about a previous aggressive behavior can have the positive consequence of inhibiting the same behavior in the future. As a whole, although all others coefficients were nonsignificant, the trends seem to indicate that shame is negatively associated with aggression among men, but positively related (or unrelated) to aggression among women. Future examinations of the possible differential effects of shame on aggression across gender are required to obtain a deeper insight into the shame-aggression link.

Our findings also supported the importance of adopting a multidimensional conceptualization of shame (Andrews et al., 2002). Indeed, over and above the influence of trait shame, characterological and bodily shame were independently associated with low self-esteem and psychological distress. Further, bodily shame was independently related to hostility. This suggests that, even after controlling for individual differences in the experience of shame in daily life, specific feelings of shame referred to one's identity or body might add to the explanation of internalizing and externalizing symptoms. As a last step, we aimed at exploring possible mechanisms linking shame feelings with maladaptive outcomes. Mediation analyses revealed that—among women—the associations of shame feelings (and, in particular, characterological shame) with hostility and psychological distress was accounted for by emotional suppression. This might indicate that both the externalization (i.e., hostility) and internalization (i.e., psychological distress) of shame feelings could be explained by poor emotion regulation, rather than being an effect of shame *per se*. In other words, shame feelings are likely to increase the individual difficulty in regulating emotions, and this in turn could lead to an increase in hostile attitudes and psychopathological symptoms (Garofalo et al., 2016; Velotti et al., 2014). On the other hand, the same pattern did not explain the association between shame and low self-esteem, suggesting that their shared variance was not accounted for by emotional suppression.

This study presented several limitations. First, the reliance on self-report questionnaires may have inflated correlations due to the spurious effect of common method variance. Second, the generalization of these results is limited by the recruitment of a convenience sample of community individuals, the majority of whom where university students. One possible problem in relying on convenience samples comprising a strong component of university students is a restriction in the variance of several demographic (e.g., Socio Economic Status) and personality (e.g., impulsive or antisocial traits) characteristics that may be linked to some of the variables examined in the present study (e.g., aggression). Third, the correlational design prevents us from drawing conclusions about the causal relations among study variables. Nevertheless, the present findings may help design longitudinal studies to test prospective associations among shame experiences and related constructs over time. Finally, the use of single measures for each construct of interest raises the possibility that results would not generalize to other operationalizations of the same constructs.

Nonetheless, we believe these findings extend current knowledge on the nomological network of shame feelings, providing novel insight on the role of specific shame experiences. Specifically, the present findings suggest that conceptualizing shame as a multidimensional construct may be helpful in delineating the associations between shame and maladaptive outcomes. Notably, our study also provides additional support for the use of the ESS as a brief multidimensional measure of shame experiences. From a clinical point of view, this is important as a focus on specific 'faces' of shame can be appropriate to target psychopathological symptoms and aggression. Finally, the current study advanced prior knowledge indicating that fostering the use of adaptive emotion regulation strategies could be an important target to prevent or reduce psychopathological symptoms and aggression.

ORCID

Carlo Garofalo (iD) http://orcid.org/0000-0003-2306-6961

References

Andrews, B., Qian, M., & Valentine, J. D. (2002). Predicting depressive symptoms with a new measure of shame: The experience of shame scale. *British Journal of Clinical Psychology, 41,* 29–42.

Balzarotti, S., John, O. P., & Gross, J. J. (2010). An Italian adaptation of the Emotion Regulation Questionnaire. *European Journal of Psychological Assessment, 26,* 61–67.

Buss, A. H., & Perry, M. (1992). The aggression questionnaire. *Journal of Personality and Social Psychology, 63,* 452–459. doi: 10.1037/0022-3514.63.3.452

Caretti, V., Craparo, G., & Schimmenti, A. (2010). Il ruolo della disregolazione affettiva, della dissociazione e della vergogna nei disturbi del comportamento alimentare. [The role of affective dysregulation, dissociation and shame in eating disorders]. In V. Caretti, & D. La Barbera (eds.), *Addiction. Aspetti Biologici e di Ricerca [Addiction. Biological and Research Aspects]* (pp. 135–165). Milano, IT: Raffaello Cortina Editore.

Cohen, J., Cohen, P., West, S. G., & Aiken, L. S. (2003). *Applied multiple regression/ correlation analysis for the behavioral sciences (3rd ed.).* Hillsdale, NJ: Erlbaum.

Cronbach, L. J., & Meehl, P. E. (1955). Construct validity in psychological tests. *Psychological Bulletin, 52(4),* 281–302.

Derogatis, L. R. (1994). *SCL-90-R, administration, scoring and procedures manual for the revised version (3rd ed.).* Minneapolis, MN: National Computer Systems.

Elison, J. (2005). Shame and guilt: A hundred years of apples and oranges. *New Ideas in Psychology, 23,* 5–32.

Elison, J., Garofalo, C., & Velotti, P. (2014). Shame and aggression: Theoretical considerations. *Aggression and Violent Behavior, 19,* 447–453.

Elison, J., Pulos, S., & Lennon, R. (2006). Shame-focused coping: An empirical study of the compass of shame. *Social Behavior and Personality, 34,* 161–168.

Farmer, E., & Andrews, B. (2009). Shameless yet angry: shame and its relationship to anger in male young offenders and undergraduate controls. *Journal of Forensic Psychiatry & Psychology, 20,* 48–65.

Fossati, A., Maffei, C., Acquarini, E., & Di Ceglie, A. (2003). Multigroup confirmatory component and factor analyses of the Italian version of the aggression questionnaire. *European Journal of Psychological Assessment, 19,* 54–65.

Garofalo, C. (2015). Emozionalità negativa ed autostima in un campione di offender detenuti: Uno studio preliminare [Negative emotionality and self-esteem in an incarcerated offender sample: Preliminary investigation]. *Giornale Italiano di Psicologia [Italian Journal of Psychology], 42,* 363–371.

Garofalo, C., Holden, C. J., Zeigler-Hill, V., & Velotti, P. (2016). Understanding the connection between self-esteem and aggression: The mediating role of emotion dysregulation. *Aggressive Behavior, 42*, 3–15.

Gilligan, J. (1996). *Violence. Reflections on a National Epidemic.* New York, NY: Vintage Books.

Gross, J. J., & John, O. P. (2003). Individual differences in two emotion regulation processes: Implications for affect, relationships, and well-being. *Journal of Personality and Social Psychology, 85*, 348–362.

Gross, J. J., & Levenson, R. W. (1993). Emotional suppression: Physiology, self-report, and expressive behavior. *Journal of Personality and Social Psychology, 64*, 970–986.

Hayes, A. F. (2013). *Introduction to mediation, moderation, and conditional process analysis: A regression-based approach.* New York, NY: Guilford Press.

Hejdenberg, J., & Andrews, B. (2011). The relationship between shame and different types of anger: A theory-based investigation. *Personality and Individual Differences, 50*, 1278–1282.

Izard, C. E., Libero, D. Z., Putnam, P., Haynes, O. M. (1993). Stability of emotion experiences and their relations to traits of personality. *Journal of Personality and Social Psychology, 64*(5), 847–860.

Lanteigne, D. M., Flynn, J. J., Eastabrook, J. M., & Hollenstein, T. (2014). Discordant patterns among emotional experience, Arousal, and expression in adolescence: Relations with emotion regulation and internalizing problems. *Canadian Journal of Behavioural Science / Revue canadienne des sciences du comportement, 46*, 29–39.

Marshall, W. L., Marshall, L. E, Serran, G. A., & O'Brien, M. D. (2009). Self-esteem, shame, cognitive distorsions and empathy in sexual offenders: Their integration and treatment implications. *Psychology, Crime & Law, 15*, 217–234.

Nyström, M. B. T., & Mikkelsen, F. (2013). Psychopathy-related personality traits and shame management strategies in adolescents. *Journal of Interpersonal Violence, 28*, 519–537.

Prezza, M., Trombaccia, F. R., & Armento, L. (1997). La scala dell'autostima di Rosenberg: Traduzione e validazione Italiana. [The Rosenberg self-esteem Scale: Italian translation and validation.]. *Bollettino di Psicologia Applicata [Applied Psychology Bulletin], 223*, 35–44.

Prunas, A., Sarno, I., Preti, E., Madeddu, F., & Perugini, M. (2012). Psychometric properties of the Italian version of the SCL-90-R: A study on a large community sample. *European Psychiatry, 27*, 591–597.

Roberton, T., Daffern, M., & Bucks, R. S. (2012). Emotion regulation and aggression. *Aggression and Violent Behavior, 17*, 72–82.

Rosenberg, M. (1965). *Society and the adolescent self-image.* Princeton, NJ: Princeton University Press.

Tangney, J. P., & Dearing, R. L. (2002). *Shame and guilt.* New York, NY: Guilford Press.

Velotti, P., Elison, J., & Garofalo, C. (2014). Shame and aggression: Different trajectories and implications. *Aggression and Violent Behavior, 19*, 454–461.

Zavattini, G. C., Garofalo, C., Velotti, P., Tommasi, M., Romanelli, R., Espirito Santo, H., & Saggino, A. (2015). Dissociative experiences and psychopathology among inmates in Italian and Portuguese prisons. *International Journal of Offender Therapy and Comparative Criminology.* Advance online publication. doi.org/10.1177/0306624X15617256.

Cognitive Alexithymia Mediates the Association Between Avoidant Attachment and Interpersonal Problems in Patients With Somatoform Disorder

Jurrijn A. Koelen, Liesbeth H.M. Eurelings-Bontekoe, and Stefan Kempke

ABSTRACT

Patients with somatoform disorder (SFD) are characterized by the presence of chronic physical complaints that are not fully explained by a general medical condition or another mental disorder. Insecure attachment patterns are common in this patient group, which are often associated with interpersonal difficulties. In the present study, the mediational role of two types of alexithymia and negative affectivity (NA) was examined in the association between attachment styles and interpersonal problems in a group of 120 patients with SFD. Patients were requested to fill out several self-report questionnaires for the assessment of attachment strategies, alexithymia, NA, and interpersonal problems. Cognitive alexithymia (i.e., the inability to identify and verbalize emotions) mediated the relationship between avoidant attachment patterns and interpersonal problems, even after controlling for NA. Preliminary findings also suggested that NA acted as a moderator of the mediator cognitive alexithymia. These results have important implications for clinical practice, as this study clearly shows that interpersonal problems do not automatically follow from insecure attachment strategies, but are contingent upon alexithymic features. It is recommended to target alexithymic features in patients with SFD, particularly in the context of negative emotions. Therefore, cognitive alexithymia may be an important therapeutic focus, specifically in the treatment of avoidant ptients with SFD.

The Diagnostic and Statistical Manual of Mental Disorders IV-TR (American Psychiatric Association, 2000) describes the main diagnostic features for somatoform disorders (SFD) as: The "presence of physical symptoms that suggest a general medical condition (…) and are not fully explained by a general medical condition, by direct effects of a substance or by another mental disorder" (p. 445). These symptoms must also result in clinically significant distress, or impairment in social, occupational, or other areas of functioning. De Waal, Arnold, Eekhof, and van Hemert (2004) reported an estimated prevalence of DSM–IV SFD of 16.1% in a Dutch general practice consulting population for moderate to severe cases of disorder, and 21.9% when mild cases were included. In the community, the prevalence rate of SFD is approximated at 6% (Wittchen et al., 2011). SFD patients are five to six times more likely to be high-users in terms of inpatient admissions or insurance-paid services (Hansen, Fink, Frydenberg, & Oxhøj,

2002). Thus, the high prevalence and associated cost of SFD underline the necessity to study the psychopathological mechanisms involved in these disorders, which may in turn suggest possibilities for treatment. This study investigates the impact of alexithymia (as a key aspect of impaired mentalization) on interpersonal problems in patients with SFD, within the context of insecure attachment relationships using mediation analysis.

Attachment, Mentalization, and Affect Regulation: A Model for Understanding Somatoform Disorder

Over recent years, attachment theory has proven to be a useful framework for understanding somatoform disorder (Kooiman & Koelen, 2012; Scheidt & Waller, 1999), particularly in terms of its consequences for affect regulation and mentalization. Mentalization is the largely unconscious mental activity that mediates the perception and interpretation of human behavior in terms of intentional mental states, such as affects, wishes, desires, and thoughts (Fonagy & Target, 2006). Secure attachment bonds between infant and caregiver facilitate the emergence of effective mentalization, and subsequently the adequate regulation of affects, because effective mentalization provides the individual with symbolized representations of internal mental and physical states (Fonagy, Gergely, Jurist, & Target, 2002). Thus, disturbance of the early attachment bond renders the individual vulnerable in the context of later social relationships, and may create vulnerabilities for psychosomatic illness (Maunder & Hunter, 2001; Scheidt & Waller, 1999).

Impaired affect regulation is a hallmark of SFD (Van Dijke et al., 2013). In this paper, we will focus on alexithymia as a key component of "affective mentalizing" (Fonagy et al., 2002). Alexithymia, that is, the inability to identify and communicate emotional states, has been regarded as a key component of SFD for many decades (De Gucht & Heiser, 2003). The ability to identify and label emotions, as well as the ability to verbalize them, helps regulate emotional as well as bodily states (Lieberman et al., 2007; Luyten & Van Houdenhove, 2013; Spaans, Veselka, Luyten, & Bühring, 2009). These are core features of alexithymia (Taylor, 1984). Interestingly, Spitzer and colleagues (Spitzer, Siebel-Jurges, Barnow, Grabe, & Freyberger, 2005) proposed that alexithymia involves a reduced capacity to use social interactions for affect regulation. Alexithymic individuals tend to distance themselves from others, and do not share emotions within a supportive relationship (Vanheule, Meganck, & Desmet, 2011). These assumptions resonate with current theorizing and treatment formulations in the field of SFD that regard impaired affective mentalizing as a key factor in the onset and perpetuation of physical symptoms, and the interpersonal problems associated with these symptoms (Luyten, Van Houdenhove, Lemma, Target, & Fonagy, 2012; Selders, Visser, Rooij, Delfstra, & Koelen, 2015). Recent studies have indeed shown that alexithymia is associated with severe interpersonal difficulties, including reduced interpersonal functioning, more severe personality problems, and impulsive aggression (Fossati et al., 2009; Nicolò et al., 2011). Together, these findings suggest that difficulties in affective mentalization, and alexithymia in particular, have an immediate impact on the ability to regulate emotions, and subsequently adversely influence the ability to function in an interpersonal context.

Insecure Attachment in Somatoform Disorder

Stuart and Noyes (1999) hypothesized that somatizing behavior, such as attempts to elicit care by continual complaints of physical illness or pain, is a form of interpersonal communication.

Such communication plays a role in maintaining somatizing behavior, for example: it triggers rejecting and unempathetic responses from family, significant others or medical personnel (Kool et al., 2010), which in turn leads somatizers to believe that care will not be available, which tends to increase their demands for care. This vicious cycle ultimately leads to feelings of frustration, helplessness, and even despair in patients, physicians and therapists (Hahn, 2001). Indeed, a pathognomonic feature of SFD is a disturbed pattern of health care behavior, leading to excessive consumption of medical resources (Waller, Scheidt, & Hartmann, 2004).

The prevalence of insecure attachment appears to be high in SFD: Two studies yielded rates of over 75% (Gil, Scheidt, Hoeger, & Nickel, 2008; Waller et al., 2004). Waller et al. (2004) examined a group of 35 patients with SFD according to ICD-10 criteria. In comparison with 20 healthy matched controls, patients with SFD had significantly higher rates of insecure (both preoccupied and dismissing) attachment. Gil et al. (2008) found even higher rates (88%) of insecure attachment among 76 patients with SFD based on DSM-IV interviews. In both these studies, dismissing attachment was more prevalent than preoccupied attachment styles. In yet another study among 134 normal subjects and 30 patient with somatoform disorder, significantly higher rates of anxious attachment were found in the patient group (Kim, Song, Bahn, Kim, & Shin, 2005). Despite disagreement on the specific attachment style, these studies converge to suggest that insecure attachment is common in patients with SFD.

Somewhat lower rates of insecure attachment styles were observed among patients with fibromyalgia; a disorder that is often comorbid with SFD. Two studies reported rates of approximately 50% (Davies, Macfarlane, McBeth, Morriss, & Dickens, 2009; Govender, Cassimjee, Schoeman, & Meyer, 2009). However, these prevalence rates of insecure attachment are hardly above those observed in the general population, that is, approximately 40% (Bakermans-Kranenburg & van IJzendoorn, 2009). This indicates that the attachment model may be more pertinent for studying strictly defined SFD according to stringent diagnostic criteria.

Attachment and Interpersonal Difficulties in SFD

According to Brennan, Clark, and Shaver (1998) there are two fundamental dimensions of insecure attachment: attachment *anxiety* (fear of intimacy and rejection) and attachment *avoidance* (avoidance of intimate relationships). Several studies have found associations between both these dimensions of attachment and interpersonal difficulties (Crawford et al., 2006; Haggerty, Hilsenroth, & Vala-Stewart, 2009; Hill et al., 2011). Haggerty et al., for example, found that both dimensions had a significant positive correlation with interpersonal distress, as measured with the IIP-64. Crawford et al. (2006), in turn, found that both insecure attachment dimensions were moderately correlated with various types of personality disorders. Another study showed that, specifically, the preoccupied attachment style (high anxiety, low avoidance), as measured with the Revised Adult Personality Functioning Assessment, correlated positively with interpersonal problems in romantic relationships (Hill et al., 2011).

In sum, interpersonal problems, which are key problems in SFD (Noyes et al., 2001), are strongly associated with insecure attachment patterns, suggesting that many interpersonal difficulties observed in SFD patients, may stem from underlying attachment disturbances (Waller et al., 2004). According to attachment theory, underlying working models of attachment tend to guide feelings, expectations, thoughts and behavior toward others, and therefore may quite easily disrupt interpersonal functioning among individuals with insecure attachment systems (Meyer & Pilkonis, 2005). In addition, disturbed attachment patterns may also explain the pathological help-seeking behavior that characterizes many SFD patients (Noyes, Stuart, & Watson, 2008; Waller et al., 2004).

Inadequate Emotion Regulation and Affective Mentalization as Mediator

It is important in research to move beyond merely quantifying direct linear associations between variables in favor of the identification of underlying mediating or moderating mechanisms that could be targeted in treatment, such as impaired emotion regulation strategies. Hence, this study focuses on the identification of potential mediators that may explain the relationship between insecure attachment strategies and interpersonal problems among patients with SFD with a focus on affective mentalizing or alexithymia in particular, as well as the presence of negative affectivity.

Several clinical and nonclinical studies have shown that impaired emotion regulation and emotional awareness play a key role in the relationship between insecure attachment patterns and the presence of both symptomatic distress and interpersonal problems. A study by Wearden, and colleagues (Wearden, Cook, & Vaughan-Jones, 2003) among 201 female undergraduate students, for example, suggested that both alexithymia and negative affectivity (NA) mediated the link between insecure (in particular avoidant) attachment and symptom reporting on the one hand, and emotional coping, on the other. The authors suggest that alexithymic individuals tend to dwell on emotions that cannot be readily identified, thus increasing distress and exacerbating a negative emotional reaction to symptoms (Wearden et al., 2003). In another study by the same group among 142 male and female undergraduates, it was found that alexithymia partially mediated the relationship between fearful attachment (high avoidance, high anxiety) and symptom reporting (Wearden, Lamberton, Crook, & Walsh, 2005). For the link between preocuccupied attachment and symptom reporting, only NA, and not alexithymia, turned out to be a significant mediator.

The hypothesis that alexithymia mediates the relationship between insecure attachment and interpersonal problems was supported by a study among 54 adolescent patients with borderline personality disorder (BPD) and 51 matched nonclinical controls (Deborde et al., 2012). This study showed that alexithymia mediated the relationship between both secure and fearful attachment styles and symptoms of borderline personality in adolescents. A partial mediation effect of alexithymia was found between secure attachment and borderline symptom severity: Secure attachment predicted low levels of BPD severity, but this was no longer the case when alexithymia was taken into account. Alexithymia was found to fully mediate the relationship between fearful attachment and borderline symptom severity. This indicates that fearful attachment is not directly associated with the expression of borderline symptoms, but only through high levels of alexithymia.

In a highly relevant study, the mediating role of impaired emotion regulation in the relation between insecure attachment and interpersonal problems was explored among 229 undergraduate college students (Wei, Vogel, Ku, & Zakalik, 2005). For the assessment of avoidant and anxious attachment strategies, the Experiences in Close Relationships scale (Fraley, Waller, & Brennan, 2000) was used. It was hypothesized that distinct patterns of emotion regulation apply to individuals with different patterns of insecure attachment. The results of their study supported the hypothesis that the link between anxious attachment and interpersonal distress was mediated by emotional reactivity, implying that anxiously attached individuals experience interpersonal problems only when they are overwhelmed by their emotions. Conversely, emotional cutoff (a construct akin to alexithymia reflecting a tendency to isolate oneself from others as well as from emotions) mediated the association between avoidant attachment and interpersonal problems, indicating that avoidantly attached individuals experience interpersonal problems only when they tend to distance themselves from internal emotional experiences (Wei et al., 2005). As this important study indicates, individuals with distinct insecure attachment patterns are at risk for problematic interpersonal interactions, but the underlying processes in terms of impaired emotion regulation are notably different, and congruent with their attachment strategies.

In sum, there is growing evidence for the mediating role of impaired emotion regulation, and alexithymia in particular, in the relationship between insecure attachment and interpersonal problems. Yet, several questions remain unanswered. First, although several studies report impaired emotional awareness as a mediator, NA has also been reported as a mediator. Second, it appears that the process through which interpersonal problems arise differs as a function of diverse attachment strategies, but this needs further study. Third, most of the studies in this area focused on nonclinical samples and it is not clear whether these findings extrapolate to patient samples. Last, the findings are in need of replication in a clinical sample using measures for both emotional and cognitive aspects of impaired emotion regulation. Therefore, in this study, we investigated whether impaired emotional awareness mediated the association between attachment strategies and interpersonal problems using two types of alexithymia. Bermond, Vorst, and Moormann (2006) have proposed that different ways of processing emotions can be identified based on an affective and a cognitive alexithymia dimension. The affective dimension reflects a reduced ability to experience emotional feelings, whereas the cognitive dimension measures the ability to explicitly process and verbalize emotional states (Vorst & Bermond, 2001). The cognitive dimension reflects the "core" alexithymia construct, while the affective dimension is a complementary construct that is in need of further study.

Objectives of the Present Study

The main aim of this study is to examine whether alexithymia mediates the relationship between insecure attachment strategies and interpersonal problems in SFD patients. This study focuses on two dimensions of alexithymia—affective and cognitive alexithymia—as well as NA as putative mediators of the attachment—interpersonal problems link in a sample of severely disturbed patients with SFD. Based on previous findings reviewed above, we expected that cognitive alexithymia positively mediates the relationship between avoidant attachment and interpersonal problems. Since affective alexithymia reflects a mirror construct to the "emotional reactivity" construct (Wei et al., 2005), we expected that affective alexithymia negatively mediates the link between anxious attachment and interpersonal problems.

Given the positive association between NA and attachment (Wearden et al., 2003, 2005), and the fact that NA has also been reported as a mediator of the association under study, we will include NA in the mediation models as a control variable, to test whether the alexithymia variables mediate the association between insecure attachment (avoidant or anxious) and interpersonal problems, even after controlling for the (mediating) impact of NA. Finally, we tested whether NA acted as a moderator of the tested mediator, to explore whether the mediation effect holds in subsamples with low and high NA.

Thus, in sum, four mediation models were tested based on these considerations:

Model 1. Cognitive alexithymia as mediator of the association between avoidant attachment and interpersonal problems;

Model 2. Cognitive alexithymia as mediator of the association between avoidant attachment and interpersonal problems, controlled for negative affectivity;

Model 3. Affective alexithymia as a mediator of the association between anxious attachment and interpersonal problems;

Model 4. Affective alexithymia as a mediator of the association between anxious attachment and interpersonal problems, controlled for negative affectivity.

The focus on alexithymia is important, because alexithymic patients are less responsive to treatment, and present clinicians with a challenge because of patients' seeming reluctance to discuss emotions (Ogrodniczuk, Piper, & Joyce, 2004; Stingl et al., 2008; Viinamäki et al., 2002). Studying its correlates and potential impact on other treatment targets, such as interpersonal functioning, may provide new insights into potentially helpful treatment strategies.

Method

Participants

The initial sample included 173 patients referred to Altrecht Psychosomatic Medicine Eikenboom, one of the largest treatment centres in the Netherlands that specializes in the treatment of severe SFD. Eikenboom provides inpatient programs, day hospital programs, and outpatient care for patients with undifferentiated SFD, conversion disorder, pain disorder, and somatization disorder (Van der Boom & Houtveen, 2014). Patients admitted to Altrecht Psychosomatic Medicine Eikenboom have generally suffered from their complaints for a mean duration of 10 years (Van der Boom & Houtveen, 2014). Patients at Eikenboom were consecutively included, that is, each individual patient was included in the study at the moment of his/her individual referral.

Of the initial 173 patients, 45 patients did not meet DSM-IV criteria for SFD, as diagnosed by the treating psychiatrist, so that the final study sample comprised 128 patients with SFD (undifferentiated SFD; $N = 60$; somatization disorder: $N = 3$; pain disorder: $N = 42$; conversion disorder: $N = 23$). Most patients were women ($N = 90$; 70%). The average age of the patients was 41.3 ($SD = 10.7$) years. Length of education was high (12–18 years) for 63% of the patients, and low (< 12 years) for 37%. Of the 128 cases, 8 cases (6%) were excluded from all further analyses due to incomplete data. Therefore, the final sample comprised 120 patients meeting DSM-IV criteria for SFD.

Design and Procedures

The research aims of the present study were addressed utilizing a cross-sectional design with one assessment point at intake. All patients were screened for inclusion by trained psychologists and the diagnosis was confirmed by the resident psychiatrist. The main inclusion criterion was the presence of a somatoform disorder according to DSM-IV(TR) citeria. Each eligible participant underwent a standard psychological assessment procedure, including the administration of a number of self-report measures between January 2009 and June 2010. The psychological assessment, which took on average two hours, was held on site. Trained clinical staff, with a minimum of a master's degree in psychology, was in charge of conducting the assessment procedure. The study was approved by the scientific and ethical committe of Altrecht. Informed consent was required from each participant before inclusion in the study.

Measures

Experiences in Close Relationships

The ECR (Fraley et al., 2000) consists of two subscales reflecting the two adult attachment dimensions—*avoidance* of intimacy and *anxiety* of rejection and separation—each covering 18 items. Participants have to rate statements using a 7-point Likert scale, which ranges from 1 ("strongly disagree") to 7 ("strongly agree"). Internal consistencies of these two dimensions are excellent ($\alpha > .93$) (Sibley & Liu, 2004). Exploratory and confirmatory factor analyses have generally replicated the theoretical two-factor structure (Conradi, Gerlsma, Duijn, & Jonge, 2006), and structural equation modeling showed that both dimensions were remarkably stable over a 6-week period (Sibley & Liu, 2004). According to a study by Conradi et al. in two Dutch and one American sample, correlations of the two ECR dimensions were theoretically coherent, and consistent with other attachment measures, indicating adeqate convergent validity. In the current study, the Dutch translation of the ECR-R was used (Luyten, Lowyck, & Vliegen, 2007).

Inventory of Interpersonal Problems–32 Item Version

The IIP-32 (Barkham, Hardy, & Startup, 1996) consists of eight subscales (domineering/controlling, vindictive/self-centered, cold/distant, socially inhibited, nonassertive, overly accommodating, self-sacrificing, intrusive/needy), and a total of 32 items. Each items is rated on a 5-point Likert scale: 0 (not at all), 1 (a little bit), 2 (moderately), 3 (quite a bit), and 4 (extremely). The 32-item version (Barkham et al., 1996) is a short version of the 64-item version, which in turn was derived from the original 127-item Inventory of Interpersonal Problems (IIP) (Horowitz, Rosenberg, Baer, Ureño, & Villaseñor, 1988). Factorial analysis by Horowitz et al. (1988) showed six subscales which had high internal consistency and high test-retest reliability. In a study among patients and students that compared the IIP-64 and IIP-32, similar results were obtained, showing adequate psychometric properties (Vanheule, Desmet, & Rosseel, 2006). Various versions of the IIP have been examined in relation to personality disorders and attachment styles, generally supporting the convergent validity (Horowitz, Alden, Wiggins, & Pincus, 2000). The IIP-32 total score ranges from 0 to 128. A higher score reflects greater distress related to interpersonal problems. In this study, the Dutch version of the IIP-32 was used (Vanheule et al., 2006). Following Wei et al. (2005), we used the total sum score. In the present study, the coefficient alpha for the IIP-32 total score was .91, indicating that the scale reflects a homogeneous construct.

Bermond-Vorst Alexithymia Questionnaire

The BVAQ (Vorst & Bermond, 2001) is a 40-item questionnaire that assesses two dimensions (affective and cognitive) of the alexithymia construct across five subscales. The subscales of "identifying," "verbalizing," and "analyzing" compose the "cognitive" dimension of alexithymia, which measures the verbal-explicit features of the alexithymia construct. The facets of fantasizing, and emotionalizing, represent the "affective" dimension of alexithymia that measures the reduced ability to experience emotional feelings, and reduced imaginative capacity (Moorman et al., 2008). Each item is rated on a 5-point Likert scale ranging from 1 ("This definitely applies") to 5 ("This in no way applies"). High scores are indicative of high levels of alexithymia. Several studies have supported the psychometric features of the BVAQ (Vorst & Bermond, 2001; Zech, Luminet, Rime, & Wagner, 1999). The differentiation between a cognitive and an affective dimension has been validated by factor analyses in six languages and seven populations (Bermond et al., 2007). Alpha coefficients for the subscales are generally above .70. In this study, the higher order dimensions of affective and cognitive alexithymia are used.

Negativism Subscale of the Dutch Short Form of the MMPI (DSFM)

The Negativism subscale of the DSFM (Luteijn & Kok, 1985) measures NA, and contains 22 items derived from the MMPI Psychopathic Deviation- (PD), Mania- (MA), Lie- (L), Depression-(D), Masculine/Feminine- (M/F), and Schizophrenia- (SC) domains. Negativism measures subjective feelings of discontent, disappointment, apathy, resistance, irritation, and distrust. Respondents with a high score on this scale are dissatisfied with their lives and have a hostile attitude toward others. They often feel tense and are self-defensive and irritable. Items are rated as true (2) or false (0). Participants have the option to respond with a question mark (1) when in doubt about their answer, but are requested to choose as few question marks as possible. The internal consistency of this scale is good (Cronbach's $\alpha = .80$) (Kline, 2000). Concerning the validity of the scale, Bramsen, Dirkzwager, and Van der Ploeg (2000) found Negativism to be a positive predictor of posttraumatic stress disorder symptom severity among former United Nations peacekeepers. Bodde et al. (2007) studied factors involved in the long-term prognosis of psychogenic nonepileptic seizures in a 4 to 6 years follow-up study. Negativism showed high temporal stability, and negatively predicted long-term seizure improvement.

Statistical Analysis

First, zero-order (Pearson) correlations were calculated between attachment strategies, interpersonal problems, cognitive and affective alexithymia, and NA. Before being able to run regressions that are required to calculate mediation effects, potential violations were examined. Hence, regression assumptions of linearity, homoscedasticity, independence of errors, and normality of error distribution were checked. No violations were observed. Also, there was no evidence for multicollinearity. All variance inflation factor (VIF) values were below 2.5. Demographic variables (age, gender, and education) were explored for potential associations with the dependent variable to see if any demographic variable should be controlled for in the regressions. For this purpose, Cohen's (1988) effect size d was included where pertinent.

The presence of mediation was tested further by using mediational path analysis in accordance with Baron and Kenny's (1986) recommendations. This entails, first, that there must be a significant relationship between the independent variable and the dependent variable (total effect c in Figure 1). Second, a significant association is required between the independent variable and the proposed mediator (path a in Figure 1). Third, the proposed mediator must be significantly associated with the dependent variable after controlling for the independent variable (path b in Figure 1). Fourth, the relationship between the independent variable and the dependent variable must be significantly reduced when the putative mediator is added to the model (direct effect c' in Figure 1). In other words, the total effect c (step 1) should be reduced to a level of non-significance after controlling for the indirect effect ab (steps 2 and 3). Since contemporary approaches tend to focus on the indirect effect, a more direct test of indirect effects was employed using the Sobel (1982) test. A p-value of $< .05$ was considered significant (two-tailed). This was followed by a bootstrapping procedure using 5,000 re-samples and

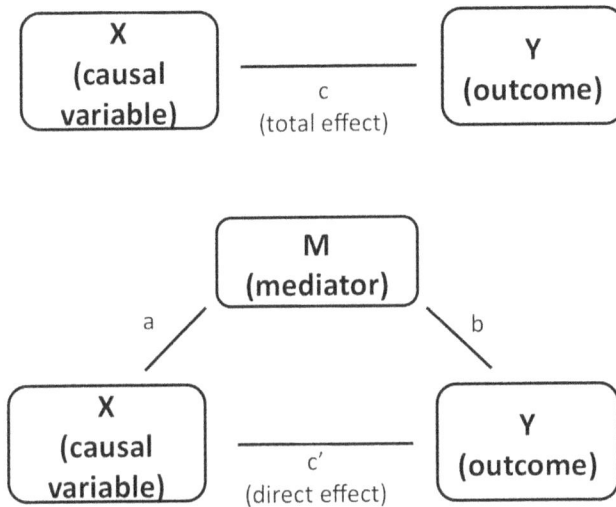

Figure 1. Unmediated model (above), showing the total effect c of variable X on variable Y, and the mediation model (below), showing the direct effect c' of variable X on variable Y, after the intervening variable M has been taken into account. a and b in combination denote the indirect effect ab.

a 95% confidence interval (CI) (Preacher & Hayes, 2004, 2008). The indirect effect was considered significant if the 95% CI did not include zero.

Fritz and MacKinnon (2007) propose that in case of medium effect size betas ($\beta = .39$) for paths a and b, a sample size of approximately $N = 400$ is required to test for the presence of full mediation (i.e., the direct effect should be equal to zero) using Baron and Kenny's (1986) approach, whereas a sample size of approximately $N = 120$ is needed to test for partial mediation (i.e., the direct effect is not reduced to zero) using this approach. However, tests of the indirect effect, such as bootstrapping, are more robust and require a smaller sample size than the Sobel test and Baron and Kenny's recommended testing (Fritz & MacKinnon, 2007). Accordingly, a sample size of approximately $N = 78$ is required using the percentile bootstrap approach, where medium effect sizes are concerned. Therefore, we expect that our sample ($N = 120$) has sufficient power to detect medium mediation effects. In the relevant mediation steps, that is, the steps that are associated with the indirect effect (paths a and b), R^2 change and f^2 are reported as indication of explained variance, and effect size, respectively. f^2 was calculated from R^2 using the formula: $f^2 = R^2 / (1 - R^2)$, where $f^2 = .02$ is considered small, $f^2 = .15$ medium, and $f^2 = .35$ large (Cohen, 1988). For the effect size of the indirect effect (ab), Preacher and Kelley's (2011) kappa-squared method was used. It is analogous in interpretation to R^2 (Field, 2013)—with 0.01, 0.09 and 0.25 representing small, medium and large effects respectively. Kappa-squared expresses the proportion of the observed indirect effect to the maximum possible indirect effect that could have been observed given the study design. It may vary between 0 (no indirect effect) to 1 (maximum possible indirect effect). Kappa-squared was presented with its associated 95% CI. The Kappa-squared method is available only for simple mediation models, i.e., for mediation models in which no additional control variables are included (Hayes, 2013). We also exploratively tested for moderated mediation with NA acting as a moderator of the mediation effect, using the same steps as previously described, but this time in two subsamples with low (below average ≤ 19) or high (above average ≥ 28) NA, following norm scores for psychiatric patiens (Luteijn & Kok, 1985).

Results

Demographic Characteristics and Zero-Order Correlations

Demographic features were examined for potential associations with the dependent variable (interpersonal problems) to see if any demographic variable should be controlled for in the regressions. This was not the case. Age was not associated with interpersonal problems (r (120) = 0.12, n.s.). Independent samples t-tests showed that gender was also not associated with interpersonal problems (t(118) = 0.96, n.s.; d = 0.20). Last, the level of education was unrelated to interpersonal problems (t(117) = 0.26, n.s.; d = 0.05). Zero-order correlations between the main variables are presented in Table 1. As can be seen in this table, NA is significantly associated with one of the proposed mediators, that is, affective alexithymia (r (120) = -.42, $p < .01$). Also, NA is associated with the main variable of interest, i.e., interpersonal problems (r(120) = .44, p < .01). This justifies running separate mediation models with NA as a control variable. Finally, anxious attachment was positively correlated with interpersonal problems (r(120) = .54, $p < .01$), and avoidant attachment was positively associated with interpersonal problems (r(120) = .22, $p < .01$). Based on Baron and Kenny' guidelines, this implies that the first prerequisite for mediation (a significant association between the independent and the dependent variable) is met.

Mediation Analyses

Four *a priori* mediation models were tested. The first two models tested cognitive alexithymia as a mediator with respect to avoidant attachment, and the latter two models tested affective alexithymia as a mediator with respect to anxious attachment.

Model 1: Cognitive Alexithymia as a Mediator

In the first step, avoidant attachment was significantly related to interpersonal problems (β = .22, $p < .05$). In the second step, avoidant attachment was also related to the mediator cognitive alexithymia [β = .42, $p < .001$; R^2 change = .17, f^2 = .21 (medium)]. In the third step, cognitive alexithymia was significantly associated with interpersonal problems, after controlling for the influence of avoidant attachment [β = .32, $p < .001$; R^2 change = .09, f^2 = .10 (small)]. In the final step, the association between avoidant attachment and interpersonal problems was rendered nonsignificant after cognitive alexithymia was added to the model (β = .08, ns). Consistent with these findings, the Sobel test revealed a significant

Table 1. Correlations between interpersonal problems, anxious attachment, avoidant attachment, cognitive alexithymia, affective alexithymia, and negative affectivity (N = 120).

	IIP	ECR-Anx	ECR-Avoid	BVAQ-Cogn	BVAQ-Aff	NA
ECR-Anx	.54**	1.00				
ECR-Avoid	.22**	.49**	1.00			
BVAQ-Cogn	.36**	.14	.42**	1.00		
BVAQ-Aff	-.25 **	-.27**	.02	.15	1.00	
NA	.44**	.58**	.18*	.15	-.42**	1.00

Note. Significant correlations are highlighted in bold; IIP: interpersonal problems; ECR-Anx: anxious attachment; ECR-Avoid: avoidant attachment; BVAQ-Cogn: cognitive alexithymia; BVAQ-Aff : affective alexithymia; NA: negative affectivity.
$^*p < .05$. $^{**}p < .01$.

mediation effect ($z = 2.82, p < .01$). Results from bootstrapping also yielded a significant indirect effect [B = .15, 95% CI (.07, .28)]. According to the kappa-squared method, the effect size of the indirect effect was $\kappa^2 = .13$ (.06–.22), which corresponds to a medium effect size.

Model 2: Cognitive Alexithymia as a Mediator Controlling for NA

In the second model, we tested whether cognitive alexithymia was still a significant mediator after controlling for NA. This was indeed the case. The total effect was reduced from $\beta = .15$ ($p < .10$), to $\beta = .03$ (n.s.), after inclusion of both NA and cognitive alexithymia in the model, indicating full mediation. The effect size of path a was $f^2 = .19$ (medium), and the effect size of path b was $f^2 = .07$ (small). Sobel's test was still highly significant ($z = 2.71, p < .01$). Bootstrapping also showed a significant indirect effect [B = .13, 95% CI (.06, .23)].

Model 3: Affective Alexithymia as a Mediator

In the first step, anxious attachment was significantly related to interpersonal problems ($\beta = .54, p < .001$). In the second step, anxious attachment was negatively, yet significantly, related to the mediator affective alexithymia ($\beta = -.27, p < .001$; R^2 change $= .07, f^2 = .08$). In the third step, affective alexithymia was not significantly associated with interpersonal problems, after controlling for the influence of anxious attachment ($\beta = -.12, p =$ n.s.; R^2 change $= .01, f^2 = .01$). In the final step, the association between anxious attachment and interpersonal problems was still highly significant after affective alexithymia was added to the model ($\beta = .50, p < .01$), indicating that affective alexithymia was not a mediator in this model. Consistent with these findings, the Sobel test revealed a nonsignificant mediation effect ($z = 1.31, p < .10$). Results from bootstrapping also indicated a nonsignificant indirect effect [B = .03, 95% CI (−.01, .09)]. Kappa-squared was equivalent to a small effect size [$\kappa^2 = .04$ (.00–.11)].

Model 4: Affective Alexithymia as a Mediator Controlling for NA

In the fourth and final a priori model, we tested whether the combined effect of NA and affective alexithymia yielded a significant mediation model. This was not the case. The total effect was not reduced after inclusion of affective alexithymia as mediator and NA as covariate into the model. The direct tests for the indirect effect (β path $a = -.05$, n.s.; R^2 change $< .01, f^2 < .01$, and β path $b = -.07$, n.s.; R^2 change $< .01, f^2 < .01$) were both nonsignificant (Sobel: $z = 0.38$, n.s.; bootstrapping: B $< .01$, 95% CI (−.01, .04).

Moderated Mediation in Subgroups with Low and High NA

Given the combined influence of NA and cognitive alexithymia on the association between avoidant attachment and interpersonal problems, we exploratively tested for moderated mediation with NA moderating the mediating effect of cognitive alexithymia. The steps for mediation analysis were repeated in two subsamples with low ($N = 48$) and high ($N = 29$) NA. Results indicated that NA indeed moderated the mediation effect reported above: In the subgroup with high NA, cognitive alexithymia turned out to be a mediator of the association between avoidant attachment and interpersonal problems [Sobel: $z = 2.00, p < .05$; Bootstrapping: B = .22, 95% CI (.07, .51)], but not in the subgroup with low NA [Sobel: $z = 1.04$, ns; Bootstrapping: B = .09, 95% CI (−.07, .26)].

In conclusion, results supported models 1 and 2, but not models 3 and 4. Cognitive alexithymia is a mediator of the association between avoidant attachment and interpersonal problems, even after controlling for the influence of NA. This implies that for those patients with SFD reporting concerns over intimacy and autonomy (avoidant attachment), interpersonal problems are more likely to arise when they are struggling with the identification and verbal expression of emotions. Explorative testing of moderated mediation indicated that this mediation effect may hold specifically in subgroups of patients with high levels of NA. The models for affective alexithymia were not significant.

Discussion

This study clearly shows that interpersonal problems do not automatically follow from insecure attachment strategies, but are contingent upon alexithymic features. Patients with SFD tend to have great difficulties recognizing negative emotions, because they are less likely to interpret physical sensations as negative emotional states (Dendy, Cooper, & Sharpe, 2001). However, when patients do experience high levels of negative emotion, they may be at risk for decreased social functioning if they are unable to verbalize and hence communicate their mental distress. One might question how patients can report high levels of negative affect, while at the same time being unable to recognize and identify these as emotions. It is not uncommon in patients with SFD to report high levels of negative affect. From a psychological perspective, this may reflect a tendency to ruminate, that is, a vicious cycle of activation of generic negative experience, while being unable to recruit top-down regulatory mechanisms, such as the conscious recognition and awareness of specific emotions at the moment of distress (Lane, 2008).

Results of this study offer an important target for intervention. Avoidant individuals, particularly those experiencing a broad range of negative emotions, such as anger, irritation, frustration, and sadness, may be stimulated to actively engage in the identification, awareness, and communication of these emotions, particularly those that are elicited in treatment. This calls for an interpersonal approach, during which the therapist is emotionally present for the patient, and is transparent about his/her own emotional reactions. In this context, it is relevant that alexithymic patients tend to evoke negative reactions in therapists, because these patients also express relatively few positive emotions (Ogrodniczuk, Piper, & Joyce, 2011). Therefore, the focus in treatment should certainly not be limited to the expression of negative emotions (both on the part of therapist and patient), particularly in working with patients that experience high levels of negative emotions.

This interpersonal focus is congruent with recent interpersonal mentalization-based approaches to the treatment of somatoform pathology (Arbeitskreis PISO, 2012; Luyten et al., 2012). These treatments focus on the restoration of the link between bodily distress and emotional states, and how these relate to dysfunctional interpersonal (attachment) patterns that are often associated with the onset and perpetuation of physical symptoms (Arbeitskreis PISO, 2012; Luyten & Van Houdenhove, 2013). Our findings are also consistent with previous reports showing that impaired „theory of mind", a construct akin to alexithymia and mentalization, was associated with decreased social functioning in patients with chronic fatigue syndrome (Oldershaw et al., 2011). In sum, findings from both empirical research and clinical practice converge to suggest that interpersonal functioning in patients suffering from SFD could be improved by enhancing capacities for emotional awareness and reflection in the context of insecure attachment relationships (Luyten & Van Houdenhove, 2013).

The strong link between (avoidant) attachment and cognitive alexithymia observed in the current study is consistent with the mentalization-based approach to development, that posits that the early attachment bond between caregiver and child facilitates the development of an internalized representational system for the regulation of affects (Fonagy & Target, 2006). Furthermore, the findings in the present study are in line with recent theoretical formulations, which contend that the cacapity to understand interactions and relationships in terms of mental states is critically challenged when stress or negative affects increase (Fonagy & Luyten, 2009). Avoidant individuals are relatively resilient, but when stress levels increase disproportionately, or when experiencing chronic stress, these individuals suffer from a breakthrough of previously warded off negative emotions, that are subsequently difficult to regulate, mentalize, and verbalize, which (further) undermines their interpersonal functioning (Fonagy & Luyten, 2009; Mikulincer, Dolev, & Shaver, 2004). Therefore, future studies should ideally focus on the combined presence of negative affects, and cognitive alexithymia, and its treatment implications, particularly among SFD patients with avoidant attachment strategies.

Limitations

This study has several limitations, which need to be considered when interpreting the results. First, the cross-sectional design of the study does not allow to identify causal relationships, but reflects only an assessment of the relationships between variables. Yet, the presence of mediation does give us some indication of the direction of associations between the main variables and may pave the way for longitudinal research into the role of emotion dysregulation as a function of attachment strategies in the causation of interpersonal problems. It seems particularly indicated to test the validity of cognitive alexithymia as a putative mechanism of change in psychotherapy, particularly in case interpersonal difficulties are considered a relevant outcome domain. Second, only self-report measures were used in this study. As people with alexithymia tend to have impaired emotional awareness and self-reflection, the validity of the BVAQ, in particular, may fall short for patients lacking some rudimentary level of self-reflection. Observer-based or performance-based measures of alexithymia such as clinician's ratings or computerized tasks might be useful for future research on this subject (e.g., the Toronto Structured Interview for Alexithymia; Bagby, Taylor, Parker, & Dickens, 2006). Furthermore, some of the findings may have been influenced by shared-method variance. Third, the model with affective alexithymia (models 3 and 4) did not reach significance, which may have been due to the limited sample size. Affective alexithymia was not a significant mediator, but the kappa-squared test indicated that the indirect effect was equivalent to a small effect size, suggesting that more power was needed to potentially reveal significant mediation in this model. At the same time, it seems highly unlikely that a type II error occured given that the final beta weights hardly changed. Fourth, findings from the present study may not necessarily generalize to other samples, since the current sample was characterized by high levels of trauma (Van Dijke et al., 2011). Fifth, our study findings can be generalized only to patients with DSM-IV(-TR) somatoform disorder, and not to patients with DSM-5 "Somatic Symptom Disorder"." Although high overlap can be expected, given the more lenient DSM-5 criteria for somatic symptom disorder, and the rejection of the dualistic assumption of psyche and soma which was implicit in DSM-IV, the DSM-5 group would be broader, and thus findings must be replicated using the renewed diagnostic criteria. Sixth, the high percentage (47%) of patients in our sample fulfilling the criteria for "undifferentiated somatoform disorder" was somewhat atypical. De Waal et al. (2004), for example, reported a prevalence estimate of 13.1% for undifferentiated SFD in general practice. However, our sample was recruited at a highly specialized treatment centre, which is likely representative of other specialized inpatient treatment facilities. Nevertheless, this calls into question the validity of this "wastebasket category," which has now been replaced with "Unspecified Somatic Symptom and Related Disorder" in DSM-5. Last, although our results suggest that cognitive alexithymia may be a risk factor for interpersonal problems in avoidantly attached patients, it cannot be ruled out that another (unmeasured) variable strongly associated with alexithymia, such as reduced empathy, is responsible for our findings. Several studies have implied that alexithymic individuals have reduced empathic abilities, and a reduced capacity to take the perspective of others, which is likely to have a profound impact on interpersonal functioning (Grynberg, Luminet, Corneille, Grèzes, & Berthoz, 2010; Moriguchi et al., 2006). In other words, reduced empathy is bound to cause conflicts and interpersonal problems. Future studies should study alexithymia while controlling for empathy.

Conclusion

This study has shown that cognitive alexithymia mediates the relationship between avoidant attachment and interpersonal problems in patients with somatoform disorder. More specifically, results from the present study indicate that the combined presence of both high levels of NA, and cognitive alexithymia are potential risk factors for complicated patterns of interpersonal relationships, and possibly as a result, a chronic course for SFD. Therefore, treatments may need to focus on impaired emotion regulation in SFD, i.e., the identification and expression of both negative and positive affects. Future studies should clarify and extend these findings by continuing to examine the role of different types of emotion regulation deficits as putative mediators between insecure attachment and interpersonal difficulties in both clinical and non-clinical samples, preferably using longitudinal designs. Last, studies should focus on emotion regulation deficits, such as alexithymia, as putative mechanisms of change in psychotherapy, particularly for patients with SFD, who often show severely impaired interpersonal functioning.

References

American Psychiatric Association. (2000). *Diagnostic and statistical manual of mental disorders, Fourth edition, text revision.* Washington, DC: American Psychiatric Press.
Arbeitskreis PISO. (2012). *Somatoforme Störungen. Psychodynamisch-Interpersonelle Therapie (PISO).* Göttingen, Germany: Hogrefe.

Bagby, R. M., Taylor, G. J., Parker, J. D. A., & Dickens, S. E. (2006). The development of the Toronto structured interview for Alexithymia: Item selection, factor structure, reliability and concurrent validity. *Psychotherapy and Psychosomatics, 75*(1), 25–39.

Bakermans-Kranenburg, M. J., & van IJzendoorn, M. H. (2009). The first 10,000 Adult Attachment Interviews: Distributions of adult attachment representations in clinical and non-clinical groups. *Attachment & Human Development, 11*(3), 223–263.

Barkham, M., Hardy, G. E., & Startup, M. (1996). The IIP-32: A short version of the Inventory of Interpersonal Problems. *The British Journal of Clinical Psychology / the British Psychological Society, 35*(Pt 1), 21–35.

Baron, R. M., & Kenny, D. A. (1986). The moderator-mediator variable distinction in social psychological research: Conceptual, strategic, and statistical considerations. *Journal of Personality and Social Psychology, 51*(6), 1173–1182.

Bermond, B., Clayton, K., Liberova, A., Luminet, O., Maruszewski, T., Bitti, P. E. R.,…Wicherts, J. (2007). A cognitive and an affective dimension of alexithymia in six languages and seven populations. *Cognition & Emotion, 21*(5), 1125–1136. http://doi.org/10.1080/02699930601056989

Bermond, B., Vorst, H. C. M., & Moormann, P. P. (2006). Cognitive neuropsychology of alexithymia: Implications for personality typology. *Cognitive Neuropsychiatry, 11*(3), 332–360.

Bodde, N. M. G., Janssen, A. M. A. J., Theuns, C., Vanhoutvin, J. F. G., Boon, P. A. J. M., & Aldenkamp, A. P. (2007). Factors involved in the long-term prognosis of psychogenic nonepileptic seizures. *Journal of Psychosomatic Research, 62*(5), 545–551.

Bramsen, I., Dirkzwager, A. J. E., & Van Der Ploeg, H. M. (2000). Predeployment personality traits and exposure to trauma as predictors of posttraumatic stress symptoms: A prospective study of former peacekeepers. *American Journal of Psychiatry, 157*(7), 1115–1119.

Brennan, K. A., Clark, C. L., & Shaver, P. R. (1998). Self-Report measures of adult attachment: An integrative overview. In J. A. Simpson & W. S. Rholes (Eds.), *Attachment theory and close relationships* (pp. 46–76). New York: The Guildford Press.

Cohen, J. (1988). *Statical Power Analysis for the Behavioral Sciences* (2nd ed.). Hillsdale, NJ: Lawrence Erlbaum.

Conradi, H., Gerlsma, C., Duijn, M. van, & Jonge, P. de. (2006). Internal and external validity of the experiences in close relationships questionnaire in an American and two Dutch samples. *The European Journal of Psychiatry, 20*(4), 258–269.

Crawford, T. N., Shaver, P. R., Cohen, P., Pilkonis, P. A., Gillath, O., & Kasen, S. (2006). Self-reported attachment, interpersonal aggression, and personality disorder in a prospective community sample of adolescents and adults. *Journal of Personality Disorders, 20*(4), 331–351.

Davies, K. A., Macfarlane, G. J., McBeth, J., Morriss, R., & Dickens, C. (2009). Insecure attachment style is associated with chronic widespread pain. *Pain, 143*(3), 200–205.

De Gucht, V., & Heiser, W. (2003). Alexithymia and somatisation: A quantitative review of the literature. *Journal of Psychosomatic Research, 54*(5), 425–434.

De Waal, M. W. M., Arnold, I. A., Eekhof, J. A. H., & van Hemert, A. M. (2004). Somatoform disorders in general practice: Prevalence, functional impairment and comorbidity with anxiety and depressive disorders. *The British Journal of Psychiatry: The Journal of Mental Science, 184*, 470–476. http://doi.org/10.1192/bjp.184.6.470

Deborde, A.-S., Miljkovitch, R., Roy, C., Bigre, C. D.-L., Pham-Scottez, A., Speranza, M., & Corcos, M. (2012). Alexithymia as a mediator between attachment and the development of Borderline Personality Disorder in adolescence. *Journal of Personality Disorders, 26*(5), 676–688.

Dendy, C., Cooper, M., & Sharpe, M. (2001). Interpretation of symptoms in chronic fatigue syndrome. *Behaviour Research and Therapy, 39*(11), 1369–1380.

Field, A. (2013). *Discovering statistics using IBM SPSS statistics* (4th ed.). Washington, DC: Sage.

Fonagy, P., Gergely, G., Jurist, E., & Target, M. (2002). *Affect regulation, mentalization and the development of the Self.* New York, NY: Other Press.

Fonagy, P., & Luyten, P. (2009). A developmental, mentalization-based approach to the understanding and treatment of borderline personality disorder. *Development and Psychopathology, 21*(4), 1355–1381.

Fonagy, P., & Target, M. (2006). The mentalization-focused approach to self pathology. *Journal of Personality Disorders, 20*(6), 544–576.

Fossati, A., Acquarini, E., Feeney, J. A., Borroni, S., Grazioli, F., Giarolli, L. E., Franciosi, G., & Maffei, C. (2009). Alexithymia and attachment insecurities in impulsive aggression. *Attachment & Human Development, 11*(2), 165–182.

Fraley, R. C., Waller, N. G., & Brennan, K. A. (2000). An item response theory analysis of self-report measures of adult attachment. *Journal of Personality and Social Psychology, 78*(2), 350–365.

Fritz, M. S., & MacKinnon, D. P. (2007). Required sample size to detect the mediated effect. *Psychological Science, 18*(3), 233–239. doi:10.1111/j.1467-9280.2007.01882.x

Gil, F. P., Scheidt, C. E., Hoeger, D., & Nickel, M. (2008). Relationship between attachment style, parental bonding and alexithymia in adults with somatoform disorders. *International Journal of Psychiatry in Medicine, 38*(4), 437–451.

Govender, C., Cassimjee, N., Schoeman, J., & Meyer, H. (2009). Psychological characteristics of FMS patients. *Scandinavian Journal of Caring Sciences, 23*(1), 76–83. http://doi.org/10.1111/j.1471-6712.2007.00592.x

Grynberg, D., Luminet, O., Corneille, O., Grèzes, J., & Berthoz, S. (2010). Alexithymia in the interpersonal domain: A general deficit of empathy? *Personality and Individual Differences, 49*(8), 845–850.

Haggerty, G., Hilsenroth, M. J., & Vala-Stewart, R. (2009). Attachment and interpersonal distress: Examining the relationship between attachment styles and interpersonal problems in a clinical population. *Clinical Psychology and Psychotherapy, 16*(1), 1–9.

Hahn, S. R. (2001). Physical symptoms and physician-experienced difficulty in the physician-patient relationship. *Annals of Internal Medicine, 134*(9 II SUPPL.), 897–904.

Hansen, M. S., Fink, P., Frydenberg, M., & Oxhøj, M.-L. (2002). Use of health services, mental illness, and self-rated disability and health in medical inpatients. *Psychosomatic Medicine, 64*(4), 668–675.

Hayes, A.F. (2013). *Introduction to Mediation, Moderation, and Conditional Process Analysis.* New York: The Guilford press.

Hill, J., Stepp, S. D., Wan, M. W., Hope, H., Morse, J. Q., Steele, M., Steele, H, & Pilkonis, P. A. (2011). Attachment, Borderline Personality, and Romantic Relationship Dysfunction. *Journal of Personality Disorders, 25*(6), 789–805.

Horowitz, L., Alden, L. E., Wiggins, J. S., & Pincus, A. L. (2000). *Inventory of interpersonal problems manual.* Odessa, FL: The Psychological Corporation.

Horowitz, L. M., Rosenberg, S. E., Baer, B. A., Ureño, G., & Villaseñor, V. S. (1988). Inventory of interpersonal problems: Psychometric properties and clinical applications. *Journal of Consulting and Clinical Psychology, 56*(6), 885–892. http://doi.org/10.1037/0022-006x.56.6.885

Kim, Y., Song, J. Y., Bahn, G. H., Kim, J. W., & Shin, Y. S. (2005). Characteristics of the attachment in patients with somatoform disorder. *Journal of the Korean Neuropsychiatric Association, 44*, 700–707.

Kline, P. (2000). *The handbook of psychological testing* (2nd ed.). New York, NY: Routledge.

Kooiman, C. G., & Koelen, J. A. (2012). Gehechtheid en somatisatie (attachment and somatization). *Tijdschrift Voor Psychotherapie, 38*(4), 291–309.

Kool, M. B., van Middendorp, H., Lumley, M. A., Schenk, Y., Jacobs, J. W. G., Bijlsma, J. W. J., & Geenen, R. (2010). Lack of understanding in fibromyalgia and rheumatoid arthritis: The Illness Invalidation Inventory (3*I). *Annals of the Rheumatic Diseases, 69*(11), 1990–1995.

Lane, R. D. (2008). Neural substrates of implicit and explicit emotional processes: A unifying framework for psychosomatic medicine. *Psychosomatic Medicine, 70*, 214–231.

Lieberman, M. D., Eisenberger, N. I., Crockett, M. J., Tom, S. M., Pfeifer, J. H., & Way, B. M. (2007). Putting feelings into words. *Psychological Science, 18*(5), 421–428.

Luteijn, F., & Kok, A. R. (1985). *Nederlandse Verkorte MMPI (NVM) manual, Rev. ed. [Dutch Short Form of the MMPI (DSFM)].* Lisse, the Netherlands: Swets & Zeitlinger B.V.

Luyten, P., Lowyck, B., & Vliegen, N. (2007). *Experiences in close relationships-revised.* Unpublished manuscript. Leuven, Belgium: University of Leuven.

Luyten, P., & Van Houdenhove, B. (2013). Common and specific factors in the psychotherapeutic treatment of patients suffering from chronic fatigue and pain. *Journal of Psychotherapy Integration, 23*(1), 14–27.

Luyten, P., Van Houdenhove, B., Lemma, A., Target, M., & Fonagy, P. (2012). A mentalization-based approach to the understanding and treatment of functional somatic disorders. *Psychoanalytic Psychotherapy, 26*(2), 121–140.

Maunder, R. G., & Hunter, J. J. (2001). Attachment and psychosomatic medicine: Developmental contributions to stress and disease. *Psychosomatic Medicine, 63,* 556–567.

Meyer, B., & Pilkonis, P. A. (2005). An attachment model of personality disorders. In M. F. Lenzenweger & J. F. Clarkin (Eds.), *Major theories of personality disorder* (2nd ed., pp. 231–281). New York, NY: The Guildford Press.

Mikulincer, M., Dolev, T., & Shaver, P. R. (2004). Attachment-related strategies during thought suppression: Ironic rebounds and vulnerable self-representations. *Journal of Personality and Social Psychology, 87*(6), 940–956.

Moorman, P. P., Bermond, B., Vorst, H., Bloemendaal, A. F. T., Teijn, S. M., & Rood, L. (2008). New avenues in alexithymia research: the creation of alexithymia types. In A. J. J. Vingerhoets, I. Nyklíček, & J. Denollet (Eds.), *Emotion regulation: Conceptual and clinical issues* (pp. 27–42). New York: Springer.

Moriguchi, Y., Ohnishi, T., Lane, R. D., Maeda, M., Mori, T., Nemoto, K., Matsuda, H.., & Komaki, G. (2006). Impaired self-awareness and theory of mind: An fMRI study of mentalizing in alexithymia. *NeuroImage, 32*(3), 1472–1482. doi.org/10.1016/j.neuroimage.2006.04.186

Nicolò, G., Semerari, A., Lysaker, P. H., Dimaggio, G., Conti, L., D'Angerio, S.,…Carcione, A. (2011). Alexithymia in personality disorders: Correlations with symptoms and interpersonal functioning. *Psychiatry Research, 190*(1), 37–42.

Noyes, R., Langbehn, D. R., Happel, R. L., Stout, L. R., Muller, B. A., & Longley, S. L. (2001). Personality dysfunction among somatizing patients. *Psychosomatics, 42,* 320–329. doi.org/http://dx.doi.org/10.1176/appi.psy.42.4.320

Noyes, R., Stuart, S., & Watson, D. (2008). A reconceptualization of the somatoform disorders. *Psychosomatics, 49,* 14–22.

Ogrodniczuk, J. S., Piper, W. E., & Joyce, A. S. (2004). Residual symptoms in depressed patients who successfully respond to short-term psychotherapy. *Journal of Affective Disorders, 82*(3), 469–473.

Ogrodniczuk, J. S., Piper, W. E., & Joyce, A. S. (2011). Effect of alexithymia on the process and outcome of psychotherapy: A programmatic review. *Psychiatry Research, 190*(1), 43–48.

Oldershaw, a, Hambrook, D., Rimes, K. A, Tchanturia, K., Treasure, J., Richards, S., Schmidt, U., & Chalder, T. (2011). Emotion recognition and emotional theory of mind in chronic fatigue syndrome. *Psychology & Health, 26*(8), 989–1005. doi.org/10.1080/08870446.2010.519769

Preacher, K. J., & Hayes, A. F. (2004). SPSS and SAS procedures for estimating indirect effects in simple mediation models. *Behavior Research Methods, Instruments, & Computers: A Journal of the Psychonomic Society, Inc, 36*(4), 717–731.

Preacher, K. J., & Hayes, A. F. (2008). Asymptotic and resampling strategies for assessing and comparing indirect effects in multiple mediator models. *Behavior Research Methods, 40*(3), 879–891.

Preacher, K. J., & Kelley, K. (2011). Effect size measures for mediation models: Quantitative strategies for communicating indirect effects. *Psychological Methods, 16*(2), Jun 2011, 93–115. doi.org/10.1037/a0022658

Scheidt, C. E., & Waller, E. (1999). Bindungsrepraesentation, affektregulation, und psychophsyiologische reaktionsbereitschaft. [Attachment representation, affect regulation and psychophysiological reactivity]. *Zeitschrift Fuer Psychosomatische Medizin Und Psychotherapie, 45,* 313–332.

Selders, M., Visser, R., Rooij, W. van, Delfstra, G., & Koelen, J. A. (2015). The development of a brief group intervention (Dynamic Interpersonal Therapy) for patients with medically unexplained somatic symptoms: A pilot study. *Psychoanalytic Psychotherapy, 29*(2), 182–198. doi.org/DOI:10.1080/02668734.2015.1036106

Sibley, C. G., & Liu, J. H. (2004). Short-term temporal stability and factor structure of the revised experiences in close relationships (ECR-R) measure of adult attachment. *Personality and Individual Differences, 36*(4), 969–975.

Sobel, M. E. (1982). Asymptotic confidence intervals for indirect effects in structural equation models. *Sociological Methodology, 13,* 290–312. Retrieved from http://www.jstor.org/stable/270723?origin=crossref

Spaans, J. A., Veselka, L., Luyten, P., & Bühring, M. E. F. (2009). Bodily aspects of mentalization: A therapeutic focus in the treatment of patients with severe medically unexplained symptoms. *Tijdschrift Voor Psychiatrie, 51*(4), 239–248.

Spitzer, C., Siebel-Jurges, U., Barnow, S., Grabe, H. J., & Freyberger, H. J. (2005). Alexithymia and interpersonal problems. *Psychotherapy and Psychosomatics, 74*(4), 240–246. doi.org/10.1159/000085148

Stingl, M., Bausch, S., Walter, B., Kagerer, S., Leichsenring, F., & Leweke, F. (2008). Effects of inpatient psychotherapy on the stability of alexithymia characteristics. *Journal of Psychosomatic Research, 65*(2), 173–180.

Stuart, S. P., & Noyes, R. (1999). Attachment and interpersonal communication in somatization disorder. *Psychosomatics, 40*, 34–43.

Taylor, G. J. (1984). Alexithymia: Concept, measurement, and implications for treatment. *American Journal of Psychiatry, 141*(6), 725–732.

Van der Boom, K. J., & Houtveen, J. H. (2014). Psychiatrische comorbiditeit bij ernstige somatoforme stoornissen in de derdelijn [Psychiatric comborbidity in severe somatoform disorders in tertiary care]. *Tiijdschrift Voor Psychiatrie, 56*, 743–747.

Van Dijke, A., Ford, J. D., van der Hart, O., Son, M. J. M., van Heijden, P. G. M., & Bühring, M. E. F. (2011). Childhood traumatization by primary caretaker and affect dysregulation in patients with borderline personality disorder and somatoform disorder. *European Journal of Psychotraumatology, 2*, 5628. doi.org/10.3402/ejpt.v2i0.5628

Van Dijke, A., Van Der Hart, O., Van Son, M., Bühring, M., Van Der Heijden, P., & Ford, J. D. (2013). Cognitive and affective dimensions of difficulties in emotional functioning in somatoform disorders and borderline personality disorder. *Psychopathology, 46*(3), 153–162.

Vanheule, S., Desmet, M., & Rosseel, Y. (2006). The factorial structure of the Dutch translation of the inventory of interpersonal problems: A test of the long and short versions. *Psychological Assessment, 18*(1), 112–117.

Vanheule, S., Meganck, R., & Desmet, M. (2011). Alexithymia, social detachment and cognitive processing. *Psychiatry Research, 190*(1), 49–51.

Viinamäki, H., Hintikka, J., Tanskanen, A., Honkalampi, K., Antikainen, R., Koivumaa-Honkanen, H., …Lehtonen, J. (2002). Partial remission in major depression: A two-phase, 12-month prospective study. *Nordic Journal of Psychiatry, 56*(1), 33–37.

Vorst, H. C. M., & Bermond, B. (2001). Validity and reliability of the Bermond-Vorst Alexithymia Questionnaire. *Personality and Individual Differences, 30*(3), 413–434.

Waller, E., Scheidt, C. E., & Hartmann, A. (2004). Attachment representation and illness behavior in somatoform disorders. *The Journal of Nervous and Mental Disease, 192*(3), 200–209. doi.org/10.1097/01.nmd.0000116463.17588.07

Wearden, A., Cook, L., & Vaughan-Jones, J. (2003). Adult attachment, alexithymia, symptom reporting, and health-related coping. *Journal of Psychosomatic Research, 55*(4), 341–347.

Wearden, A. J., Lamberton, N., Crook, N., & Walsh, V. (2005). Adult attachment, alexithymia, and symptom reporting: An extension to the four category model of attachment. *Journal of Psychosomatic Research, 58*(3), 279–288.

Wei, M., Vogel, D. L., Ku, T.-Y., & Zakalik, R. A. (2005). Adult attachment, affect regulation, negative mood, and interpersonal problems: The mediating roles of emotional reactivity and emotional cutoff. *Journal of Counseling Psychology, 52*(1), 14–24.

Wittchen, H. U., Jacobi, F., Rehm, J., Gustavsson, A., Svensson, M., Jönsson, B.,…Steinhausen, H. C. (2011). The size and burden of mental disorders and other disorders of the brain in Europe 2010. *European Neuropsychopharmacology, 21*(9), 655–679.

Zech, E., Luminet, O., Rime, B., & Wagner, H. (1999). Alexithymia and its measurement: confirmatory factor analyses of the 20-item Toronto Alexithymia Scale and the Bermond - Vorst Alexithymia Questionnaire. *European Journal of Personality, 13*, 511–532. doi.org/10.1002/(SICI)1099-0984 (199911/12)13:6<511::AID-PER347>3.0.CO;2-0

Impact of Economic Hardship and Financial Threat on Suicide Ideation and Confusion

Lisa Fiksenbaum, Zdravko Marjanovic, Esther Greenglass, and Francisco Garcia-Santos

ABSTRACT
The present study tested the extent to which perceived economic hardship is associated with psychological distress (suicide ideation and confusion) after controlling for personal characteristics. It also explored whether *perceived financial threat* (i.e., fearful anxious-uncertainty about the stability and security of one's personal financial situation) mediates the relationship between economic hardship and psychological distress outcomes. The theoretical model was tested in a sample of Canadian students (n = 211) and was validated in a community sample of employed Portuguese adults (n = 161). In both samples, the fit of the model was good. Parameter estimates indicated that greater experience of economic hardship increased with financial threat, which in turn increased with levels of suicide ideation and confusion. We discuss the practical implications of these results, such as for programs aimed at alleviating the burden of financial hardship, in our concluding remarks.

The 2007–2009 Great Recession had devastating consequences for the entire world economy, and for the health and welfare of those who endured it (Greenglass et al., 2014). Although no single cause was identified, in the United States, the economic downturn was triggered by policies that encouraged home ownership, access to loans, overvaluation of sub-prime mortgages, and problematic trading practice in addition to lack of capital by financial institutions to back their financial commitments (Mian & Sufi, 2014). The economic downturn resulted in massive job losses as organizations tried to restructure their labor force to cut costs and stay competitive (Reinhart & Rogoff, 2009). In May 2009 alone, Canada lost 42,000 jobs (Usalcus, 2010). In the United States, about 1 in 6 Americans lost their jobs in the period between 2007 and 2009 and in 2010, the unemployment rate hovered around 9.6%, a full year after the official end of the recession (Farber, 2011; US Bureau of Labor Statistics, 2009). Europe, too, felt the loss. 21.5 million people were unemployed as of May 2009 in the EU area (Eurostat, 2013a). The Baltic member states and Spain were particularly affected (Eurostat, 2013a). Portugal's unemployment rate reached an all-time high in 2012 at 16.90% (Trading Economics, 2013). In general, employees who retained their jobs after organizational restructuring experience cuts to their hours and wages, decreased job security, increased workload, and fewer opportunities for advancement (Amundson, Borgen, Jordan, & Erlebach, 2004; Moscarini & Postel-Vinay, 2016). Uncertain and changing employment conditions like these left many individuals confused and worried about losing their jobs.

Demographic Variation in Financial Strain

While the economic downturn affected all sectors of the population, the changes particularly affected certain demographic groups. For example, women suffered increased levels of domestic violence (Schneider, Harknett, & McLanahan, 2016), psychological distress and prescription drug use (Chen & Dagher, 2016), job loss and underemployment (Sum & Khatiwada, 2010), economic hardship (Thébaud & Sharkey, 2016), and decreased fertility (Percheski & Kimbro, 2014). The prevalence of economic loss and hardship also varied by educational achievement. In general, economic downturns negatively affect individuals with low levels of education in jobs with low-skill requirements and greater redundancy (Kirsch & Ryff, 2016). During the Great Recession, all levels of the labor market were negatively impacted, but uneducated groups were among the hardest hit (Danziger, Chavez, & Cumberworth, 2012; Hoynes, Miller, & Schaller, 2012; Kirsch & Ryff, 2016). Trends in labor market conditions, such as free-trade, globalization, and automation of industry, decreased the opportunity for less-educated individuals to obtain secure, well-paying jobs with opportunity for advancement (Board of Governors of the Federal Reserve System, 2014).

As a subset of this group, young people (i.e., 16–24 year olds) had an especially hard time due to their lack of employment experience and education/skills, redundancy, and lower wages (Bell & Blanchflower, 2011; Litwin & Sapir, 2009). Data show that in most countries, the unemployment rate for young people was approximately twice that of the national average. In 2009, the ratio of youth-to-adult unemployment rate was 2.7 (International Labour Organization (ILO), 2010). In 2010, the global youth unemployment rate was 12.6% (ILO, 2011). Long-term unemployment and underemployment can have debilitating psychological effects on young workers, which may lead young people to withdraw from the labor market altogether (ILO, 2010). Unemployment in young people may have long-term negative psychological effects. Prolonged youth unemployment can lead to reduced self-efficacy and feelings of hopelessness, and can negatively affect their plans for the future including marrying and having a family. For example, in 2011, an increasing number of young adults in the United States were living with their parents—some 19% of men between the ages of 25 and 34, up from 14% in 2005. Thus, their inability to afford independent living expenses resulted in their loss of independence (Davidson, 2014; Fry, 2013). Given the long-term repercussions of chronic unemployment, it is important to focus on the psychological aspects of unemployment in young people.

Psychophysiological Consequences of Unemployment and Economic Hardship

Unemployment and economic hardship can have profound effects on the psychological and physiological well-being of individuals (Bambra & Eikemo, 2009; Greenglass, Marjanovic, & Fiksenbaum, 2013). When people are out of work, they lose income and work-based social networks. These losses, in turn, increase psychosocial and material stress, and can strain non-work-based social relationships including those with spouses, partners, and other family members (Bolger, Patterson, & Kupersmidt, 1995; Griep et al., 2016). The main characteristic of involuntary job loss, unlike other forms of stress or transitions (e.g., retirement, return to school, maternity leave, and long-term illness) is that people do not have any control over it. To explain the negative psychological effects of unemployment, Jahoda (1987) argues that unemployment deprives individuals of more than just income, but of time structure, social contacts, work-related self-esteem, and as a result, individuals experience lower psychological health. If unemployment is prolonged, many individuals may lose the ability to pay their mortgage or rent and may face eviction, displacing families to substandard housing or even homelessness. In the United States, the financial crisis resulted in massive foreclosure rates, with California, Michigan, Ohio, and Florida having the highest foreclosure rates (Lynch, 2008). From the peak of US housing prices in early 2006–2010, home equity had lost about 50% of its value, over 7 trillion dollars (Ellen & Dastrup, 2012). This was especially difficult for some minority-group households (e.g., black, Hispanic) that were increasingly burdened by rent and experienced greater declines in homeownership. US rates of poverty similarly rose from approximately 12.5% in 2007 to roughly 15% in 2011. In the Great Recession, the young, uneducated, and minorities experienced sharper increases in poverty than their counterparts and the effects for these groups persist today (Danziger et al., 2012).

In order to conserve resources during the Great Recession, many individuals had to prioritize their needs and make difficult lifestyle choices about what was and was not necessary. Some, for example, postponed household and clothing purchases, cut back on social activities, changed transportation patterns and eating habits, and even sold possessions to make ends meet. At times, the Great Recession also motivated many people to make financially sound decisions—to increase their savings, cut their expenses, and pay down their debts (Alan, Crossley, & Low, 2012; Chakrabarti, Lee, van der Klaauw, & Zafar, 2011). However, the recession also had the effect of exacerbating rates of unemployment and economic hardship that worsened individuals' physical and mental distress (Jun, Shah, & Svoboda, 1995; Strully, 2009). Finding action-oriented solutions to financial hardship (e.g., increasing income, cutting expenses) is not always straightforward for individuals. When solutions to acute or chronic economic losses are not apparent or desirable, cognitive confusion and indecision may result in increased psychological distress and dysfunction (Ennis, Hobfoll, & Schröder, 2000). Situation-induced confusion and indecision may have the added negative effect of distracting attention from and degrading performance on actionable means to help improve personal financial conditions, thereby making it more difficult to escape poverty (Haushofer & Fehr, 2014; Sarason, Sarason, & Pierce, 1990). Increased social isolation, loss of self-esteem, malnutrition, substance abuse, and degraded cognitive function are just some of the challenges that face the unemployed and impoverished (Merline, O'Malley, Schulenberg, Bachman, & Johnston, 2004).

In general, people experiencing economic hardship report increased somatic complaints and symptoms of depression and anxiety. Weich and Lewis (1998) found that financial stress was a powerful independent predictor of both the onset and persistence of episodes of common mental disorders, even after adjusting for standard of living. More recently, Hardie and Lucas (2010) found economic hardship was associated with psychological distress, such as depression and anxiety, while Gallo and colleagues (2004) found that unemployment correlates with mortality rates and cardiovascular disease. In a comprehensive meta-analysis of 237 cross-sectional studies ($n = 458,820$), Paul and Moser (2009) found that unemployed individuals had significantly more psychological distress than the employed, with the greatest differences in men, blue-collar workers, long-term unemployed, and in countries with weak unemployment protection systems. This is consistent with research on the Great Recession. The downturn wreaked havoc on the individuals' financial stability and security, which in turn deteriorated their levels of psychological and physical well-being (Green, Felstead, Gallie, & Inanc, 2016; Margerison-Zilko, Goldman-Mellor, Falconi, & Downing, 2016; Mucci, Giorgi, Roncaioli, Perez, & Arcangeli, 2016).

Suicide is one of the severest consequences of economic hardship. Research shows that suicide rates correlate positively with unemployment rates and other markers of economic contraction. Platt and Hawton (2000) summarized the results of 165 empirical studies on this topic from the period 1984 to 1999. The risk of both suicide and self-injurious behavior increased with unemployment. Chang, Gunnell, Sterne, Luc, and Cheng (2009) found suicide rates increased between 39% and 45% in some Asian countries after the financial crisis of 1998, apparently due in large part to the resulting steep rise in unemployment rather than to changes in the divorce rate or other factors. Chen et al. (2010), using longitudinal aggregate data from Taiwan from the years 1978 to 2006, found that a 1% increase in the unemployment rate corresponded to a 4.9% increase in the suicide rate. Likewise, US data analyzed by Classen and Dunn (2012) depicted one additional death by suicide for every 4,200 men who lose their job during a mass layoff, with a lower rate for women (1:7,100), thus reflecting the well-known gender difference in suicide rates (Greenglass, 1982). Barr, Taylor-Robinson, Scott-Samuel, McKee, and Stuckler (2012) found that growing unemployment and economic hardship were important factors in more than 1,000 suicides among British people between 2008 and 2010. Including all of Europe, United States, and Canada, about 10,000 suicides between 2008 and 2010 are attributable to the Great Recession and economic factors (Reeves, McKee, & Stuckler, 2014). More recently, statistics show how closely tied suicide rates are to fluctuating economic factors. For example, from 2014 to 2015 in Alberta, Canada, suicide rates rose 30% in the wake of collapsing oil prices and widespread job loss (CBC, 2015). Related trends in Alberta were also reported such as an increased demand for mental health services. While one cannot assume cause and effect here, the robust positive association of suicide and economic hardship suggests that economic factors have a meaningful impact on suicidal intentions and behaviors.

The Mediating Role of Financial Threat

The empirical connection between economic hardships and psychological well-being is well established, robust, and conceptually sensible (e.g., Beck & Tolnay, 1990; Jahoda, 1988; McInerney, Mellor, & Nicholas, 2013; Paul & Moser, 2009). The relationship, however, is likely more complex than previously thought. Not all individuals, for example, interpret negative situational financial pressures, such as job loss, in the same way, nor do all people interpret positive financial indicators the same. Lazarus and Folkman (1984) articulated this idea in their transactional model of stress, stating that a person's perceptions of threatening stimuli are not always ground in reality, and often have more to do with their perceived danger of a stressor and their ability to cope with it than anything else. Based on this premise, researchers recently identified a powerful mediator of the economic hardship-to-psychological well-being relationship: *perceived financial threat* (Marjanovic, Greenglass, Fiksenbaum, & Bell, 2013; Marjanovic et al., 2015).

Defined as fear and anxious-uncertainty about the security and stability of one's personal finances, perceived financial threat is worsened by situational hardships (e.g., job loss, high debt load) and, to a lesser extent, by conceptually related personality traits, such as the tendency to worry and have low self-efficacy. In a recent study, researchers experimentally induced high levels of financial threat in university students by telling them their tuition was increasing in the next year and that their prospects of acquiring good jobs following their university studies were negligible (Wohl, Branscombe, & Lister, 2014). Later, these threatened students reacted ironically by engaging in significantly riskier gambling behaviors than a control group that was not provoked to experience financial threat. In related studies, researchers showed that the historical relation between economic hardship and financial threat was significantly greater among pessimists than optimists (Grezo & Sarmany-Schuller, 2015), and that individuals with a high level of personal mastery had better outcomes after economic hardships than individuals with low mastery (Pudrovska, Schiemen, Pearlin, & Nguyen, 2005). Thus, financial threat is affected by situational changes in one's environment, as well as by one's personality, general outlook, and hopefulness for the future. Financial threat, in turn, is also associated with psychological distress, such as with depression, anxiety, mood disturbance, and burnout (Marjanovic et al., 2013, 2015), and lower levels of life satisfaction (Tay, Batz, Parrigon, & Kuykendall, 2016). Importantly, when levels of financial threat are statistically controlled, the robust relationship between economic hardship and psychological distress outcomes is substantially diminished (Marjanovic et al., 2015). This suggests financial threat mediates that relationship, i.e., as economic hardship worsens, financial threat increases, which in turn relates to decreasing psychological health.

We argue financial threat merits greater consideration as a psychological construct based on the following couple of points. First, people's ability to provide for themselves and their loved ones (i.e., the base of Maslow's hierarchy of needs, food, water, security, and safety) chiefly depends on maintaining a favorable balance between income and expenses. Any potential obstacle that may upset this balance or its predictability is potentially a serious threat. Given the majority of the world's population contends with these types of accounting struggles and many are living near or below the poverty line (Hokayem & Heggeness, 2014; United Nations, 2015), we also suggest that financial threat is a widespread experience, especially in turbulent economic times. Therefore, financial threat is likely a highly generalizable psychological construct that applies similarly to diverse groups of people.

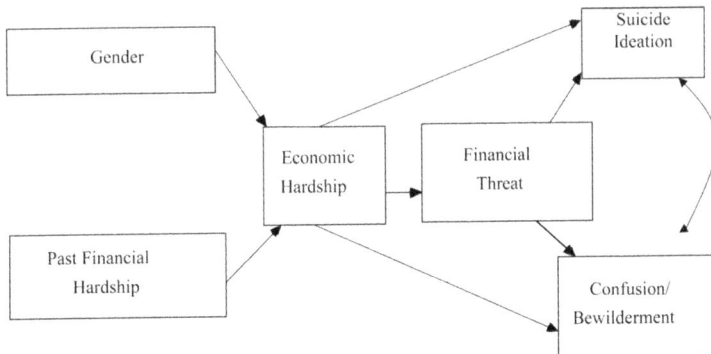

Figure 1. The proposed model relating economic hardship and financial threat on suicide ideation and confusion/bewilderment, controlling for gender, and past financial hardship. *Note.* ***$p <.001$, *$p < .05$.

Purpose of this Investigation

In this paper, we tested a hypothetical model (see Figure 1) that explores the extent to which perceived economic hardship is associated with financial threat, after controlling for personal characteristics such as gender and past financial hardships, and how financial threat is associated with psychological distress outcomes such as suicide ideation and states of reported more economic hardships. Furthermore, we examined the direct link between economic hardship and suicide ideation and states of confusion as endogenous variables (i.e., outcome variables), and the extent to which financial threat mediated that relation. We tested the model in a Canadian student sample (Study 1). Students represent a young, uneducated group with limited personal resources, who according to the above findings should be especially vulnerable to the impact of economic downturns. Student samples are ideal for testing these exploratory models given the rising costs of higher education, mounting debt levels many students incur to earn their degrees, and their tenuous employability.

In order to cross-validate the model, we tested the model in a community sample of employed, non-student, and older individuals living in Portugal (Study 2). We selected these two countries (Canada and Portugal) because of their economic-prosperity differences at the height of the downturn. In 2009, two key indicators of a country's economic prosperity (i.e., debt-to-gross domestic product ratio and unemployment rate) were substantially worse in Portugal than Canada (Eurostat, 2013b; Treasury Board of Canada Secretariat, 2011). Consequently, individuals in Portugal likely perceived their economic situation as more precarious than Canadians and may have experienced more economic hardship, financial threat, and psychological distress as a result.

Specifically, we hypothesized the following:

1. Participant variables would be associated with current economic hardship, such that women and individuals who experienced past financial hardship would experience greater current hardship.
2. Current economic hardship would be positively associated with financial threat and psychological distress (i.e., greater suicide ideation and cognitive confusion), even after controlling for participant variables.
3. Financial threat is positively associated with psychological distress.
4. Financial threat mediates the negative relationship between current economic hardship and psychological distress.

Method

Participants

We collected data from a convenience sample of undergraduate students enrolled in introductory psychology courses at a Canadian university in exchange for course credit. These data were collected in 2009, which was at the height of the economic crisis for Canada. The initial sample consisted of 292 individuals who completed an online questionnaire; however, we eliminated 81 responders from the sample due to incomplete information provided at the middle and the end of the questionnaire. The remaining sample consisted of 65 men (30.81%) and 146 women (69.19%). The age of the respondents ranged from 17 to 52 years, with an average age of 20.91 years ($SD = 4.77$). Approximately half lived alone (50.5%) and approximately two-thirds were employed (62.1%). Slightly over half of the participants worked on a part-time basis (52.1%). Just over half of the sample (57.8%) lived with relatives (e.g., mother, father, and grandparents), 5.7% lived alone, 28% lived with partner/spouse with or without children, and 8.5% lived with friends. On average, students reported a total gross annual income of $13,851.00 CAD (*SD* = 39,507), and a total debt level of $14,030 CAD (*SD* = 43,685).

Measures

Financial Threat

We measured concerns about the stability and security of one's personal financial situation with the *Financial Threat Scale* (FTS; Marjanovic et al., 2013). The FTS is a recently developed measure adapted from research on reactions to ambiguous and threatening situations/ events. This scale consists of 5 items that measure an individual's fear, uncertainty, and preoccupation with his/her current financial situation. Each item is rated on a 5-point scale, with the anchors ranging from 1 = *Not at All* to 5 = *A Great Deal/Extremely*. A sample item is "How uncertain do you feel?" Previous research has demonstrated that the FTS is a highly reliable and valid scale (Marjanovic et al., 2015). It has been strongly associated with situational variables related to economic hardship (e.g., job stability, personal income change), personality variables associated with sensitivity to threat (e.g., trait worry, self-esteem), and psychological distress variables associated with depression, anxiety, and burnout. We say these associations were "strong" with reference to Cohen's (1988) standards for interpreting effect sizes: correlations near or higher than .50 being deserving of that label.

Economic Hardship

To assess current economic hardship, respondents completed the *Economic Hardship Questionnaire* (EHQ; Lempers, Clark-Lempers, & Simons, 1989). The EHQ is a 10-item scale measuring one's inability to make ends meet, not having enough money for necessities, and making lifestyle adjustments due to financial need. Respondents were asked during the last few years, if either their family or selves made any changes to their lifestyles or cut back on activities. Each item was rated on a 4-point Likert scale, ranging from *1* (Never) to *4* (Very Often). A sample item is "Change food shopping or eating habits to save money?" The EHQ has acceptable psychometric properties (Lempers et al., 1989). In terms of reliability, the Cronbach's alpha in the current study was .89. Using a single item, respondents were also asked about past financial hardships on a 3-point scale: 1 = *Mild*, 2 = *Moderate*, and 3 = *Severe*.

Confusion

We measured confusion with the 5-item Confusion/Bewilderment subscale from the *Profile of Mood States–Short Form* (POMS-SF; Shacham, 1983). The POMS uses mood-related adjectives to measure psychological distress. Respondents were asked to indicate using a 5-point scale, ranging from 1 = *Not at all* to 5 = *Extremely*, how they felt about their current financial situation. A sample item is "Unable to concentrate."

Suicide Ideation

We measured suicide ideation with the 5-item Brief-Symptom Rating Scale (BSRS-5; Lung & Lee, 2008). This scale has been used as a screening device in both community, and general medical and psychiatric settings. Each item is rated on a 5-point Likert type scale, ranging from 1 = *Not at all* to 5 = *Extremely*. A sample item is "Had thoughts about committing suicide." The BSRS-5 has demonstrated good reliability and validity (Lung & Lee, 2008).

Demographic Information

The following demographic information was collected: sex, age, marital status, living arrangements, total annual income before taxes, and total debt level.

Procedure

We recruited students to participate in a voluntary, confidential, and anonymous online questionnaire. The questionnaire took approximately 30 minutes to complete. While we offered no monetary incentive to respondents for their participation, we informed them of the scholarly and practical use of the research, and invited them to contact the researcher about the results.

Results

We conducted tests of statistical assumptions prior to testing the theoretical model and found no univariate outliers and/or anomalies in the data. Given that the sample consisted of employed and unemployed students, we conducted several t-tests on all study measures prior to collapsing the groups and found no group differences (see Table 1). Table 2 displays correlations, means, standard deviations, and Cronbach's alphas for all study measures. In general, respondents reported moderate levels of past financial hardships, as well as financial threat, and states of confusion. They reported low-to-moderate levels of current economic hardship and suicide ideation. In terms of correlations, women reported greater economic hardship, suicide ideation, and confusion than men. Past financial hardship was positively and moderately correlated to current economic hardship, suicide ideation, and confusion. Perceived current economic hardship was positively and strongly correlated with suicide ideation, states of confusion, and financial threat. Finally, financial threat was strongly and positively related to suicide ideation and states of confusion.

    Path analysis, using structural equation modeling techniques (SEM), was used to explore the relationships among age, gender, perceived economic hardship, financial threat, and psychological distress (i.e., suicide ideation and states of confusion). Manifest variables were based on the composite of each study measure. We used AMOS version 16.0 (Arbuckle, 2005), with maximum likelihood parameter estimation, to generate path coefficients and tests of the overall goodness of fit of the model. We evaluated several fit indices in order to assess model fit. The traditional measure for evaluating overall goodness of fit of the model is the chi-square goodness-of fit statistic, which tests the difference between sample and fitted covariance matrices (Hu & Bentler, 1999). Typically, a non-significant chi-square test signifies a good model fit; however, this measure nearly always rejects the model when sample sizes are large (e.g., $n > 200$; Jöreskog & Sörbom, 1993). Consequently, researchers have sought alternative indices to assess model fit.

Table 1. Means and Standard Deviations, for Employed and Unemployed Canadian Students.

Variable	Employed (n = 127)		Unemployed (n = 80)			
	M	SD	M	SD	t	p
Past financial hardship	1.76	0.73	1.61	0.66	0.31	.151
Economic hardship	2.06	0.64	1.91	0.67	1.70	.091
Suicide ideation	11.73	5.55	10.30	5.26	1.84	.067
Confusion/bewilderment	2.30	1.05	2.07	0.95	1.62	.107

Table 2. Study 1 Correlations, Means, Standard Deviations, and Cronbach's Alphas for Canadian Students.

		1	2	3	4	5	6	α	M	SD
1.	Gender[1]	—						—	—	—
2.	Past financial hardship	.02	—					—	1.71	0.72
3.	Economic hardship	.15[a]	.27[c]	—				.89	2.00	0.65
4.	Suicide ideation	.18[a]	.30[c]	.50[c]	—			.95	11.17	5.46
5.	Confusion	.16[a]	.32[c]	.53[c]	.89[c]	—		.88	2.24	1.10
6.	Financial threat	.12	.19b	.50[c]	.57[c]	.64[c]	—	.89	3.0	1.01

Note. [1]Gender was coded 1 = male, 2 = female. [a]$p < .05$, [b]$p < .01$, [c]$p < .001$.

In line with their recommendations, we used the relative chi-square statistic to assess fit, which is less susceptible to influence by sample size. We calculate this by dividing the chi-square value by the model's degrees of freedom. If the value is less than 5, the model fit is acceptable (Schumacker & Lomax, 2004). Alternatively, we used the root mean square error of approximation (RMSEA) to assess model fit. An RMSEA value in the range of 0.05–0.10 indicates fair fit, whereas values above 0.10 indicate poor fit (MacCallum, Browne, & Sugawara, 1996). We also used the goodness-of-fit statistic (GFI), comparative fit index (CFI), Tucker Lewis Index, and incremental fit index (IFI), all of which share the cutoff of $\geq .95$ to indicate good fit (Hu & Bentler, 1999). Results of our analysis showed that the chi-square goodness-of-fit statistic (χ^2 $_{(7)} = 14.86$, $p = .038$) was significant, indicating poor model fit; however, as stated above, we attributed this to our large sample size. More importantly, the relative chi-square value (2.12) showed that the model provided an adequate fit to the data, and all of our other fit indices, RMSEA (.07), GFI (.98), CFI (.99), TLI (.97), and IFI (.99), were all in the satisfactory range. Based on these values, we were satisfied that the model fits the data. AMOS indicated that no post-hoc modifications were required.

Parameter Estimates

Hypothesized relations were assessed using parameter estimates from the model. Figure 2 presents the model with the standardized parameter estimates. All parameter estimates were

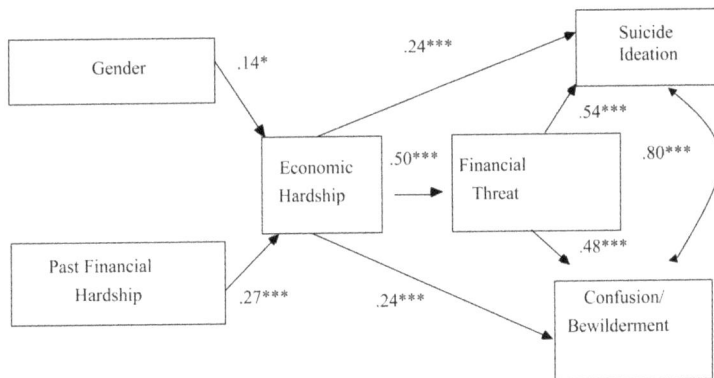

Figure 2. Canadian sample model relating economic hardship and financial threat on suicide ideation and confusion/bewilderment, controlling for gender, and past financial hardship with standardized coefficients. Note. ***$p < .001$, *$p < .05$.

significant. Women and those who had experienced severe economic hardships in the past reported current economic hardships ($\beta = .15$ and $\beta = .27$, respectively). Greater economic hardship was associated with increased financial threat ($\beta = .53$), which in turn was related to increased suicide ideation ($\beta = .54$) and confusion ($\beta = .48$). Greater economic hardship was also associated with increased suicide ideation ($\beta = .24$) and confusion ($\beta = .24$).

We tested our mediation hypothesis using the Sobel test (Sobel, 1982). The Sobel test determines the significance of the indirect effect of the mediator by testing the hypothesis of no difference between the total effect and the direct effect. Results revealed that financial threat mediated the relation between economic hardship and suicide ideation (Sobel Test Statistic z = 6.47, SE = 0.37, $p<.001$) as well as with confusion (Sobel Test Statistic z = 5.88, SE = .0.07, $p<.001$).

In sum, the results of this Study 1 supported all four of our investigation hypotheses. First, women, and individuals who suffered greater past economic hardship (i.e., participant variables), reported greater current economic hardship. This is consistent with past findings in the literature (e.g., Thébaud & Sharkey, 2016). Second, current economic hardship related to higher levels of financial threat and psychological distress, even after controlling for participant variables. Third, financial threat positively related to psychological distress, such that greater concern for one's financial stability/security linked to thoughts about suicide and cognitive indecision. Lastly, financial threat mediated the relationship between economic hardship and psychological distress. In other words, if levels of financial threat are controlled or kept constant, the well-established relationship between economic hardship and psychological distress is greatly diminished, showing the importance of financial threat in accounting for this relation.

Study 2

We selected a community-based, non-student Portuguese sample, which we tested at the height of the recession, to cross-validate our model. Compared to Canada, the downturn negatively influenced Portugal's economy more due to a large public debt, a high budget deficit, and high unemployment rates (Economist, 2010). Similar to other countries that struggled to endure the crisis, the Portuguese government was required to take a number of restrictive measures. The state severely cut the welfare system budget and decreased the social benefits to many needy families. In addition, wages of public employees (i.e., those who worked for the government) were frozen, and the budgets of other sectors were reduced (e.g., education). Even some national holidays were cut to conserve funds (Economist, 2010). In April 2011, Portugal became the third country in a row, after Greece and Ireland, to receive a bailout from the "Troika" of the European Commission, the European Central Bank, and the International Monetary Fund (IMF) (Kowsmann, 2011). For these reasons, this sample of non-student, mature Portuguese provides a good sample to cross-validate and test the generalizability of our model.

Method

Participants
Our initial convenience sample consisted of 231 individuals who completed an online survey very similar to the one used in Study 1. Data collection took place in the summer of 2011—at

the height of Portugal's economic crisis. From those, we eliminated 70 respondents from the sample due to incomplete data toward the middle and the end of the questionnaire. The remaining sample consisted of 79 men (49.07%) and 82 women (50.03%). The age of the respondents ranged from 23 to 79 years, with an average age of 39.61 years ($SD = 11.01$). A little over half of the sample (57.1%) was married or in a common law relationship, 10.6% were separated/divorced, and 32.3% were single. The majority of the respondents (59.6%) lived with a partner/spouse with or without children, 19.3% lived alone, 16.1% lived with relatives (e.g., mother, father, grandparents), and 5% lived with friends. On average, respondents reported a total annual income, before taxes, of $28,253.46 € ($SD = 31, 976.47$), and a total debt level of $51,232.98 € ($SD = 69,375.24$). The majority of the sample worked full time (70.8%), 3.7% worked part time, and 13.7% worked on a contract basis.

Measures

All the measures included in Study 1 were included in Study 2. In order to adapt the questionnaire for use in Portugal, the questionnaire was first translated to Portuguese and then back-translated to English to ensure its semantic parity.

Procedure

We invited the public to complete an anonymous questionnaire posted on the Internet through an advertisement in a Portuguese daily newspaper. Informed consent was obtained from participants by having them click a continue button to signal their agreement to participate after they had read the form. The survey took approximately 30 minutes to complete. While no monetary incentive was offered to respondents for participating, they were informed of the scholarly and practical use of the research, and were invited to contact the researcher if they wished to know the results.

Results

Table 3 displays correlations, means, standard deviations, and Cronbach's alphas for all study measures. Men reported greater past financial hardship than women, whereas women reported greater current economic hardship than men. Past financial hardship was positively and moderately related to current economic hardship, suicide ideation, and confusion. Economic hardship was positively and strongly correlated with suicide ideation, states of

Table 3. Study 2 Correlations, Means, standard deviations, and Cronbach's Alphas for Portuguese Employees.

		1	2	3	4	5	6	α	M	SD
1	Gender[1]	—						—	—	—
2	Past Financial Hardship	−.19[a]	—					—	1.65	0.68
3	Economic Hardship	.18a	.18[a]	—				.81	2.14	0.52
4	Suicide Ideation	−.09	.17	.50[c]	—			.86	10.31	4.82
5	Confusion	−.11	.16[a]	.48[c]	.86[c]	—		.84	2.09	0.92
6	Financial Threat	−.09	.10	.52[c]	.65[c]	.61c	—	.89	3.47	0.78

Note. [1]Gender was coded 1 = male, 2 = female. [c]$p < .001$, [a]$p < .05$.

confusion, and financial threat. Financial threat was strongly and positively related to suicide ideation and states of confusion.

In order to cross-validate the model tested in Study 1, path analysis with maximum likelihood method of parameter estimation was used to provide path coefficients and tests of the overall goodness of fit of the model. The χ^2 goodness-of-fit statistic (χ^2 $_{(7)}$ = 18.665, p = .009) was significant; however, the relative chi-square statistic (2.67) indicated that the model provided an adequate fit to the data, and other fit indices GFI (.96), CFI (.97), TLI (.94), IFI (.97), and RMSEA (.10) were satisfactory. No post hoc modifications to the model were indicated by AMOS.

Parameter Estimates

Hypothesized relations were assessed using parameter estimates from the model. Figure 3 presents the model with the standardized parameter estimates. All parameter estimates were significant. Women and those who had experienced more severe economic hardships in the past reported current economic hardships (β = .22 and β = .22, respectively). As hypothesized, greater economic hardship was associated with increased financial threat (β = .52), which in turn was related to increased suicide ideation (β = .54) and confusion (β = .49). Greater economic hardship was also associated with increased suicide ideation (β = .22) and confusion (β = .23). Results of the mediation analysis revealed that financial threat significantly mediated the relation between economic hardship and suicide ideation (Sobel Test Statistic z = 5.52, SE = 0.46, p < .001). Financial threat also mediated the relation between economic hardship and states of confusion (Sobel Test Statistic z = 5.10, SE = 0.09, p < .001).

Similar to Study 1, the results of Study 2 supported all four of our hypotheses. First, current economic hardship was associated with gender and past financial experiences. Second, current economic hardship linked to greater concern over one's financial stability/security and heightened psychological distress, even after controlling for participant variables. Third, financial threat strongly and positively related to psychological stress, relating to both suicidal thoughts and cognitive indecision. Finally, financial threat was a mediator of the historical and robust relationship between economic hardship and psychological distress.

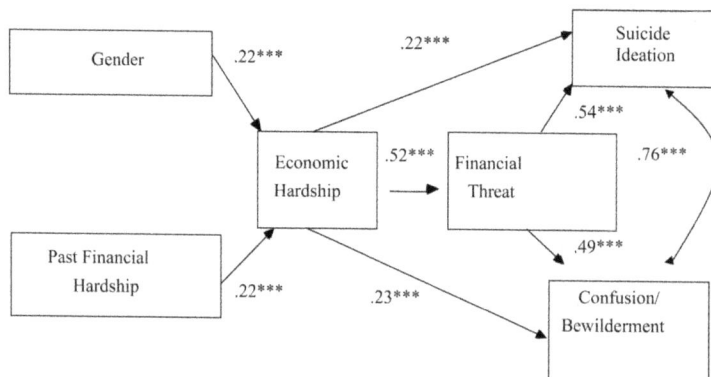

Figure 3. Portuguese sample model relating economic hardship and financial threat on suicide ideation and confusion/bewilderment, controlling for gender, and past financial hardship with standardized coefficients. *Note.* ***p <.001

Discussion

This research tested a model that examined the relationship between economic hardship, financial threat, and psychological distress (i.e., suicide ideation and cognitive confusion), while controlling for past financial hardship and gender. Results of these studies showed that in both a Canadian student sample and a Portuguese community sample, economic hardship was positively associated with financial threat, which in turn was positively associated with psychological distress. The Sobel test was used to test for mediation, and results showed that financial threat mediated the relation between economic hardship and both distress variables—suicide ideation and confusion/bewilderment. Previous research has reported results that parallel these findings, namely that financial threat was a significant mediator of the influence of self-efficacy on psychological distress (Greenglass & Mara, 2012). Individuals who had higher levels of self-efficacy appraised their financial condition as less threatening, which resulted in less psychological distress. Likewise, individuals who reported past financial hardship were more likely to experience current financial hardships, results that are expected unless there are significant changes in the person's behavior. Finally, these data revealed that in both samples, women were more likely to experience economic hardships than men; however, the magnitude of these relations was small. Additionally, gender was not directly related to psychological consequences of economic hardship: financial threat, suicide ideation, or confusion. Thus, these data suggest that the psychological impact of the economic crisis was unaffected by gender.

The results of the current study are consistent with those of a number of studies that have explored the associations between financial strain and psychological functioning (Paul & Moser, 2009). These studies suggest that individuals who experience more financial hardship are at increased risk of impaired psychological functioning. Not having enough financial means is a source of frustration, anxiety, uncertainty, and worry. Such negative feelings may threaten a person's sense of self (i.e., an individual may no longer feel competent, efficacious), which is emotionally damaging. Over time, these feelings take a significant toll on their psychological functioning. Financial hardships trigger economic strain (e.g., financial threat or insecurity). Financial threat is the anxious feeling that available resources are insufficient to meet personal needs. Financial threat subsequently increases psychological distress (e.g., depressed mood, anxiety, suicide). Thus, findings from the current study enhance our understanding of the psychological consequences of economic hardship and financial threat. Moreover, the findings that the theoretical model put forth held in two diverse national samples differentially affected by the recession, underline the robustness of the present model. Further, our data contribute to the growing body of research that investigates the role of psychological factors as related to other measures of economic hardship (Greenglass, 2016). Given the fragility of the global economy and the accompanying high unemployment rates around the world, individuals are more likely to experience worry and fear about their financial situation, and are thereby at increased risk of psychological distress.

There are a number of practical implications of this investigation. With high youth unemployment and limited job opportunities, many post-secondary students may be completing their education with scarce job prospects, or none at all. Unemployment early in a young person's work life can have enduring negative effects on future earnings, productivity, and employment opportunities (Mroz & Savage, 2001). These spiraling effects can further deepen the hardships that individuals face. Given the current unstable economic environment, individuals may choose underemployment as a means to help them deal with their expenses and mounting debt. In response, training programs could be offered to recent school graduates in order to provide them with skills necessary to become gainfully employed and ease the transition from school to the workforce.

Active labor market programs could also be implemented for those who have been employed and have, recently, found themselves unemployed. These programs, which may include resilience-building activities, should be aimed at helping people retain jobs and improve the prospects of finding gainful employment. Despite the high number of competitors for each single job advertised, and the frustration, sense of helplessness, and lack of control that this issue may have, job seekers should be encouraged and motivated to engage actively and effectively in seeking re-employment through networking and retraining. These interventions may also reduce the duration of unemployment insurance claims and social welfare benefits.

Interventions could also be targeted to individuals having difficulties satisfying many of the basic requirements of daily living (e.g., paying bills, eating nutritious meals). Programs could be designed to help them overcome the stress and strains associated with financial hardship. This may bolster one's self-esteem and self-efficacy, which in turn will have positive effects on one's emotional state, reducing thoughts of suicide and confusion. Debt relief programs, such as debt advice and access to free mental health-related services, can be effective in alleviating the adverse effects of recession on mental health. Individuals may benefit from social support offered by family and/or friends, and family and friends can be an important source of both practical assistance and material support. For example, they can offer shelter and money when needed. These individuals can also be ideal sources of emotional support. And finally, problem-solving skills, which have been shown to be important for successful re-entry into the job market (Julkunen, 2001), should be promoted.

Limitations

Results from the current study add to the literature that examines the psychological effects of economic hardship and financial threat. Nevertheless, these studies are not without limitations. Like many studies, the Canadian and Portuguese samples relied on self-report data and used convenience sampling. Future studies should utilize a multimethod approach, from multiple informants (i.e., collecting objective data and using qualitative methods). Similarly, researchers could use a longitudinal design in order to produce information about potentially causal relationships. Another limitation is that many respondents either did not know or did not want to report their current income and exact debt levels; this may have resulted in an under- or overestimation of debt and income levels for the sample. Finally, using a listwise procedure, we eliminated several responders' questionnaires in each study due to incomplete data. Because the location of these missing data was mostly at the middle and the end of the study questionnaires, we attributed this loss to the length of our questionnaire, which is a common consequence of administering surveys anonymously. Closer statistical analysis of the complete and incomplete questionnaires revealed no systematic differences between samples on important study variables, such as sex, economic hardship, or psychological distress. We conclude that researchers be mindful of such attrition when conducting research online.

Conclusion

Economic crises may have long-term psychological consequences for individuals both directly and indirectly affected. Findings from the current study showed that economic hardship was positively associated with anxiety and worry that individuals have about their current financial situation, which, in turn, were negatively associated with mental health. Given the empirical and theoretical tools of psychologists, they are well positioned to conduct research on psychological aspects of financial hardship. The findings of this research have implications not only for theoretical development within psychology but also for practical interventions that could be implemented to help people cope with economic stressors. Government and policy makers could introduce a variety of programs aimed at assisting prospective entrants to the labor force find employment as well as those who have lost their jobs.

Acknowledgments

Thanks are due to the Faculty of Health at York University and the Greenglass Lab, including Joana Katter, Melina Condren, Dean Hodge, Constance Mara, Karina Meysel, Lisa Santorelli, and Jessica Campoli for their contributions to this research.

References

Alan, S., Crossley, T., & Low, H. (2012). *Saving on a rainy day, borrowing for a rainy day*. Institute for Fiscal Studies, Working Paper no. W12/11. Retrieved from https://www.ifs.org.uk/publications/6171.

Amundson, N., Borgen, W. A., Jordan, S., & Erlebach, A. C. (2004). Survivors of downsizing: Helpful and hindering experiences. *The Career Development Quarterly, 52*, 256–271. https://doi.org/10.1002/j.2161-0045.2004.tb00647.x

Arbuckle, J. L. (2005). *Amos 6.0 user's guide*. Chicago, IL: SPSS.

Bambra, C., & Eikemo, T. (2009). Welfare state regimes, unemployment and health: A comparative study of the relationship between unemployment and self-reported health in 23 European countries. *Journal of Epidemiology and Community Health, 63*, 92–98. https://doi.org/10.1136/jech.2008.077354

Barr, B., Taylor-Robinson, D., Scott-Samuel, A., McKee, M., & Stuckler, D. (2012). Suicides associated with the 2008–10 economic recession in England: Time trend analysis. *British Medical Journal, 345*, 1756–1833. https://doi.org/10.1136/bmj.e5142

Beck, E. M., & Tolnay, S. (1990). The killing fields of the deep south: The market for cotton and the lynching of Blacks, 1882–1930. *American Sociological Review, 55,* 526–539. https://doi.org/10.2307/2095805

Bell, N. F., & Blanchflower, D. G. (2011). Young people and the Great Recession. *Oxford Review of Economic Policy, 27,* 241–267. https://doi.org/10.1093/oxrep/grr011

Board of Governors of the Federal Reserve System. (2014). *In the shadow of the Great Recession: Experiences and perspectives of young workers.* Retrieved from www.federalreserve.gov/publications/default.htm

Bowers, J. R., & Segrin, C. (in press). Transitional instability, psychological health, and sexual risk taking among college students. *Journal of Student Affairs Research and Practice.*

Bolger, K. E., Patterson, C. J., & Kupersmidt, W. W. (1995). Psychosocial adjustment among children experiencing persistent and intermittent family economic hardship. *Child Development, 66,* 1107–1129. https://doi.org/10.2307/1131802

CBC News. (2015, December). *Suicide rate in Alberta climbs 30% in wake of mass oilpatch layoffs. CBC News.* Retrieved from http://www.cbc.ca/news/canada/calgary/suicide-rate-alberta-increase-layoffs-1.3353662

Chakrabarti, R., Lee, D., van der Klaauw, W., & Zafar, B. (2011). *Household debt and saving during the 2007 recession. National Bureau of Economic Research, Working Paper no. 16999.* Cambridge, MA: National Bureau of Economic Research.

Chang, S. S., Gunnell, D., Sterne, J. A. C., Luc, T. H., & Cheng, A. T. A. (2009). Was the economic crisis 1997–1998 responsible for rising suicide rates in East/Southeast Asia? A time-trend analysis for Japan, Hong Kong, South Korea, Taiwan, Singapore, and Thailand. *Social Science and Medicine, 68,* 1322–1331. https://doi.org/10.1016/j.socscimed.2009.01.010

Chen, V. C., Chou, J., Lai, T., Lee, C. T. (2010). Suicide and unemployment rate in Taiwan: A population-based study, 1978–2006. *Social Psychiatry and Psychiatric Epidemiology, 45,* 447–452. https://doi.org/10.1007/s00127-009-0083-8

Chen, J., & Dagher, R. J. (2016). Gender and race/ethnicity differences in mental health care use before and during the Great Recession. *Journal of Behavioral Health Services and Research, 43,* 187–199. https://doi.org/10.1007/s11414-014-9403-1

Classen, T. J., & Dunn, R. A. (2012). The effect of job loss and unemployment duration on suicide risk in the United States: A new look using mass-layoffs and unemployment duration. *Health Economics, 21,* 338–350. https://doi.org/10.1002/hec.1719

Cohen, J. (1988). *Statistical power analysis for the behavioral sciences* (2nd ed.). Hillsdale, NJ: Lawrence Earlbaum Associates.

Danziger, S., Chavez, K., & Cumberworth, E. (2012). *Poverty and the Great Recession.* Stanford, CA: Stanford Center on Poverty and Inequality.

Davidson, A. (2014, June 20). *It's official: The boomerang kids won't leave. The New York Times.* Retrieved from http://www.nytimes.com

Economist. (2010). *Europe's economic woes: The PIIGS that won't fly. A guide to the euro-zone's troubled economies.* Retrieved on March 1, 2013 from http://www.economist.com/node/15838029

Ellen, I. G., & Dastrup, S. (2012). *Housing and the Great Recession.* Stanford, CA: Stanford Center on Poverty and Inequality.

Ennis, N. E., Hobfoll, S. E., & Schröder, K. E. E. (2000). Money doesn't talk, it swears: How economic stress and resistance resources impact inner-city women's depressive mood. *American Journal of Community Psychology, 28,* 149–173. https://doi.org/10.1023/A:1005183100610

Eurostat. (2013a, March 1). *Portugal Age 25-74 Underemployment.* Retrieved from https://ycharts.com/indicators/portugal_age_2574_underemployment

Eurostat. (2013b, March 1). *Euro area unemployment rate at 12%.* Retrieved from http://epp.eurostat.ec.europa.eu/statistics_explained/index.php/Unemployment_statistics

Farber, H. (2011). *Job loss in the Great Recession: Historical perspective from the Displaced Workers Survey, 1984–2010. National Bureau of Economic Research, Working Paper No. 17040.* Cambridge, MA: National Bureau of Economic Research.

Fry, R. (2013). *A rising share of young adults live in their parents' home: A record 21.6 million in 2012.* Retrieved from http://www.pewsocialtrends.org/2013/08/01/a-rising-share-of-young-adults-live-in-their-parents-home/

Gallo, W. T., Bradley, E. H., Falba, T. A., Dubin, J. A., Cramer, L. D., Bogardus, S. T., Jr., & Kasl, S. V. (2004). Involuntary job loss as a risk factor for subsequent myocardial infarction and stroke: Findings from the Health and Retirement Survey. *American Journal of Industrial Medicine, 45*, 408–416. https://doi.org/10.1002/ajim.20004

Green, F., Felstead, A., Gallie, D., & Inanc, H. (2016). Job-related well-being through the Great Recession. *Journal of Happiness Studies, 17*, 389–411. https://doi.org/10.1007/s10902-014-9600-x

Greenglass, E. (1982). *A world of difference: Gender roles in perspective.* Toronto: Wiley.

Greenglass, E. R. (2016). Importance of cross-national and interdisciplinary research for the study of financial stress: A Comment on Sinclair and Cheung. Invited commentary. *Stress and Health, 32*, 199–200.

Greenglass, E., Antonides, G., Christandl, F., Foster, G., Katter, J. K. Q., Kaufman, B. E., & Lea, S. E. G. (2014). The financial crisis and its effects: Perspectives from economics and psychology. *Journal of Behavioral and Experimental Economics, 50*, 10–12. https://doi.org/10.1016/j.socec.2014.01.004

Greenglass, E., & Mara, C. A. (2012). Self-efficacy as a psychological resource in difficult economic times. In K. A. Moore, K. Kaniasty, & P. Buchwald (Eds.), *Stress and anxiety: Application to economic hardship, occupational demands, and developmental challenges* (pp. 29–38). Berlin: Logos Verlag.

Greenglass, E., Marjanovic, Z., & Fiksenbaum, L. (2013). The impact of the recession and its aftermath on individual health and well-being. In A. S. G. Antoniou, & C. Cooper (Eds.), *The psychology of the recession in the workplace* (pp. 42–58). Cheltenham, UK: Edward Elgar.

Grezo, M., & Sarmany-Schuller, I. (2015). Coping with economic hardship: A broader look on the role of dispositional optimism. *Journal of Psychology, 2*(2), 6–14.

Griep, Y., Kinnunen, U., Nätti, J., De Cuyper, N., Mauno, S., Mäkinkangas, A., & De Witte, H. (2016). The effects of unemployment and perceived job insecurity: A comparison of their association with psychological and somatic complaints, self-rated health and life satisfaction. *International Archives of Occupational and Environmental Health, 89*, 147–162. https://doi.org/10.1007/s00420-015-1059-5

Hardie, J. H., & Lucas, A. (2010). Economic factors and the relationship quality among young couples: Comparing cohabitation and marriage. *Journal of Marriage and Family, 72*, 1141–1154.

Haushofer, J., & Fehr, E. (2014). On the psychology of poverty. *Science, 344*, 862–867.

Hokayem, C., & Heggeness, M. L. (2014). *Living in near poverty in the United States: 1966–2012.* Current Population Reports. Suitland, MD: U.S. Census Bureau.

Hoynes, H., Miller, D. L., & Schaller, J. (2012). Who suffers during recessions? *Journal of Economic Perspectives, 26*, 27–47. https://doi.org/10.1257/jep.26.3.27

Hu, L. T., & Bentler, P. M. (1999). Cutoff criteria for fit indexes in covariance structure analysis: Conventional criteria versus new alternatives. *Structural Equation Modeling, 6*(1), 1–55.

International Labour Organization. (2010, August). *Global employment trends for youth 2010: Special issue on the impact of the global economic crisis on youth.* Geneva: International Labour Office.

International Labour Organization. (2011, January). *Global employment trends 2011: The challenge of a jobs recovery.* Geneva: International Labour Office.

Jahoda, M. (1987). Unemployed men at work. In D. M. Fryer, & P. Ullah (Eds.), *Unemployed people: Social and psychological perspectives* (pp. 1–73). London: Open University Press.

Jahoda, M. (1988). Economic recession and mental health: Some conceptual issues. *Journal of Social Issues, 44*(4), 13–23. https://doi.org/10.1111/j.1540-4560.1988.tb02089.x

Jöreskog, K., & Sörbom, D. (1993). *LISREL 8: Structural equation modeling with the SIMPLIS command language.* Chicago, IL: Scientific Software International Inc.

Julkunen, I. (2001). Coping and mental well-being among unemployed youth. A Northern European perspective. *Journal of Youth Studies, 4*, 261–278. https://doi.org/10.1080/13676260120075419

Jun, R. L., Shah, C. P., & Svoboda, T. J. (1995). The impact of unemployment on health: A review of the evidence. *Canadian Medical Association Journal, 153*, 529–540. https://doi.org/10.2307/3343311

Kirsch, J. A., & Ryff, C. D. (2016). Hardships of the Great Recession and health: Understanding varieties of vulnerability. *Health Psychology Open*, *3*(1), 1–15. https://doi.org/10.1177/2055102916652390

Kowsmann, P. (2011). *Portugal bailout plan detailed*. Retrieved from https://www.wsj.com/articles/SB10001424052748703937104576302883922114642

Lazarus, R. S., & Folkman, S. (1984). *Stress, appraisal, and coping*. New York, NY: Springer.

Lempers, J. D., Clark-Lempers, D., & Simons, R. L. (1989). Economic hardship, parenting, and distress in adolescence. *Child Development*, *60*, 25–39.

Litwin, H. F. A., & Sapir, E. V. (2009). Perceived income adequacy among older adults in 12 countries: Findings from the survey of health, ageing, and retirement in Europe. *Gerontologist*, *49*, 397–406. https://doi.org/10.1093/geront/gnp036

Lung, F. W., & Lee, M. B. (2008). The five-item Brief-Symptom Rating Scale as a suicide ideation screening instrument for psychiatric inpatients and community residents. *BMC Psychiatry*, *8*, 53–61.

Lynch, S. (2008). *Metro US. home prices fall on higher foreclosures*. Retrieved from http://www.bloomberg.com

MacCallum, R. C., Browne, M. W., & Sugawara, H. M. (1996). Power analysis and determination of sample size for covariance structure modeling. *Psychological Methods*, *1* (2), 130–149.

Margerison-Zilko, C., Goldman-Mellor, S., Falconi, A., & Downing, J. (2016). Health impact of the Great Recession: A critical review. *Current Epidemiology Reports*, *3*, 81–91. https://doi.org/10.1007/s40471-016-0068-6

Marjanovic, Z., Greenglass, E. R., Fiksenbaum, L., & Bell, C. M. (2013). Psychometric evaluation of the Financial Threat Scale (FTS) in the context of the Great Recession. *Journal of Economic Psychology*, *36*, 1–10. https://doi.org/10.1016/j.joep.2013.02.005

Marjanovic, Z., Greenglass, E. R., Fiksenbaum, L., De Witte, H., Garcia-Santos, F., Buchwald, P., Peiró, J. M., & Mañas, M. A. (2015). Further psychometric evaluation of the Financial Threat Scale (FTS) in four European, non-student samples. *Journal of Behavioral and Experimental Economics*, *55*, 72–80.

McInerney, M., Mellor, J. M., & Nicholas, L. H. (2013). Recession depression: mental health effects of the 2008 stock market crash. *Journal of Health Economics*, *32*, 1090–1104. https://doi.org/10.1016/j.jhealeco.2013.09.002

Merline, A. C., O'Malley, P. M., Schulenberg, J. E., Bachman, J. G., & Johnston, L. D. (2004). Substance use among adults 35 years of age: Prevalence, adulthood predictors, and impact of adolescent substance use. *American Journal of Public Health*, *94*, 96–102.

Mian, A., & Sufi, A. (2014). *House of debt: How they (and you) caused the Great Recession and how we can prevent it from happening again*. Chicago, IL: University of Chicago Press.

Moscarini, G., & Postel-Vinay, F. (2016). Did the job ladder fail after the Great Recession? *Journal of Labor Economics*, *34*, S1. https://doi.org/10.1086/682366

Mroz, T. A., & Savage, T. H. (2001). The long term-effects of youth unemployment. *Journal of Human Resources*, *41*, 259–293.

Mucci, N., Giorgi, G., Roncaioli, M., Perez, J. F., & Arcangeli, G. (2016). The correlation between stress and economic crisis: A systematic review. *Neuropsychiatric Disease and Treatment*, *12*, 983–993. https://doi.org/10.2147/NDT.S98525

Paul, K., & Moser, K. (2009). Unemployment impairs mental health: Meta-analyses. *Journal of Vocational Behavior*, *74*, 264–282.

Percheski, C., & Kimbro, R. (2014). How did the Great Recession affect fertility? *Focus*, *30* (2), 26–30.

Platt, S., & Hawton, K. (2000). Suicidal behaviour and the labour market. In K. Hawton, & K. van Heeringen (Eds.), *International handbook of suicide and attempted suicide* (pp. 309–384). London: Wiley.

Pudrovska, T., Schiemen, S., Pearlin, L. I., & Nguyen, K. (2005). The sense of mastery as a mediator and moderator in the association between economic hardship and health in late life. *Journal of Aging and Health*, *17*, 634–660.

Reeves, A., McKee, M., & Stuckler, D. (2014). Economic suicides in the Great Recession in Europe and North America. *British Journal of Psychiatry*, *205*, 246–247.

Reinhart, C. M., & Rogoff, K. S. (2009). *The aftermath of financial crises. National Bureau of Economic Research, Working Paper no. 14656.* Cambridge, MA: National Bureau of Economic Research.

Sarason, I. G., Sarason, B. R., & Pierce, G. R. (1990). Anxiety, cognitive interference, and performance. *Journal of Social Behavior and Personality, 5* (2), 1–18.

Schneider, D., Harknett, K., & McLanahan, S. (2016). Intimate partner violence in the great recession. *Demography, 53,* 471–505.

Schumacker, R. E., & Lomax, R. G. (2004). *A beginner's guide to structural equation modeling* (2nd ed.). Mahwah, NJ: Lawrence Erlbaum Associates.

Shacham, S. (1983). A shortened version of the Profile of Mood States. *Journal of Personality Assessment, 47,* 305–306. https://doi.org/10.1207/s15327752jpa4703_14

Sobel, M. E. (1982). Asymptotic intervals for indirect effects in structural equations models. In S. Leinhart (Ed.), *Sociological methodology 1982* (pp. 290–312). San Francisco: Jossey-Bass.

Strully, K. W. (2009). Job loss and health in the U.S. labor market. *Demography, 46,* 221–246.

Sum, A., & Khatiwada, I. (2010). The Nation's underemployed in the "Great Recession" of 2007–09. *Monthly Labor Review, November, 133*(11), 3–15.

Tay, L., Batz, C., Parrigon, S., & Kuykendall, L. (2016). Debt and subjective well-being: The other side of the income-happiness coin. *Journal of Happiness Studies, 17,* 1–35. https://doi.org/10.1007/s10902-016-9758-5

Thébaud, S., & Sharkey, A. J. (2016). Unequal hard times: The influence of the Great Recession on gender bias in entrepreneurial financing. *Sociological Science, 3,* 1–31. https://doi.org/10.15195/v3.a1

Trading Economics. (2013). *Portugal unemployment rate.* Retrieved from http://www.tradingeconomics.com/portugal/unemployment-rate

Treasury Board of Canada Secretariat. (2011). *Canada's performance the year in review: Annual report to parliament 2010–11.* Retrieved from http://www.tbs-sct.gc.ca/reports-rapports/cp-rc/2010-2011/cp-rc-eng.pdf

United Nations. (2015). *The millennium development goals report 2015.* Retrieved from http://unstats.un.org/unsd/mdg/Host.aspx?Content=Products/ProgressReports.htm

U. S. Bureau of Labor Statistics. (2009). *Unemployment rate in May 2009.* Retrieved from http://www.bls.gov/opub/ted/2009/jun/wk2/art02.htm

Usalcus, J. (2010). *Labour market review 2009.* Retrieved from http://www.statcan.gc.ca/pub/75-001-x/2010104/pdf/11148-eng.pdf

Weich, S., & Lewis, G. (1998). Poverty, unemployment, and common mental disorders: population based cohort study. *British Medical Journal, 317,* 115–119.

Wohl, M. J. A., Branscombe, N. R., & Lister, J. J. (2014). When the going gets tough: Economic threat increases financial risk-taking in games of chance. *Social Psychological and Personality Science, 5,* 211–217.

Part II

The Effect of Psychopathology on Everyday Life

The Role of Vulnerable and Grandiose Narcissism in Psychological Perpetrated Abuse Within Couple Relationships: The Mediating Role of Romantic Jealousy

Lucia Ponti ⓘD, Simon Ghinassi ⓘD, and Franca Tani ⓘD

ABSTRACT
The aim of this study was to analyze the direct and indirect relationships between the two phenotypes of narcissism, vulnerable and grandiose, and the tendency to perpetrate psychological abuse, exploring the mediating role of romantic jealousy. Our sample included 473 participants (213 males), aged 18–30 years ($M = 22.74$; $SD = 2.81$), involved in a stable romantic relationship. A structural equation modeling was conducted to test our model and a multi-group analysis was performed to test gender differences. Results show that the two forms of narcissism are both linked to psychological perpetrated abuse, but in different ways. Vulnerable narcissism was linked to psychological abuse only indirectly, through the role of romantic jealousy. On the contrary, grandiose narcissism was positively and directly associated with psychological abuse within the romantic relationship. Moreover, the model was invariant across genders. Limitations, strengths, and theoretical and clinical implications are discussed.

Literature has shown that narcissism is typically associated to dysfunctions in interpersonal relationships due to grandiose sense of self-importance and antagonistic behaviors (American Psychiatric Association, 2013), which significantly influence the tendency to act out on a number of behaviors, including interpersonal aggression, vengeance, and overbearing and vindictive conducts (Brown, 2004; Ogrodniczuk, Piper, Joyce, Steinberg, & Duggal, 2009; Reidy, Foster, & Zeichner, 2010). All these behaviors are strictly linked to the quality of romantic relationship and, in particular, to different forms of perpetration psychological abuse within the couple relationship. To our knowledge, no studies have explored the role of narcissism on this topic. The present study aims to fill this void, exploring the possible mediator variables involved in onset and maintenance of psychological abuse. In particular, the main focus of this study was to study the role played by romantic jealousy, since it is linked to narcissism (Barelds, Dijkstra, Groothof, & Pastoor, 2017; Chin, Atkinson, Raheb, Harris, & Vernon, 2017), and is often indicated as one of the main causes of psychological abuse in couple relationships (Buss, 2000; Collibee & Furman, 2016).

Theoretical Framework

Narcissism

Most studies carried out to date on the effect of narcissism on the quality of romantic relationship have studied narcissism as a unitary dimension (Barelds et al., 2017; Chin et al., 2017; Gormley & Lopez, 2010). However, as clinical and theoretical research has highlighted, narcissism consists of two different components, vulnerable and grandiose (Campbell & Foster, 2007; Lapsley & Aalsma, 2006; Miller et al., 2011; Pincus & Lukowitsky, 2010; Rose, 2002; Zeigler-Hill, Clark, & Pickard, 2008). These two forms of narcissism share some traits: grandiose fantasies, sense of entitlement, and the exploit-ation of others (Pincus et al., 2009). However, they differ on relevant aspects that allow us to imagine different correlations and outcomes associated with each. In particular, grandiose narcissistic individuals are characterized by arrogance, grandiosity, egoism, lack empathy, and use maladaptive strategies to increase their opinions of themselves (Dickinson & Pincus, 2003; Pincus, Cain, & Wright, 2014). Therefore, when they feel threatened, they try to keep their self-esteem high with explicit self-praise and devalu-ation of others who menace their self-esteem (Pincus et al., 2014). However, these strat-egies are illusive and self-defending, since grandiose narcissists need continuous approval and confirmation (Miller & Campbell, 2008; Rose, 2002). This form of narcis-sism tends to be more frequent in males than females. On the contrary, no significant gender differences emerge in vulnerable narcissism (Grijalva et al., 2015).

Vulnerable narcissistic individuals tend to be timid, embarrassed, and anxious, with a frail self-esteem that is influenced and regulated by the responses of others (Dickinson & Pincus, 2003; Given-Wilson, McIlwain, & Warburton, 2011). Moreover, they tend to be more inclined, compared to the grandiose narcissist, to experience negative emotions as a result of a threat to their romantic relationship (Besser & Priel, 2009, 2010). This form of narcissism correlates with reduced happiness and satisfaction with life (Miller & Campbell, 2008; Rose, 2002), psychopathological problems like depression, anxiety and paranoia (Dickinson & Pincus, 2003; Miller et al., 2011), and tends to be associated with anxious romantic attachment and rejection sensitivity (Besser & Priel, 2009).

Based on specific characteristics of the two forms of narcissisms previously described, it is possible to hypothesize that grandiose and vulnerable narcissism may be associated differently to psychological abuse within couple relationships. However, to our know-ledge, no study has explored the relationship between narcissism and psychological abuse taking in account these two forms of narcissism. Our study aims to verify the role that grandiose and vulnerable narcissism have on psychological abuse perpetration.

Psychological Perpetrated Abuse

Psychological perpetrated abuse is a form of interpersonal violence that is implemented through a wide variety of acts and behaviors ranging from dominance, control, isola-tion, physical threats, and criticism, which entail significant and negative consequences for psychological, physical and relational wellbeing of abused subjects (Bonechi & Tani, 2011a, 2011b; Follingstad & DeHart, 2000; Ro & Lawrence, 2007). This form of abuse is very common and has a great incidence in Western cultures (Antônio & Hokoda, 2009;

Falconier, 2010; Menesini & Nocentini, 2008) with percentages ranging from 70% to 90% (Kar & Garcia-Moreno, 2009), compared to Eastern cultures, where the percentages range from 5% to 59% (Hou, Yu, Ting, Sze, & Fang, 2011; Tiwari et al., 2009). It is equally distributed among men and women (Hamel & Nicholls, 2006; Pimlott-Kubiak & Cortina, 2003), and is especially frequent in college dating romantic relationships and during transition to adulthood (Jose & O'Leary, 2009; Milletich, Kelley, Doane, & Pearson, 2010; Schnurr, Lohman, & Kaura, 2010).

Considering the prevalence and negative outcomes of psychological perpetrated abuse, the aim of this study was to explore the possible risk factors involved in its onset and maintenance. Among these, we focused on the role played by romantic jealousy, which resulted to be a significant predictor of psychological abuse perpetration in couple relationships.

Romantic Jealousy

Romantic jealousy is a common and frequent feeling within the couple relationship that can be defined by multiple emotional, cognitive and behavioral manifestations (Pfeiffer & Wong, 1989). The tendency to experience feelings of jealousy within romantic relationships significantly varies by gender: females tend to experience more frequent and intense feelings of jealousy than males (Aumer, Bellew, Ito, Hatfield, & Heck, 2014; Elphinston, Feeney, & Noller, 2011; Tani & Ponti, 2016).

When jealousy is experienced at a high level, becomes excessively frequent, manifests strongly and/or arises in response to unfounded or imaginary situations, it can induce a wide range of effects, significantly influencing the well-being of the individuals (Kingham & Gordon, 2004; White, 1981) and it can have a negative impact on overall life satisfaction and the quality of romantic relationship (Barelds & Barelds-Dijkstra, 2007; Guerrero & Eloy, 1992; Pfeiffer & Wong, 1989, Zusman & Knox, 1998). Numerous studies have widely documented that excessive jealousy can lead to acts of physical, sexual and psychological violence toward partner (Babcock, Costa, Green, & Eckhardt, 2004; Stith, Smith, Penn, Ward, & Tritt, 2004; Wigman, Graham-Kevan, & Archer, 2008), or even cases of murder and suicide (O'Leary, Smith-Slep, & O'Leary, 2007). The aim of the present study was to verify the role played by romantic jealousy on the relationship between narcissism and psychological abuse perpetration within couple relationships.

The Current Study

Starting with the above considerations, the main focus of this study was to verify the different roles of the two forms of narcissism on psychological perpetrated abuse, exploring the possible mediator role of romantic jealousy, taking in account gender differences. In particular, our aim was to: 1) analyze gender differences and relationships in all variables considered; 2) test the theoretical model shown in Figure 1; 3) explore gender differences in influencing the complex relations among these variables.

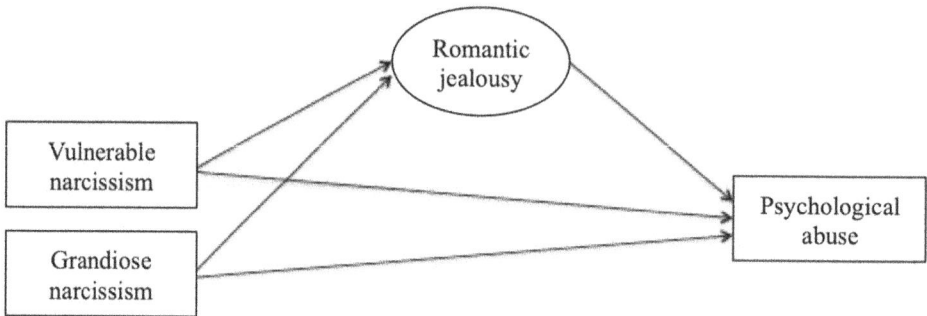

Figure 1. Hypothesized model.

Methods

Participants and Procedure

A convenience sample of 473 participants involved in a romantic relationship (213 males and 260 females), aged 18–30 years ($M = 22.74$; SD $= 2.81$), was recruited among university students (School of Psychology, Political Science and Law) in Florence (Italy).

The study was conducted in compliance with the ethical principles of research published by the American Psychological Association and approval of the study was obtained by the ethics committee of the University of Florence (n.35/7th November 2018). All subjects were fully informed about the goals of the survey. They were told that their participation was voluntary, and they could drop out at any time without incurring in any consequences. The inclusion criterion to participate in the survey was to be involved in a stable and heterosexual romantic relationship for at least one year. Written informed consent was obtained for all participants before data collection. Two trained researchers recruited participants. Specifically, they presented our research project during classes of several university courses and asked students to participate in the study. About the 10% of students approached declined the invitation without providing any explanation. Students who accepted were invited to a meeting room at the university to complete the questionnaires in small groups, and the researcher recommended that participants fill in all items. After signing the informed consent form, participants anonymously completed a battery of questionnaires designed to gather information about personal and demographic data, measure their level of vulnerable and grandiose narcissism, romantic jealousy, and their tendency to perpetrate psychological abuse. The order of the questions was randomized in order to control possible bias related to tiredness. No monetary reward was given for participation.

Measures

In order to assess the level of vulnerable narcissism, the Italian version of the *Hypersensitive Narcissism Scale* (HSNS: Fossati et al., 2009; Hendin & Cheek, 1997) was used. The HSNS is a self-report questionnaire composed of 10 items, rated on a 5-point Likert-type scale from 1 (very uncharacteristic or untrue) to 5 (very characteristic or true), which measures vulnerable narcissism using statements regarding feelings of narcissistic hypersensitivity (example of item: "I often interpret the remarks of others in a personal way"). The HSNS has demonstrated a good reliability and validity in several studies (e.g. Miller et al., 2011; Pincus et al., 2009), both in clinical and non-clinical samples (Fossati et al., 2009). Higher scores on the HSNS indicate higher levels of vulnerable narcissism. In the present study, the alpha coefficient was .67. Although this alpha value is questionable (George & Mallery, 2003), it is consistent with the reliability value reported by the authors of the original scale (Hendin & Cheek, 1997) and by the authors of the Italian version (Fossati et al., 2009).

To assess grandiose narcissism, the Italian version of the *Narcissistic Personality Inventory* (NPI-16; Ames, Rose, & Anderson, 2006; Fossati, Borroni, & Maffei, 2008) was used. This scale is a self-report questionnaire and it is a shorter, unidimensional measure of the NPI-40. The NPI-16 contains 16 pairs of items, each consisting of two opposing statements which the participant chooses according to his/her beliefs and feelings (example of a pair of items, "I am more capable than other people" and "There is a lot that I can learn from other people"). Also in this case, higher scores on the NPI-16 reflect higher levels of grandiose narcissism. In the present study, the Alpha coefficients was .76.

Participants' romantic jealousy was assessed by using the Italian version of the *Short Form of the Multidimensional Jealousy Scale* (SF-MJS: Elphinston et al., 2011; Tani & Ponti, 2016). The SF-MJS is a self-report questionnaire consisting of 17 items that assesses a global score on three main dimensions of romantic jealousy. In particular, the first dimension, *cognitive jealousy*, refers to the subject's tendency to have suspicions, thoughts and doubts related to the partner's fidelity (e.g. "I suspect that my partner is secretly seeing someone else of the opposite sex"). The second dimension, emotional jealousy, refers to the affective responses of the subject to possible threats to their own relationship (e.g. "Your partner comments to you on how great looking a particular member of the opposite sex is"). Finally, the third dimension, behavioral jealousy, assesses the presence of control and intrusion behaviors implemented by the subject (e.g. "I look through my partner's drawers, handbag, or pockets").

Each item is rated on a 7-point Likert-type scale from 1 to 7: from 1 (all the time) to 7 (never) for cognitive and behavioral dimensions, and from 1 (very pleased) to 7 (very upset) for emotional dimension. Higher scores correspond to a higher presence of feelings of romantic jealousy. The *ISF-MJS* has demonstrated a good factorial structure and internal consistency, both in dimension and global score (Tani & Ponti, 2016). In the present study, the global score of jealousy was used and its Cronbach's alpha value was .83.

Finally, the perpetration subscale of the Italian version of the *Multidimensional Measure of Emotional Abuse* (Bonechi & Tani, 2011b; MMEA Murphy & Hoover, 1999; Murphy, Hoover, & Taft, 1999) was used to assess the presence of perpetrated psychological abuse. It is a self-report scale containing 28 items rated on a 7-point Likert-type scale from 0 (never) to 6 (more than 20 times). Participants were asked to report the frequency with which forms of psychological abuse were perpetrated within their own romantic relationship within the past six months. In particular, the MMEA assesses a global score of perpetrated psychological abuse or four main dimensions of this construct: 1) Restrictive Engulfment, which includes coercive acts or behaviors that isolate, restrict, monitor, and control the partner's activities and social contacts, or represent displays of jealousy or possessiveness that increase the partner's dependency and avail-ability (e.g. "Tried to stop your partner from seeing certain friends or family mem-bers"); 2) Denigration, which comprises actions or verbal attacks that reduce the partner's self-esteem, through denigration and humiliation (e.g. "Called your partner a loser, failure, or similar term"); 3) Hostile Withdrawal, which consists of behaviors that are intended to punish the partner or increase anxiety or insecurity about the relation-ship, such as cold and punitive avoidance during conflict, withholding emotional con-tact and availability (e.g. "Intentionally avoided your partner during a conflict or disagreement"); 4) Dominance/Intimidation, which includes behaviors that produce fear or submission through the use of aggression, such as threats, property destruction, and intense verbal aggression (e.g. "Threw, smashed, hit, or kicked something in front of your partner"). Higher scores on the perpetration subscale of the MMEA indicate higher levels of psychological abuse perpetrated in couple relationship. In the present study, the global score of psychological abuse was used and its internal consistency was .85.

Data Analysis

Descriptive analyses and bivariate correlations among all the variables were calculated for all participants. To examine gender differences with regards to vulnerable and grandiose narcissism, romantic jealousy and psychological abuse, a series of univari-ate analyses of variance (ANOVA) was employed. In order to test the theoretical hypothesized model, structural equation modeling was conducted, using the MPLUS statistical program (Muthén & Muthén, 1998–2007). To evaluate the model, several indices were reported, including the χ^2, the Comparative Fit Index (CFI, Bentler, 1990), the Tucker & Lewis Index (TLI, Tucker & Lewis, 1973), the Root Mean Square Error of Approximation (RMSEA; Browne & Cudeck, 1993), and the Standardized Root Mean Square Residual (SRMR; Bentler, 1995). Cutoff values for fit were consid-ered adequate if CFI and TLI values were ≥.90, and RMSEA and SRMR values were ≤.05, (Blunch, 2008). In order to examine the indirect effects, the bootstrapping method and bias-corrected 95% confidence intervals were used, with 2,000 boot-strap samples.

Finally, to test the invariance of the theoretical model, a multigroup analysis was per-formed. We started from an unconstrained structural path in order to obtain a baseline χ^2 value. This baseline model does not assume any equality constraint for the parame-ters in males and females. If the model fits, the structural paths of the tested model were constrained across sex. Invariance was tested by comparing the baseline model with the constrained one (Meredith, 1993). No significant outcome between the two models suggested invariance across groups.

Results

Descriptive and Bivariate Correlations Data

Referring to the socio-demographical characteristics of the sample, more than 95% of the participants were Caucasian, and 72% of them came from central Italy.

Table 1. Descriptive Statistics, Correlations Values and Skewness and Kurtosis Values of the Two Forms of Narcissism, the Three Dimensions of Romantic Jealousy, and the Psychological Abuse.

	Range	M	SD	Skewness	Kurtosis	1	2	3	4
1. Vulnerable narcissism	10–50	27.02	5.75	−.305	−.176	–	.08	.26**	.13*
2. Grandiose narcissism	0–16	3.37	2.96	.957	.375	.16*	–	.15*	.43**
3. Romantic jealousy	17–119	54.87	14.14	.296	.419	.32**	.08	–	.35**
4. Psychological abuse	0–196	27.32	18.32	.921	.700	.24**	.23**	.36**	–

Note. *$p<.01$; **$p<.001$; referring to correlation values, below the diagonal are reported the values for males, above the diagonal the values for females.

Overall, participants came from families of middle or high socio-economic status (SES), with more than 79% of the fathers and 83% of the mothers having a high school diploma or university degree. The duration of the couple relationship ranged from 12 to 51 months ($M_{months}=25.80$; SD $= 9.65$). Ninety-four couples (19.9%) were cohabitants, none were married.

Significant differences emerged between cohabitants and non-cohabitants with respect to the duration of romantic relationship ($t(469)=6.60$; $p=.000$) and the level of romantic jealousy ($t(469)=-2.88$; $p=.004$) with cohabitants having a longer relationship and reporting lower levels of jealousy towards their partners. However, no significant differences emerged between cohabitants and non-cohabitants in reference to the level of psychological abuse ($t(469)=-.40$; $p=.686$), vulnerable narcissism ($t(469)=-.76$; $p=.448$), and grandiose narcissism ($t(469)=1.33$; $p=.185$).

Moreover, we controlled the role of the age, romantic relationship length, ethnicity, and SES on the level of psychological perpetrated abuse. Results of linear regression showed that neither the age nor the duration of couple relationship affected the level of perpetrated abuse (age: $\beta=.06$; $p = 194$; length relationship: $\beta=-.06$; $p = 162$). Moreover, no significant differences emerged with respect to ethnicity ($t(471)=-1.01$; $p=.311$). Finally, we created a score of high vs. low SES, considering as high a family in which both parents have at least a high school diploma or more. We found 115 participants (24.3%) with a family characterized by a low SES and 358 (75.7%) by a high SES. Also for this variable, no significant difference emerged in reference to the level of psychological perpetrated abuse ($t(471)=-.16$; $p=.887$).

Overall, the levels of the tendency to perpetrate psychological abuse within couple relationships were high. Almost all participants ($n = 478$; 98.9%) reported that some form of psychological abuse had taken place in their couple relationships within the preceding six months.

Table 1 reports the descriptive statistics and bivariate correlations among all the variables, the last separately for gender. Referring to bivariate correlations, in accordance with the criteria provided by Hinkle, Wiersma, and Jurs (2003), that a coefficient value less than .30 is negligible, results highlighted significant and positive correlations between psychological abuse and behavioral jealousy for both genders. Moreover, only for females, psychological abuse also showed significant and positive correlations with grandiose narcissism. Finally, only for males, vulnerable narcissism was positively correlated with romantic jealousy. Males who reported high levels of romantic jealousy presented higher levels of vulnerable narcissism and psychological abuse in their romantic relationships. Females who reported high levels of psychological abuse presented higher levels of grandiose narcissism and romantic jealousy.

Table 2. Descriptive Statistics and Univariate Analyses Results by Gender.

	Males		Females					95% CI	
	M	SD	M	SD	F(1,471)	p	η^2	Lower	Upper
Vulnerable narcissism	26.53	6.05	27.42	5.47	2.75	.098	.01	−1.92	.16
Grandiose narcissism	4.20	3.23	2.69	2.52	32.69	.000	.07	.993	2.03
Romantic jealousy	52.01	14.84	57.20	13.12	16.27	.000	.03	−7.72	−2.67
Psychological abuse	26.64	19.97	27.89	16.87	.544	.461	.00	−4.58	2.08

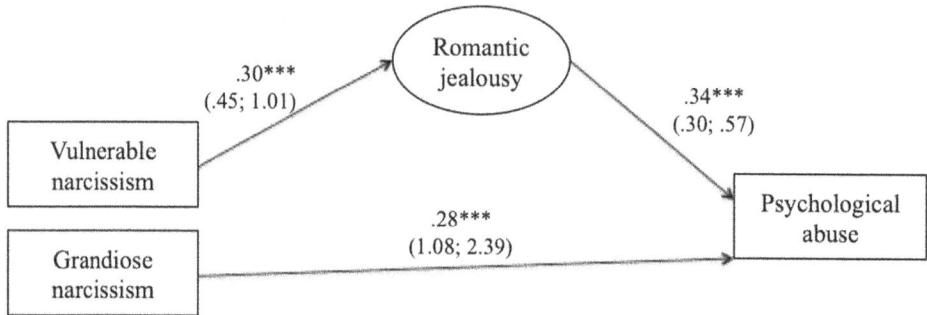

Figure 2. Results of tested model and its standardized solution (95% CI are shown in parentheses).

Gender Differences

Table 2 reports the mean and standard deviations of the variables under study by gender, and the results of the univariate comparisons obtained with ANOVAs.

As shown in the table, there are significant differences between males and females on the level of grandiose narcissism and the level of romantic jealousy. In particular, males reported higher levels of grandiose narcissism and lower levels of jealousy towards their partners than females. On the contrary, males and females did not differ regarding vulnerable narcissism and level of psychological abuse.

Model Testing

We tested the hypothesized model using the Maximum Likelihood estimator (ML, Muthén & Muthén, 1998–2007), because all variables have univariate skewness and kurtoses within the range ±1.

Results showed that two path coefficients were not statistically significant: 1) vulnerable narcissism on psychological perpetrated abuse, and 2) grandiose narcissism on romantic jealousy. Therefore, we proceeded to remove these paths and repeated the analysis on the modified model reported in Figure 2.

The modified model fit the data very well: $\chi^2=3.238$, $df=2$; $p=.151$; CFI=.99, TLI=.98; RMSEA=.04; SRMR=.02). The findings revealed significant effects of grandiose narcissism on the level of psychological abuse. A high level of this form of narcissism was positively linked to the tendency to act out psychological abuse in the romantic relationship. On the contrary, vulnerable narcissism was positively linked to romantic jealousy and this, in turn, showed a significant and positive link with psychological abuse. Finally, psychological abuse was predicted in an indirect way by the level of vulnerable narcissism ($\beta=.10$, $p<.001$; CI 95%: .16, .48).

Table 3. Results of the Invariance Tests and Their Goodness of Fit Indices.

	χ^2	df	χ^2/df	CFI	TLI	RMSEA	SRMR	Δdf	$\Delta\chi^2$
Baselined model	8.637	4	2.16	.97	.93	.07	.4	–	–
Constrained model	15.945	7	2.28	.94	.92	.07	.06	3	ns

Squared multiple correlation coefficients from the model indicated that 20% of the variance in observed variable of psychological abuse, and 9% of the variance in romantic jealousy, were accounted for. In Figure 1, all statistical coefficients of direct effect are reported.

Invariance Across Gender

Results of the invariance test across the male and female sample resulted in a non-significant change in χ^2 value, showing that the model was invariant in males and females. Results of the invariance analysis are shown in Table 3.

Discussion

The main aim of this study was to examine the associations of vulnerable and grandiose narcissism with the perpetration of psychological abuse and analyze the potential mediating role of romantic jealousy, taking into consideration the gender effect. Most literature found a significant relationship between narcissism and psychological abuse, however, to our knowledge, no studies have investigated this relationship taking into consideration the different forms of both vulnerable and grandiose narcissism and the possible role played by romantic jealousy.

Therefore, the present study expands on current literature, implementing a structural equation model to test a complex theoretical model regarding the link between vulnerable and grandiose narcissism separately, romantic jealousy, and the level of psychological abuse perpetrated in romantic relationships. Moreover, the role of gender differences was also explored.

First, results demonstrated that some of the variables we studied showed sex differences. In line with previous studies, we found that females reported higher levels of romantic jealousy than males (Aumer et al., 2014; Elphinston et al., 2011; Tani & Ponti, 2016). Regarding the two forms of narcissism, results showed that gender differences arise only for the grandiose form, where men reported higher levels than women (Grijalva et al., 2015), while no differences emerged in vulnerable narcissism and psychological abuse. As previous studies have shown, grandiose narcissism reflects specific psychological characteristics that are more typical in the male population, such as aggressiveness, leadership, or unethical and abusive behaviors (Brunell, Staats, Barden, & Hupp, 2011; Grijalva et al., 2015). On the contrary, in line with the social role theory (Eagly & Wood, 2011), women face tougher sanctions when displaying dominant and aggressive behaviors in comparison to men, making the adoption of grandiose narcissism less adaptive for women.

Referring to psychological abuse, results have shown that these behaviors were equally perpetrated by males and females, in line with previous studies which highlighted that this specific form of abuse can be implemented by both members of the couple (Archer,

2000; Bonechi & Tani, 2011b; Hamel & Nicholls, 2006; Pimlott-Kubiak & Cortina, 2003). Moreover, results showed that behaviors of psychological perpetrated abuse are very common in our sample. It is probable that the high prevalence of abuse is linked to specific characteristics of our participants. In fact, they were Western university students, mostly non-cohabitants. These results are consistent with previous national (Bonechi & Tani, 2011a), and international studies (Kar & Garcia-Moreno, 2009), carried out on similar samples in terms of age, status of romantic relationship and ethnicity, and in general with extensive literature showing that psychological abuse perpetration is very frequent in romantic dating relationships during the transition to adulthood in Western cultures (Jose & O'Leary, 2009; Milletich et al., 2010; Schnurr et al., 2010).

In reference to the second aim, our results showed that the two forms of narcissism are linked to the perpetration of psychological abuse in different ways. In particular, vulnerable narcissism was indirectly linked to psychological perpetrated abuse through romantic jealousy: participants who reported high levels of this dimension tend to feel a high level of jealousy toward their partners and, in turn, this feeling is a significant risk factor to act out psychological abuse. These results can be understood by taking into consideration previous studies, which have highlighted that vulnerable narcissists experience high anxiety within interpersonal relationships, are highly sensitive to separation signals, and feel greater distress at the time of separation (Besser & Priel, 2009, 2010). These individual characteristics, in turn, could reflect higher vigilance to potential threats to their own romantic relationships, consequently increasing their jealousy feelings.

On the contrary, results highlighted that grandiose narcissism was directly related to the tendency to be psychologically abusive towards partners. In other words, grandiose narcissistic individuals that are indifferent regarding their partner's feelings and have difficulty understanding the impact of their behaviors on others (Miller, Campbell, & Pilkonis, 2007) tend to implement psychological abuse through behaviors such as isolation, denigration, disdain, and control of the partner, in order to keep their own self-image high and maintain dominance in the relationship (Pincus et al., 2014).

This explicative tested model resulted invariant between males and females. Therefore, despite the above-mentioned gender differences in the level of jealousy and grandiose narcissism, the relations among all the investigated variables were uniform across gender.

There are some limitations to the present study. First, research relied only on self-report measures. Despite the limitations of a self-report questionnaire and the need to confirm the pattern of relations with other study designs, the individuals' perception of their close relationships and feelings represents an important source of information that should not be neglected (Cunningham & Barbee, 2000). Second, we did not consider any measure of social desirability. This could be a problem especially for the MMEA, where students may have had difficulty admitting to psychological abuse in their couple relationships. Third, we assessed only psychological perpetrated abuse. It would also be interesting to examine the relationship between the two forms of narcissism and the tendency to be victims of psychological abuse in couple relationships and explore the possible differences in the relationship between vulnerable and grandiose narcissism on victimization vs perpetration of psychological abuse. Fourth, given the cross-sectional study design, it is impossible to infer casual relations and determine the direction of the observed effects. Moreover, we investigated only heterosexual relationships. It would be interesting to explore the role that these variables play in other types of relationships. Another limitation is the convenience sample used in this study. Future research should extend the recruitment to a stratified sample (e.g. stratified SES, provenience, and culture), since the results of the present study are based on a sample constituted only by young university students, for the most part Italian and with a romantic relationship status as a non-cohabitant. Finally, the tested model is not exhaustive, and other variables can certainly play a significant role in the interaction between these constructs. For example, regarding vulnerable narcissism, Besser and Priel (2009) found a significant role played by anxious romantic attachment in mediating the relationship between vulnerable narcissism and romantic jealousy.

Despite these limitations, this study has important theoretical and clinical implications. From a theoretical point of view, our study enriches the understanding of the complex construct of narcissism and the different outcomes that it has for the individual and his/her relational life. In fact, our results confirm the necessity to separately analyze the two forms of narcissism, grandiose and vulnerable, for the different associations and implications that they have with several psychological and relational variables.

From a clinical point of view, these findings could have important implications for clinicians who deal with couples and victims of abuse. In fact, greater knowledge of the role that the different phenotypes of narcissism have on implementation of psychological abuse, and the role that romantic jealousy has in this relationship, can be useful knowledge to prevent abuse in the relationship, or to more effectively help those who are involved in violent relationships.

ORCID

Lucia Ponti http://orcid.org/0000-0001-8255-5672
Simon Ghinassi http://orcid.org/0000-0002-7451-1861
Franca Tani http://orcid.org/0000-0002-6795-6520

References

American Psychiatric Association. (2013). *Diagnostic and statistical manual of mental disorders* (5th ed.). Washington, DC: American Psychiatric Publishing.

Ames, D. R., Rose, P., & Anderson, C. P. (2006). The NPI-16 as a short measure of narcissism. *Journal of Research in Personality*, 40(4), 440–450. doi:10.1016/j.jrp.2005.03.002

Antônio, T., & Hokoda, A. (2009). Gender variations in dating violence and positive conflict resolution among Mexican adolescents. *Violence & Victims*, 24(4), 533–545. doi:10.1891/0886-6708.24.4.533

Archer, J. (2000). Sex differences in aggression between heterosexual partners: A meta-analytic review. *Psychological Bulletin*, 126(5), 651–680. doi:10.1037//0033-2909.126.5.651

Aumer, K., Bellew, W., Ito, B., Hatfield, E., & Heck, R. (2014). The happy green eyed monogamist: Role of jealousy and compersion in monogamous and non-traditional relationships. *Electronic Journal of Human Sexuality*, 17(1), 77–88.

Babcock, J. C., Costa, D. M., Green, C. E., & Eckhardt, C. I. (2004). What situations induce intimate partner violence? A reliability and validity study of the Proximal Antecedents to Violent Episodes (PAVE) scale. *Journal of Family Psychology*, 18(3), 433–442. doi:10.1037/0893-3200.18.3.433

Barelds, D. P. H., & Barelds-Dijkstra, P. (2007). Relations between different types of jealousy and self and partner perceptions of relationship quality. *Clinical Psychology & Psychotherapy*, 14, 176–188. doi:10.1002/cpp.532

Barelds, D. P. H., Dijkstra, P., Groothof, H. A. K., & Pastoor, C. D. (2017). The Dark Triad and three types of jealousy: Its relations among heterosexuals and homosexuals involved in a romantic relationship. *Personality & Individual Differences*, 116, 6–10. doi:10.1016/j.paid.2017.04.017

Bentler, P. M. (1990). Comparative fit indexes in structural models. *Psychological Bulletin*, 107(2), 238–246. doi:10.1037/0033-2909.107.2.238

Bentler, P. M. (1995). *EQS structural equations program manual*. Encino, CA: Multivariate Software.

Besser, A., & Priel, B. (2009). Emotional responses to a romantic partner's imaginary rejection: The roles of attachment anxiety, covert narcissism, and self-evaluation. *Journal of Personality*, 77(1), 287–325. doi:10.1111/j.1467-6494.2008.00546.x

Besser, A., & Priel, B. (2010). Grandiose narcissism versus vulnerable narcissism in threatening situations: Emotional reactions to achievement failure and interpersonal rejection. *Journal of Social & Clinical Psychology*, 29(8), 874–902. doi:10.1521/jscp.2010.29.8.874

Blunch, N. J. (2008). *Introduction to structural equation modeling*. London, UK: SAGE.

Bonechi, A., & Tani, F. (2011a). Le ferite invisibili: L'abuso psicologico nelle relazioni di coppia [The invisible injures: The psychological abuse in intimate relationships]. *Psicologia Clinica Dello Sviluppo*, 15(3), 491–524. doi:10.1449/35885

Bonechi, A., & Tani, F. (2011b). Italian adaptation of the multidimensional measure of emotional abuse (MMEA). *TPM-Testing, Psychometrics, Methodology in Applied Psychology*, 18(2), 65–86.

Brown, R. P. (2004). Vengeance is mine: Narcissism, vengeance, and the tendency to forgive. *Journal of Research in Personality*, 38(6), 576–584. doi:10.1016/j.jrp.2003.10.003

Browne, M. W., & Cudeck, R. (1993). Alternative ways of assessing model fit. *Sociological Methods & Research*, 21, 230–258. doi:10.1177/0049124192021002005

Brunell, A. B., Staats, S., Barden, J., & Hupp, J. M. (2011). Narcissism and academic dishonesty: The exhibitionism dimension and the lack of guilt. *Personality & Individual Differences*, 50(3), 323–328. doi:10.1016/j.paid.2010.10.006

Buss, D. M. (2000). *The dangerous passion: Why jealousy is as necessary as love and sex*. New York, NY: The Free Press.

Campbell, W. K., & Foster, J. D. (2007). The narcissistic self: Background, an extended agency model, and ongoing controversies. In C. Sedikides & S. J. Spencer (Eds.), *The self* (pp. 115–138). New York, NY: Psychology Press.

Chin, K., Atkinson, B. E., Raheb, H., Harris, E., & Vernon, P. A. (2017). The dark side of romantic jealousy. *Personality & Individual Differences, 115*, 23–29. doi:10.1016/j.paid.2016.10.003

Collibee, C., & Furman, W. (2016). Chronic and acute relational risk factors for dating aggression in adolescence and young adulthood. *Journal of Youth & Adolescence, 45*(4), 763–776. doi:10.1007/s10964-016-0427-0

Cunningham, M. R., & Barbee, A. P. (2000). Social support. In C. Hendrick & S. S. Hendrick (Eds.), *Close relationships: A sourcebook* (pp. 273–285). Thousand Oaks, CA: SAGE.

Dickinson, K. A., & Pincus, A. L. (2003). Interpersonal analysis of grandiose and vulnerable narcissism. *Journal of Personality Disorders, 17*(3), 188–207. doi:10.1521/pedi.17.3.188.22146

Eagly, A. H., & Wood, W. (2011). Social role theory. *Handbook of theories in social psychology* (Vol. 2, pp. 458–476). New York, NY: SAGE. doi:10.4135/9781446249222.n49

Elphinston, R. A., Feeney, J. A., & Noller, P. (2011). Measuring romantic jealousy: Validation of the multidimensional jealousy scale in Australian samples. *Australian Journal of Psychology, 63*(4), 243–251. doi:10.1111/j.1742-9536.2011.00026.x

Falconier, M. K. (2010). Female anxiety and male depression: Links between economic strain and psychological aggression in Argentinean couples. *Family Relations, 59*(4), 424–438. doi:10.1111/j.1741-3729.2010.00613.x

Follingstad, D. R., & DeHart, D. (2000). Defining psychological abuse of husbands toward wives: Contexts, behaviors, and typologies. *Journal of Interpersonal Violence, 15*(9), 891–920. doi:10.1177/088626000015009001

Fossati, A., Borroni, S., Grazioli, F., Dornetti, L., Marcassoli, I., Maffei, C., & Cheek, J. (2009). Tracking the hypersensitive dimension in narcissism: Reliability and validity of the Hypersensitive Narcissism Scale. *Personality & Mental Health, 3*(4), 235–247. doi:10.1002/pmh.92

Fossati, A., Borroni, S., & Maffei, C. (2008). Proprietà Psicometriche della Versione Italiana del Narcissistic personality inventory [Psychometric properties of the Italian version of the Narcissistic Personality Inventory]. *Rivista di Psicologia Clinica, 1*, 96–115.

George, D., & Mallery, P. (2003). *SPSS for Windows step by step: A simple guide and reference. 11.0 update* (4th ed.). Boston, MA: Allyn & Bacon.

Given-Wilson, Z., McIlwain, D., & Warburton, W. (2011). Meta-cognitive and interpersonal difficulties in overt and covert narcissism. *Personality & Individual Differences, 50*(7), 1000–1005. doi:10.1016/j.paid.2011.01.014

Gormley, B., & Lopez, F. G. (2010). Correlates of psychological abuse perpetration in college dating relationships. *Journal of College Counseling, 13*(1), 4–16. doi:10.1002/j.2161-1882.2010.tb00044.x

Grijalva, E., Newman, D. A., Tay, L., Donnellan, M. B., Harms, P. D., Robins, R. W., & Yan, T. (2015). Gender differences in narcissism: A meta-analytic review. *Psychological Bulletin, 141*(2), 261. doi:10.1037/a0038231

Guerrero, L. K., & Eloy, S. V. (1992). Relationship satisfaction and jealousy across marital types. *Communication Reports, 5*(1), 23–31. doi:10.1080/08934219209367540

Hamel, J., & Nicholls, T. (2006). *Family interventions in domestic violence: A handbook of gender-inclusive theory and treatment.* New York, NY: Springfield Publishing.

Hendin, H. M., & Cheek, J. M. (1997). Assessing hypersensitive narcissism: A reexamination of Murray's narcissism scale. *Journal of Research in Personality, 31*(4), 588–599. doi:10.1006/jrpe.1997.2204

Hinkle, D. E., Wiersma, W., & Jurs, S. G. (2003). *Applied statistics for the behavioral sciences* (5th ed.). Boston, MA: Houghton Mifflin.

Hou, J., Yu, L., Ting, S. M. R., Sze, Y. T., & Fang, X. (2011). The status and characteristics of couple violence in China. *Journal of Family Violence, 26*(2), 81–92. doi:10.1007/s10896-010-9343-3

Jose, A., & O'Leary, K. D. (2009). Prevalence of partner aggression in representative and clinic samples. In K. D. O'Leary & E. M. Woodin (Eds.), *Psychological and physical aggression in couples: Causes and interventions* (pp. 15–35). Washington, DC: American Psychological Association.

Kar, H. L., & Garcia-Moreno, C. (2009). Partner aggression across cultures. In K. D. O'Leary & E. M. Woodin (Eds.), *Psychological and physical aggression in couples: Causes and interventions* (pp. 59–75). Washington, DC: American Psychological Association.

Kingham, M., & Gordon, H. (2004). Aspects of morbid jealousy. *Advances in Psychiatric Treatment, 10*(3), 207–215. doi:10.1192/apt.10.3.207

Lapsley, D. K., & Aalsma, M. C. (2006). An empirical typology of narcissism and mental health in late adolescence. *Journal of Adolescence, 29*(1), 53–71. doi:10.1016/j.adolescence.2005.01.008

Menesini, E., & Nocentini, A. (2008). Comportamenti aggressivi nelle prime esperienze sentimentali in adolescenza [Aggressive behaviors in early sentimental experiences in adolescence]. *Giornale Italiano di Psicologia, 35*(2), 407–434.

Meredith, W. (1993). Measurement invariance, factor analysis, and factorial invariance. *Psychometrika, 58*(4), 525–543. doi:10.1007/BF02294825

Miller, J. D., & Campbell, W. K. (2008). Comparing clinical and social-personality conceptualizations of narcissism. *Journal of Personality, 76*(3), 449–476. doi:10.1111/j.1467-6494.2008.00492.x

Miller, J. D., Campbell, W. K., & Pilkonis, P. A. (2007). Narcissistic personality disorder: Relations with distress and functional impairment. *Comprehensive Psychiatry, 48*(2), 170–177. doi:10.1016/j.comppsych.2006.10.003

Miller, J. D., Hoffman, B. J., Gaughan, E. T., Gentile, B., Maples, J., & Keith Campbell, W. (2011). Grandiose and vulnerable narcissism: A nomological network analysis. *Journal of Personality, 79*(5), 1013–1042. doi:10.1111/j.1467-6494.2010.00711.x

Milletich, R. J., Kelley, M. L., Doane, A. N., & Pearson, M. R. (2010). Exposure to interparental violence and childhood physical and emotional abuse as related to physical aggression in undergraduate dating relationships. *Journal of Family Violence, 25*(7), 627–637. doi:10.1007/s10896-010-9319-3

Murphy, C. M., & Hoover, S. A. (1999). Measuring emotional abuse in dating relationships as a multifactorial construct. *Violence & Victims, 14*(1), 39–53. doi:10.1891/0886-6708.14.1.39

Murphy, C. M., Hoover, S. A., & Taft, C. (1999, November). *The multidimensional measure of emotional abuse: Factor structure and subscale validity.* Paper presented at the Annual Meeting of the Association for the Advancement of Behavior Therapy, Toronto, ON, Canada.

Muthén, L. K., & Muthén, B. O. (1998–2007). *Mplus user's guide* (7th ed.). Los Angeles, CA: Muthén & Muthén.

O'Leary, K. D., Smith Slep, A. M., & O'Leary, S. G. (2007). Multivariate models of men's and women's partner aggression. *Journal of Consulting & Clinical Psychology, 75*(5), 752. doi:10.1037/0022-006X.75.5.752

Ogrodniczuk, J. S., Piper, W. E., Joyce, A. S., Steinberg, P. I., & Duggal, S. (2009). Interpersonal problems associated with narcissism among psychiatric outpatients. *Journal of Psychiatric Research, 43*(9), 837–842. doi:10.1016/j.jpsychires.2008.12.005

Pfeiffer, S. M., & Wong, P. T. P. (1989). Multidimensional jealousy. *Journal of Social & Personal Relationships, 6*(2), 181–196. doi:10.1177/026540758900600203

Pimlott-Kubiak, S., & Cortina, L. M. (2003). Gender, victimization, and outcomes: Reconceptualizing risk. *Journal of Consulting & Clinical Psychology, 71*(3), 528–539. doi:10.1037/0022-006X.71.3.528

Pincus, A. L., Ansell, E. B., Pimentel, C. A., Cain, N. M., Wright, A. G., & Levy, K. N. (2009). Initial construction and validation of the Pathological Narcissism Inventory. *Psychological Assessment, 21*(3), 365. doi:10.1037/a0016530

Pincus, A. L., Cain, N. M., & Wright, A. G. (2014). Narcissistic grandiosity and narcissistic vulnerability in psychotherapy. *Personality Disorders: Theory, Research, & Treatment, 5*(4), 439–443. doi:10.1037/per0000031

Pincus, A. L., & Lukowitsky, M. R. (2010). Pathological narcissism and narcissistic personality disorder. *Annual Review of Clinical Psychology, 6*(1), 421–446. doi:10.1146/annurev.clinpsy.121208.131215

Reidy, D. E., Foster, J. D., & Zeichner, A. (2010). Narcissism and unprovoked aggression. *Aggressive Behavior, 36*(6), 414–422. doi:10.1002/ab.20356

Ro, E., & Lawrence, E. (2007). Comparing three measures of psychological aggression: Psychometric properties and differentiation from negative communication. *Journal of Family Violence*, 22(7), 575–586. doi:10.1007/s10896-007-9109-8

Rose, P. (2002). The happy and unhappy faces of narcissism. *Personality & Individual Differences*, 33(3), 379–391. doi:10.1016/S0191-8869(01)00162-3

Schnurr, M. P., Lohman, B. J., & Kaura, S. A. (2010). Variation in late adolescents' reports of dating violence perpetration: A dyadic analysis. *Violence & Victims*, 25(1), 84. doi:10.1891/0886-6708.25.1.84

Stith, S. M., Smith, D. B., Penn, C. E., Ward, D. B., & Tritt, D. (2004). Intimate partner physical abuse perpetration and victimization risk factors: A meta-analytic review. *Aggression & Violent Behavior*, 10(1), 65–98. doi:10.1016/j.avb.2003.09.001

Tani, F., & Ponti, L. (2016). The romantic jealousy as multidimensional construct: A study on the Italian Short Form of the Multidimensional Jealousy Scale. *The Open Psychology Journal*, 09(1), 111–120. doi:10.2174/1874350101609010111

Tiwari, A., Wong, J., Brownridge, D. A., Chan, K. L., Fong, D. Y., Leung, W. C., & Ho, P. C. (2009). Psychological intimate partner abuse among Chinese women: What we know and what we still need to know. *The Open Social Science Journal*, 2(1), 32–36. doi:10.2174/1874945300902010032

Tucker, L. R., & Lewis, C. (1973). A reliability coefficient for maximum likelihood factor analysis. *Psychometrika*, 38(1), 1–10. doi:10.1007/BF02291170

White, G. L. (1981). A model of romantic jealousy. *Motivation & Emotion*, 5(4), 295–310. doi:10.1007/BF00992549

Wigman, S. A., Graham-Kevan, N., & Archer, J. (2008). Investigating sub-groups of harassers: The roles of attachment, dependency, jealousy and aggression. *Journal of Family Violence*, 23(7), 557–568. doi:10.1007/s10896-008-9171-x

Zeigler-Hill, V., Clark, C. B., & Pickard, J. D. (2008). Narcissistic subtypes and contingent self-esteem: Do all narcissists base their self-esteem on the same domains? *Journal of Personality*, 76(4), 753–774. doi:10.1111/j.1467-6494.2008.00503.x

Zusman, M. E., & Knox, D. (1998). Relationship problems of casual and involved university students. *College Student Journal*, 32, 606–609.

Personality Change in Middle Adulthood: With Focus on Differential Susceptibility

Tetsuya Kawamoto (iD)

ABSTRACT

Little attention has been paid to middle adulthood in research on personality stability and change. In addition, previous research on individual differences in personality change has not fully explained its variability. This study focused on the differential susceptibility model, which suggests that individual susceptibility interacts with environmental factors and produces variability in outcomes, and investigated individual differences in personality change with a middle adult sample. A total of 1051 Japanese middle adults ($M = 41.61$ years; SD = 5.31; range 30–50 years; 534 females) participated in this two-wave short-term longitudinal study. Latent change score model analyses revealed substantial mean-level declines in Agreeableness and Honesty–Humility. Moreover, the results showed that the influences of some life events on personality change are moderated for better and for worse by individual susceptibility to one's environment. These findings suggest that the trends of personality development may differ between Western and non-Western countries and that differential susceptibility model may play an important role in deriving individual differences in personality stability and change.

Research on personality development has revealed the normative trajectories and life-long malleability of the human personality (for a meta-analytic review, see Roberts, Walton, & Viechtbauer, 2006). In life-span personality development, personality can be influenced by various environmental factors resulting in both stability and change. Empirical studies have examined personality change due to environmental factors, such as life events, and showed their socialization effects (Hudson, Roberts, & Lodi-Smith, 2012; Kandler, Bleidorn, Riemann, Angleitner, & Spinath, 2012; Le, Donnellan, & Conger, 2014; Lüdtke, Roberts, Trautwein, & Nagy, 2011; Roberts, Caspi, & Moffitt, 2003; Vaidya, Gray, Haig, & Watson, 2002). Behavioral genetic studies examining personality development have revealed robust environmental contributions to personality change (Hopwood et al., 2011; Kandler et al., 2010; Kawamoto & Endo, 2019). Thus, environmental factors may play a major role in personality change. However, environmental events may affect individuals differently and even serve to accentuate individual differences (Belsky, 1997, 2005), an issue that has received limited attention in research on personality development. This study drew on life history (LH) theory, which explains how organisms' resources are distributed in response to their fluctuating environmental conditions (Ellis, Figueredo, Brumbach, & Schlomer, 2009), and examined personality change from life events in middle adults with focus on individual susceptibility.

Patterns of Personality Stability and Change

Many studies in Western countries have examined rank-order personality stability, which refers to stable relative rankings of individual personality levels over time, and mean-level personality change, which refers to changes in average personality scores over time. Some reviews or meta-analyses on rank-order personality stability have concluded that rank-order stability linearly increases with age until at least 50 years (e.g. Ardelt, 2000; Ferguson, 2010; Roberts & DelVecchio, 2000). This increase of rank-order personality stability with age is termed *cumulative-continuity principle* (Roberts, Wood, & Caspi, 2008).

However, many longitudinal and cross-sectional studies have presented evidence of the developmental trajectories of personality (e.g. Donnellan & Lucas, 2008; Lucas & Donnellan, 2009; Soto, John, Gosling, & Potter, 2011; Specht, Egloff, & Schmukle, 2011; Terracciano, McCrae, Brant, & Costa, 2005). Findings that are largely concordant with a meta-analytic summary of mean-level changes in longitudinal samples (Roberts et al., 2006). These findings are mainly based on the Big Five model, which measures personality in five broad domains: Extraversion, Agreeableness, Conscientiousness, Neuroticism, and Openness (Goldberg, 1993). Generally, Agreeableness and Conscientiousness increase across the life course, but Conscientiousness may decline in later life. Neuroticism increases in adolescence and gradually declines; however, some studies have failed to support this pattern (Donnellan & Lucas, 2008). Extraversion and Openness tend to decline across the life span. In short, people become socially desirable across the life course. The association between trajectories of personality trait changes and functional advantages that people work toward (Roberts & Wood, 2006), are referred to as the *maturity principle* (Roberts et al., 2008). According to this principle, people have come to possess qualities that serve to facilitate functioning in society, including social relationships, work, and family activities.

As described above, these findings have been mostly derived from the five-factor framework. However, one additional domain—Honesty–Humility—was recently suggested, as the sixth trait to be added to the model which is now referred to as 'HEXACO' (Ashton & Lee, 2007). According to Ashton, Lee, and de Vries (2014), Extraversion, Conscientiousness, and Openness in the HEXACO model are closely similar to those in the Big Five model. Agreeableness and Emotionality in HEXACO moderately reflect Agreeableness and Neuroticism in the Big Five model. Honesty–Humility is slightly correlated with Agreeableness in the Big Five model; it also shows relative independence from the previous five broad personality domains. With the HEXACO model, we might be able to identify important developmental trends in personality that have not been observed previously. Despite the cross-sectional age trends, Ashton and Lee (2016) showed some inconsistency in Agreeableness with the previous results in the Big Five model.

Personality Stability and Change During Middle Adulthood in Western and Non-Western Countries

Although middle adulthood has been perceived as a time of quiet and stabilization, in many cases, middle adulthood is a rather dynamic developmental stage (Brim, Ryff, & Kessler, 2004). People in middle adulthood belong to multiple communities related to friends, neighborhood, workplace, leisure-time activities, religions, and culture. They play multiple roles and build social relationships in the communities (Antonucci, Akiyama, & Merline, 2001), resulting in their well-being or sense of generativity (MacDermid, Franz, & De Reus, 1998). Research on the normative developmental trends of personality in middle adulthood has revealed, in terms of rank-order personality stability, that stability coefficients range around 0.6 (Roberts & DelVecchio, 2000) or around 0.8 after controlling for measurement error (Ferguson, 2010). These findings show that relative rankings of personality traits are highly stable but not completely consistent.

As for mean-level change in personality, the meta-analytic study by Roberts et al. (2006) suggested that people showed an increase on measures of social dominance, Conscientiousness, and emotional stability after the age of 30. Other studies have also indicated an increase in emotional stability (Allemand, Zimprich, & Hertzog, 2007; Helson, Jones, & Kwan, 2002; Helson & Soto, 2005; Mroczek & Spiro, 2003; van Aken, Denissen, Branje, Dubas, & Goossens, 2006). However, the findings are contradictory regarding the increase in Agreeableness (Allemand et al., 2007) and social dominance (Helson et al., 2002; Helson & Soto, 2005), and a decrease in social vitality (Helson et al., 2002).

While these findings are obtained from studies conducted in the Western countries, very few studies are conducted in non-Western countries. Research on cross-sectional age differences in the Big Five has suggested that the rough sketches of personality development during middle adulthood in Japan (Kawamoto et al., 2015), Korea (McCrae et al., 1999), and Vietnam (Walton et al., 2013) are basically consistent with those in Western countries. However, some differences have been noted. For example, McCrae et al. (1999) showed that social dominance in the Korean sample was not associated with age, whereas in Western samples social dominance increased with age (Roberts et al., 2006). In a study by Walton et al. (2013), Openness was positively associated with age, though previous research in Western countries showed that Openness tends to decline (Donnellan & Lucas, 2008) or remain stable (Roberts et al., 2006). The study in Japan showed that Extraversion and Openness were not associated with age (Kawamoto et al., 2015). Thus, there might be some cultural differences especially in Extraversion and Openness between Western and non-Western countries, whereas Agreeableness, Conscientiousness, and Neuroticism show highly similar developmental trends both in Western and non-Western countries. Such differences and similarities indicate the need to examine personality development in non-Western countries.

Individual Differences in Personality Change

Although the meta-analytic review of mean-level personality change has shown that people experience changes in personality trait levels (Roberts et al., 2006), those of rank-order stability have suggested that the relative rankings of personality trait levels are not completely maintained over time (Ardelt, 2000; Ferguson, 2010; Roberts & DelVecchio, 2000). Not everyone shows the same patterns of mean-level change in personality traits across their life course, rather each person shows different developmental patterns.

These individual differences have been investigated with a focus on life experiences. For example, levels of some personality traits can be increased or decreased based on work involvement and investment (Hudson et al., 2012; Le et al., 2014; Roberts et al., 2003) and various life events (Kandler et al., 2012; Lüdtke et al., 2011; Vaidya et al., 2002). These studies have demonstrated the importance of various environmental experiences for personality change; however, they have not adopted the viewpoint of person–environment interaction. Bleidorn, Kandler, and Caspi (2014) pointed out that gene–environment interaction may be involved in shaping the developmental trajectories of personality traits, a research issue in personality development that should be examined in the future. To shed light on individual differences in personality change, attention should be paid to the interaction between the person and environment.

Person–Environment Interaction and Differential Susceptibility Theory

Although personality psychologists have historically paid little attention to the evolutionary framework, the evolutionary perspective argues that individual differences are adaptive. Changes in personality traits over time are caused by changes in environmental conditions across the human lifespan (Lewis, 2015), supporting the view of plasticity of personality traits. However, within an evolutionary framework, not everyone adapts to an environmental condition. Belsky (1997, 2005) in particular has discussed individual differences in susceptibility or sensitivity to environmental influences, and has suggested the concept of differential susceptibility referring to intra-individual characteristics maintained in evolutionary history.

Differential susceptibility theory insists that certain characteristics, which are partly determined by genetic factors, interact with environmental factors and engender individual differences. Environmental factors have a different impact on individuals with different characteristics, and function to accentuate individual differences (Ellis et al., 2011). Individuals who are high in susceptibility demonstrate an enhanced reactivity to both negative (stressful) and positive (nurturing) environments and are therefore more likely to experience developmental changes in response to environmental influences. The gist of differential susceptibility is person–environment interactions in development (Belsky, 1997, 2005; Ellis et al., 2011), which is a significant phenomenon for personality change (Bleidorn et al., 2014). Thus, susceptible individuals are liable to show increases and decreases in personality trait levels through positive and negative life experiences.

Although studies examining the differential susceptibility model in relation to adults are relatively few, some studies have shown its effectiveness in later adulthood. For example, young adults with insecure attachment were more susceptible to life experiences, and the influences of daily life experiences on personality change were more pronounced for them (Kawamoto, 2016). Moreover, young adults with greater amygdala reactivity to facial expressions were more susceptible to socioeconomic resources (Gard,

Shaw, Forbes, & Hyde, 2018). In a longitudinal study of young to middle adulthood mothers and fathers, parents who were high in negative affect and constraint were more susceptible to their marital relationship quality and experienced changes in their parental sensitivity for better and for worse (Jessee et al., 2010). Cao et al. (2018) found evidence for the moderating effects of a serotonin-related gene (*5-HTT*) in an adult sample. Young and middle-aged adults with the TT genotype proved to be more responsive to both the detrimental effects of higher stress and the beneficial effects of lower stress compared to those with the G allele. These findings provide support for the differential susceptibility model in adulthood, in that individual differences in susceptibility to environmental contexts might play a decisive role in personality change.

Evolutionary LH theory (Wilson, 1975) explains how organisms allocate their total bioenergetic and material resources between somatic and reproductive efforts depending on their local environments. Based on this theory, researchers have hypothesized that individuals evolving and developing in predictable and controllable environments strategically adapt to stable and specific conditions, whereas those evolving and developing in unpredictable and uncontrollable environments strategically maximize their flexibility in migrating between different conditions (Figueredo, Woodley, Brown, & Ross, 2013). LH theory suggests that LH traits inter-correlate with each other, which include characteristics related to the growth, reproduction, and survivorship of organisms, such as reproductive years, fecundity, and dispositions associated with how one allocates one's resources. Therefore, variability in LH traits is captured by a unidimensional, common factor, the *K*-factor (Figueredo et al., 2005). Individual differences in the *K*-factor can be roughly measured with the Mini-K scale, which has good validity (Figueredo et al., 2006, 2014). According to Figueredo et al. (2013), high-*K* individuals strategically differentiate their LH traits to adapt to their local environments; hence, their LH traits show temporal stability. Conversely, low-*K* people strategically integrate their LH traits to adapt to changing, unstable, and unpredictable environments; hence, their LH traits are temporarily less stable. This phenotype of low-*K* individuals is considered to function as the susceptible characteristics noted in differential susceptibility theory. Therefore, we can expect that when facing various life events, low-*K* individuals undergo more changes in their personality traits, whereas high-*K* individuals remain stable.

The Present Study

This study had two aims. First, this study investigated personality change in middle adults in a non-Western country using a longitudinal design and the HEXACO model. Previous research has mainly been from Western countries using the Big Five model. The few studies from non-Western countries show cross-sectional age differences in the Big Five scores and suggest the possibility of some cultural differences in personality development. Thus, more research is needed from non-Western countries using a longitudinal design and theoretical model other than the Big Five. Second, this study examined individual differences in personality change focusing on differential susceptibility. According to Figueredo et al. (2013), low-*K* individuals are liable to change on measures of personality traits from positive and negative life events, whereas high-*K* people tend to remain stable. Hence, this study investigated the influence of positive and negative life events on personality change between high-K and low-K individuals.

Material and Methods

Participants and Procedures

This study conducted a two-wave longitudinal survey. Both survey waves were conducted in a web-based questionnaire format. All of the participants were members of an online research panel service provided by MyVoice Communications (http://www.myvoice.co.jp/index.html). People in the panel were Japanese residents who had provided their participation consent. The distribution of demographic variables including household annual income and labor status among the members of this research panel was shown to be substantially representative compared with that of the general population in Japan. An invitation for this study was emailed to panel registrants who were 30–50 years old on July 11, 2014. This email contained information regarding informed consent and a hyperlink to the web-based survey. The company collected data for 2000 participants (1000 female) on July 11–15, 2014 and then sent the data to the author without any individual identifying information. The mean age of all participants was 40.94 years (SD = 5.35, range 30–49 years; $M = 41.67$, SD = 5.07 for males; $M = 40.21$, SD = 5.52 for females). In the second survey wave, the invitation was emailed on January 9, 2015 to the people who participated in the first survey. The assessment interval was 6 months. The company collected data for 1273 participants (606 females) on January 9–14, 2015 and then sent the data to the author without any individual identifying information. As some participants answered the questionnaire with a very perfunctory attitude, they were excluded from the analyzed data. Thus, remaining 1051 participants (534 female) were analyzed. The mean age of these participants was 41.61 years (SD = 5.31, range 30–50 years; $M = 42.32$, SD = 5.01 for males; $M = 40.92$, SD = 5.51 for females).

Measures

First Survey

The questionnaire used in the first survey was composed of the following three sections: personality traits, human LH tendency, and demographic information.

    A. Personality traits were measured with the Japanese version of the 60-item HEXACO Personality Inventory-Revised (HEXACO-PI-R; Ashton & Lee, 2009; Wakabayashi, 2014). This scale measures the six domains of personality, namely, Extraversion, Agreeableness, Conscientiousness, Emotionality, Openness to experience, and Honesty–Humility, with 10 items for each domain. Each domain scale includes four facet scales, which reflect narrower personality characteristics. The answer format is a five-point Likert scale ranging from strongly disagree (1) to strongly agree (5). Internal reliability was acceptable (α = 0.79 for Extraversion; α = 0.66 for Agreeableness; α = 0.68 for Conscientiousness; α =

0.70 for Emotionality; $\alpha = 0.72$ for Openness to experiences; $\alpha = 0.66$ for Honesty–Humility).

B. The *K*-factor, which underlies various LH traits, was measured with the Japanese version of the Mini-K scale (Mini-K-J; Figueredo et al., 2006; Kawamoto, 2015). Item examples of the Mini-K-J are as follows: "I have a close and warm romantic relationship with my sexual partner" and "I often find the bright side to a bad situation." The Mini-K-J contains 20 items, and the answer format is a seven-point Likert scale that ranges from disagree strongly (-3) to agree strongly (3). Internal reliability was good ($\alpha = 0.83$).

C. Demographic information was asked about the participants' age and sex (i.e., 0: Male, 1: Female).

Second Survey

The questionnaire used in the second survey included the following two sections: personality traits and life events check list.

A. Personality traits were measured with the HEXACO-PI-R (Ashton & Lee, 2009; Wakabayashi, 2014), which is the same measure in the first survey. Internal reliability was acceptable ($\alpha = 0.80$ for Extraversion; $\alpha = 0.68$ for Agreeableness; $\alpha = 0.70$ for Conscientiousness; $\alpha = 0.68$ for Emotionality; $\alpha = 0.72$ for Openness to experiences; $\alpha = 0.67$ for Honesty–Humility).

B. The occurrence of life events were measured by a 30-item life event checklist (see Table 1) similar to that used by Plomin, Lichtenstein, Pedersen, McClearn, and Nesselroade (1990) and Kandler et al. (2012). Response categories were (-3) very negative, (-2) negative, (-1) rather negative, (0) nor, (1) rather positive, (2) positive, (3) very positive, and (9) no experienced. The participants rated the

Table 1. Percentage of Individuals for Whom an Event Occurred and Valence of Each Life Event.

	Life events	Frequency in %	Positive valence
1	Change of address	6.18	**0.58**
2	Death of a person close to you	10.94	0.18
3	Separation from spouse for an extended period	6.28	0.30
4	Major improvement in financial status	25.50	**0.61**
5	Traffic or job related accident	11.42	0.22
6	Major deterioration in financial status	34.92	0.23
7	Major conflict with neighbors	9.61	0.29
8	Starting a new hobby or sport	16.65	**0.73**
9	Major conflict with close relatives	6.47	0.26
10	Changing to a new work place	4.66	**0.55**
11	Serious illness or injury (self)	7.33	0.20
12	Quitting a hobby or sport	17.60	0.31
13	Development of mental health problem	32.83	0.24
14	Increase of snack and meal	31.97	0.36
15	Child in trouble	1.81	0.30
16	Promotion in the work place	5.80	**0.69**
17	Serious illness or injury of a person close to you	9.80	0.15
18	Engaging in sexual relations without emotional commitment	2.47	**0.62**
19	Entering into a serious new romantic relationship	3.62	**0.75**
20	Birth of own child	1.81	**0.89**

Self-rated valence was adapted to take values between 0 and 1. Higher values indicate more positive events. Values above 0.50 are shown in boldface.

items that have happened within the past 6 months on a –3 to 3 scale, and then rated the items that have not happened within the past 6 months as 9. In the analyses of this study, the categories were reduced to never experienced (0) and at least one-time (1).

In accordance with previous studies (Kandler et al., 2012), the mean values of each life event item valence were linearly transformed to range from 0 to 1. According to the transformed valence scores, the 20 life events were classified into two clusters (cutoff = 0.50): positive life events (PLE: items 1, 4, 8, 10, 16, 18, 19, 20), and negative life events (NLE: items 2, 3, 5, 6, 7, 9, 11, 12, 13, 14, 15, 17).

Data Analyses

To examine mean-level change in personality and individual differences in personality change, this study applied the latent change score model (McArdle, 2009) to each HEXACO-PI-R domain (see Figure 1). Each domain scale was estimated as a latent variable by using the four facet scores. This model enabled estimation of the means and variances of the changes of the latent scale scores and testing of these estimates as statistically significant. This study utilized three fit indices to evaluate model fit: (a) the comparative fit index (CFI; Bentler, 1990), (b) Tucker–Lewis index (TLI; Tucker &

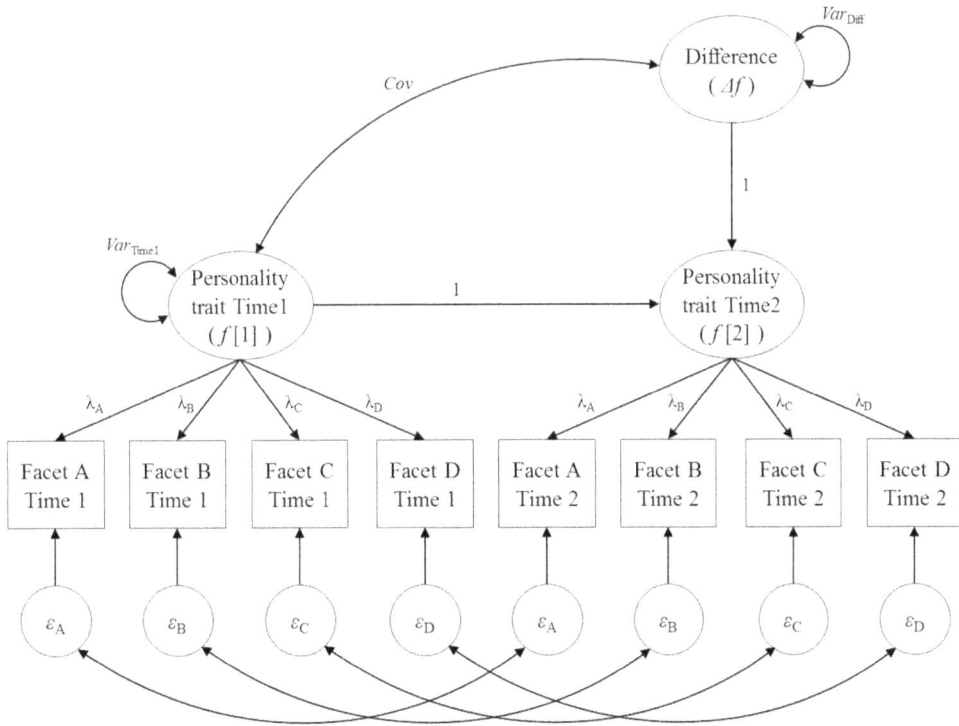

Figure 1. Latent change score model for investigating mean-level change in personality and individual differences in personality change.

Lewis, 1973), and (c) the root mean square error of approximation (RMSEA; Steiger, 1990). According to Hu and Bentler (1999), values of CFI > 0.95, TLI > 0.95, and RMSEA < 0.06 are considered as good fit. In addition, values of CFI > 0.90, TLI > 0.90, and RMSEA < 0.08 are considered as acceptable fit. The latent change score model was then estimated as a multi-group model to test for differences in the path coefficients between high-K and low-K groups. Analyses began with a baseline model that allowed all paths to vary freely across the groups, similar to what would be obtained if separate models were conducted for each group, except the one group was examined simultaneously in a single model. Subsequently, equality constraints were imposed to determine whether constraining the coefficients to be equal across the moderator subgroups would degrade the fit of the multi-group model, as indicated by an increase in chi-squared over that of the baseline model with degrees of freedom equal to the number of parameters constrained. A significant difference in chi-squared would indicate a moderation effect. These analyses were conducted with Mplus ver. 7 (Muthén & Muthén, 2012).

Results

Attrition Analyses

Approximately 64% of the Time 1 participants completed the questionnaires at Time 2 in this study. Attrition effects were inspected for split samples by comparing mean age, sex, personality scores at Time 1, and Mini-K-J score at Time 1 between participants who completed the questionnaires at both assessments and those who completed it at Time 1 but did not take part at the next assessment. For demographic variables, no differences were found in age ($t = 1.51$, $df = 1968.3$, $p = 0.13$), and sex ($\chi^2 = 0.51$, $df = 1$, $p = 0.47$). Uncorrected for multiple testing effects, no differences were revealed in four personality trait scores and the Mini-K-J score ($ts = 0.13$–1.29, $ps > 0.20$). However, statistically significant differences were observed in the remaining personality traits ($t = 4.26$, $df = 1991.8$, $p < 0.001$, Cohen's $d = 0.19$ for Conscientiousness; $t = 2.72$, $df = 1991.7$, $p = 0.01$, Cohen's $d = 0.12$ for Honesty–Humility). Therefore, the participants who participated in both assessments in this study had slightly higher levels of Conscientiousness and Honesty–Humility. However, the effect sizes of the two personality traits were not large. Hence, this study considered that the difference between them were not substantial.

Rank-Order Stability and Mean-Level Change in the HEXACO Personality

This study investigated rank-order stability in the HEXACO personality. The results showed high rank-order stability of the HEXACO-PI-R ($rs = 0.75 - 0.82$, $ps < 0.001$). The detailed stability coefficients were given in Table 2. For an illustration of mean-level changes of the HEXACO-PI-R scales, the study fitted the latent change score model with measurement invariance to the two-wave longitudinal data (see Figure 1). Based on the criteria of fit indices (Hu & Bentler, 1999), the present latent change score model adequately fitted to the data for all the HEXACO scores (CFI > 0.97; TLI > 0.96; RMSEA < 0.07). The latent scores of Agreeableness and Honesty–Humility significantly

Table 2. Results of Rank-Order Stability and Mean-Level Change in the HEXACO Scales.

Personality traits	Rank-order stability		Mean-level change				Model Fit			
	r	99% CI	Mean	99% CI	Variance	99% CI	CFI	TLI	RMSEA	90% CI
Extraversion	0.82	[0.80, 0.85]	−0.02	[−0.11, 0.08]	0.48	[0.29, 0.66]	0.97	0.97	0.07	[0.06, 0.08]
Agreeableness	0.75	[0.71, 0.78]	−0.07	[−0.12, −0.02]	0.11	[0.05, 0.16]	0.99	0.99	0.03	[0.02, 0.04]
Conscientiousness	0.75	[0.72, 0.78]	−0.04	[−0.11, 0.02]	0.20	[0.10, 0.30]	0.97	0.96	0.06	[0.05, 0.07]
Emotionality	0.76	[0.72, 0.79]	0.04	[−0.06, 0.13]	0.41	[0.20, 0.61]	0.99	0.99	0.03	[0.02, 0.05]
Openness	0.82	[0.79, 0.84]	−0.02	[−0.09, 0.05]	0.26	[0.15, 0.38]	1.00	1.00	0.02	[0.00, 0.03]
Honesty–Humility	0.74	[0.70, 0.77]	−0.08	[−0.15, −0.01]	0.15	[0.05, 0.26]	1.00	1.00	0.01	[0.00, 0.03]

$N = 1051$. The estimates which are significant at $p < .01$ level are in boldface.

declined over the interval. The remaining trait scores remained stable. The variances of the latent difference scores of all the HEXACO-PI-R scales were statistically significant, indicating broad individual differences in them. The detailed parameter estimates and fit indices were shown in Table 2.

Moderation Effects of Latent Life History Construct on Life Events

To investigate the moderation effects of latent LH construct on life events, this study conducted multi-group latent change score model analyses. The participants were divided into two groups: high-K and low-K groups. The cutoff score was the mean of the Mini-K-J score.

Extraversion

The effects of three life events on the latent change scores of Extraversion significantly differed between the high-K and low-K groups. The three life events were items 5 ('traffic or job related accident': $\Delta\chi^2(1) = 5.33$, $p = .02$), 8 ("starting a new hobby or sport": $\Delta\chi^2(1) = 4.52$, $p = 0.03$), and 18 ('engaging in sexual relations without emotional commitment': $\Delta\chi^2(1) = 5.32$, $p = 0.02$). Among the three, item 5 was rated as a negative life event. With respect to the two positive items (item 8 and 18), low-K individuals were more affected on the level of Extraversion in a positive direction by experiencing these life events compared with high-K individuals. They are also more influenced in a negative direction by having experiencing traffic- or job-related accidents. The detailed results are given in Table 3.

Agreeableness

As for Agreeableness, the effect of one life event on the latent change score was significantly moderated by the Mini-K-J score. The life event, item 15 ('child in trouble': $\Delta\chi^2(1) = 4.70$, $p = .03$), was rated as a negative life event. The results showed that low-K individuals were more affected on the level of Agreeableness in a negative direction by having problems related to their children ($\beta = -0.17$ [99% CI: −0.37 to 0.03], $p = 0.03$) but that high-K individuals were not significantly influenced ($\beta = 0.06$ [99% CI: −0.15 to 0.27], $p = 0.45$).

Table 3. Results of Multi Group Moderation Analyses for Extraversion.

Life event	Model	Subgroup	β	99 % CI	Model comparison
			Path coefficient (β_6)		
Item 5					
Traffic or job related accident	Baseline	High-K	−0.06	[−0.25, 0.13]	$\Delta\chi^2(1) = 5.33$
		Low-K	−0.23	[−0.41, −0.05]	$p = 0.02$
	Constraint		−0.14*	[−0.29, 0.01]	
Item 8					
Starting a new hobby or sport	Baseline	High-K	−0.07	[−0.25, 0.12]	$\Delta\chi^2(1) = 4.52$
		Low-K	0.15*	[−0.03, 0.33]	$p = 0.03$
	Constraint		0.06	[−0.11, 0.18]	
Item 18					
Engaging in sexual relations without emotional commitment	Baseline	High-K	−0.07	[−0.26, 0.12]	$\Delta\chi^2(1) = 5.32$
		Low-K	0.22	[0.04, 0.40]	$p = 0.02$
	Constraint		0.03	[−0.11, 0.16]	

All models include control variables for age and gender. β refers to standardized path coefficient.
*Refers to being statistically significant at $p < 0.05$.

Table 4. Results of Multigroup Moderation Analyses for Emotionality.

Life event	Model	Subgroup	β	99% CI	Model comparison
			Path coefficient (β_6)		
Item 1					
Change of address	Baseline	High-K	−0.03	[−0.25, 0.18]	$\Delta\chi^2(1) = 4.37$
		Low-K	0.20	[0.00, 0.40]	$p = 0.04$
	Constraint		0.08	[−0.07, 0.24]	
Item 14					
Increase of snack and meal	Baseline	High-K	0.02	[−0.19, 0.22]	$\Delta\chi^2(1) = 6.49$
		Low-K	0.29	[0.10, 0.49]	$p = 0.01$
	Constraint		0.15	[0.00, 0.30]	

All models include control variables for age and gender. β refers to standardized path coefficient.

Conscientiousness

With respect to Conscientiousness, the difference in chi-squared values on each life event was not statistically significant. That is, there were no interaction effects.

Emotionality

The effects of two life events on the latent change scores of Emotionality significantly differed between high-K and low-K groups: items 1 ('change of address': $\Delta\chi^2(1) = 4.37$, $p = 0.04$) and 14 ("increase of snack and meal": $\Delta\chi^2(1) = 6.49$, $p = 0.01$). Item 1 was rated as a positive life event, whereas item 14 was rated as a negative life event. The results indicated that low-K individuals were more affected on the level of Emotionality in a negative direction by experiencing these life events. The detailed results are given in Table 4.

Openness

As for Openness, the effects of three life events on the latent change scores significantly differed between high-K and low-K groups: items 5 ('traffic or job-related accident': $\Delta\chi^2(1) = 6.00$, $p = 0.01$), 11 ('serious illness or injury (self)': $\Delta\chi^2(1) = 5.23$, $p = 0.02$), and 19 ('entering into a serious new romantic relationship': $\Delta\chi^2(1) = 4.94$, $p = 0.03$).

Table 5. Results of Multi Group Moderation Analyses for Openness.

Life event	Model	Subgroup	β	99 % CI	Model comparison
			\multicolumn{2}{c}{Path coefficient (β_6)}	
Item 5					
Traffic or job related accident	Baseline	High-K	0.10	[−0.10, 0.30]	$\Delta\chi^2(1) = 6.00$
		Low-K	−0.17*	[−0.36, 0.03]	$p = 0.01$
	Constraint		−0.04	[−0.30, 0.21]	
Item 11					
Serious illness or injury (self)	Baseline	High-K	0.01	[−0.20, 0.21]	$\Delta\chi^2(1) = 5.23$
		Low-K	−0.22	[−0.41, −0.03]	$p = 0.02$
	Constraint		−0.11	[−0.26, 0.05]	
Item 19					
Entering into a serious new romantic relationship	Baseline	High-K	−0.10	[−0.30, 0.10]	$\Delta\chi^2(1) = 6.75$
		Low-K	0.18*	[−0.01, 0.37]	$p = 0.01$
	Constraint		0.03	[−0.14, 0.19]	

Notes. All models include control variables for age and gender. β refers to standardized path coefficient.
*Refers to being statistically significant at $p < 0.05$.

Table 6. Results of Multi Group Moderation Analyses for Honesty–Humility.

Life event	Model	Subgroup	β	99 % CI	Model comparison
			\multicolumn{2}{c}{Path coefficient (β_6)}	
Item 3					
Separation from spouse for an extended period	Baseline	High-K	−0.04	[−0.27, 0.13]	$\Delta\chi^2(1) = 5.06$
		Low-K	−0.28	[−0.49, −0.07]	$p = 0.02$
	Constraint		−0.16*	[−0.34, 0.01]	
Item 6					
Major deterioration in financial status	Baseline	High-K	0.30	[0.10, 0.50]	$\Delta\chi^2(1) = 5.87$
		Low-K	0.03	[−0.20, 0.26]	$p = 0.02$
	Constraint		0.16	[0.01, 0.31]	
Item 18					
Engaging in sexual relations without emotional commitment	Baseline	High-K	0.09	[−0.13, 0.31]	$\Delta\chi^2(1) = 5.89$
		Low-K	−0.21*	[−0.42, 0.00]	$p = 0.02$
	Constraint		−0.06	[−0.22, 0.09]	

All models include control variables for age and gender. β refers to standardized path coefficient. * refers to being statistically significant at $p < 0.05$.

Among these three life events, item 19 was rated as a positive life event. With respect to the two negative items, low-K individuals were more influenced on the levels of Openness in a negative direction by experiencing these events. In addition, they were more affected in a positive direction by entering into a serious new romantic relationship. The detailed results are shown in Table 5.

Honesty–Humility

With respect to Honesty–Humility, the effects of three life events on the latent change scores were significantly moderated by the Mini-K-J score: items 3 ('separation from spouse for an extended period': $\Delta\chi^2(1) = 5.06$, $p = 0.02$), 6 ('major deterioration in financial status': $\Delta\chi^2(1) = 5.87$, $p = 0.02$), and 18 ('engaging in sexual relations without emotional commitment': $\Delta\chi^2(1) = 5.89$, $p = 0.02$). Among these three life events, items 3 and 6 were rated as negative life events. The results showed that low-K individuals were more affected on the level of Honesty–Humility by separation from their spouses for an extended period (item 3) and engaging in sexual relations without emotional commitment (item 18). However, with respect to item 6, high-K individuals were significantly influenced on the level of Honesty–Humility by a major deterioration in financial status. The detailed results are given in Table 6.

Discussion

This study investigated short-term personality change in middle adulthood. First, the study examined rank-order stability and mean-level change in personality traits. The results showed relatively high rank-order stability of HEXACO personality traits and small mean-level declines in Agreeableness and Honesty–Humility. Second, the analysis results also showed that all latent change scores included substantial between-individual variances that refer to individual differences in personality change. Finally, this study investigated whether LH tendencies (K-factor) amplify or suppress the effects of life events. The results indicated that some effects from positive and negative life events were moderated by the Mini-K-J score, which reflects latent LH constructs. These findings regarding the moderation effects of LH are vital and unique points of this study.

The general patterns of rank-order personality stability found in this study were consistent with the cumulative continuity principles (Roberts et al., 2008). The stability coefficient estimates in this study were approximately 0.80. The estimates are similar to a recent meta-analysis result (Ferguson, 2010) but relatively higher than that in other meta-analytic studies (e.g., Roberts & DelVecchio, 2000). This variation is because the assessment interval was relatively short. According to Ardelt (2000), stability coefficients are negatively associated with retest intervals. Therefore, this study obtained relatively high coefficients.

In terms of mean-level change in personality, these results showed that the scores of Agreeableness and Honesty–Humility in Japanese middle adults slightly declined. On the other hand, the other four scores of the HEXACO personality traits did not significantly change. According to the maturity principle (Roberts et al., 2008), people gradually come to possess desirable qualities that serve to facilitate functioning in society. In other words, people tend to become nicer, more responsible, and self-disciplined, and more emotionally stable with age. A meta-analytic study in Western countries showed that people increase in measures of social dominance, Conscientiousness, and emotional stability after age 30 years (Roberts et al., 2006). Other empirical studies in Western countries have also indicated increases in emotional stability (Allemand et al., 2007; Helson & Soto, 2005; Helson et al., 2002; Mroczek & Spiro, 2003; van Aken et al., 2006), Agreeableness (Allemand et al., 2007), and social-dominance (Helson & Soto, 2005; Helson et al., 2002), and decline in social vitality (Helson et al., 2002). In non-Western countries, previous research on cross-sectional age differences in personality has also shown that levels of Agreeableness, Conscientiousness, and emotional stability linearly increase with age (Kawamoto et al., 2015; McCrae et al., 1999; Walton et al., 2013). Therefore, these results of declines in Agreeableness and Honesty–Humility are inconsistent with those earlier works in Western and non-Western countries.

One possible explanation to this inconsistency is scale specificity. This study used the HEXACO-PI-R (Ashton & Lee, 2009; Wakabayashi, 2014), which suggests that human personality is composed of six basic domains. As the HEXACO model adds a sixth personality trait, Honesty–Humility, to the Big Five model, each domain in the HEXACO model may be slightly different from those in the Big Five model. Especially, Agreeableness in the HEXACO personality inventory certainly correlates with Agreeableness as assessed by the NEO Five-Factor Inventory, a well-established questionnaire based on the Five-Factor Model of personality, but the correlation coefficients are smaller compared with other corresponding domains (Ashton et al., 2014; Wakabayashi, 2014). Agreeableness in the HEXACO model may be slightly different from that in the Big Five.

Meanwhile, sample specificity may also be a possible cause. A large number of the previous related studies were conducted in Western countries. Personality development is tapered by the contextual demands of people's circumstances (Roberts et al., 2008; Wood & Denissen, 2015). If the circumstances change, then the contextual demands change as well. For example, the work–life environment is very close to adults and influences adults' well-being and health (Helson & Soto, 2005). The work–life environment in Japan differs drastically from that in Western countries (Hobson, 2013). Japan has traditionally followed Confucian ideology. Compared with other Western countries, employees in Japan are often forced to work for a much longer time (Chandra, 2012). In addition, employed men are often required to be breadwinners in their family, whereas women are often required to be full-time homemakers, regardless of their will. Therefore, Japanese middle adults are likely to experience strong work–life conflict. Moreover, in recent Japan, it has been often pointed out that social relationships in communities have become weakened (Toyama, 2016). Middle adults usually play multiple roles and develop social relationships in their multiple communities, which could positively affect their well-being or sense of generativity (Antonucci et al., 2001; MacDermid et al., 1998). However, considering the weak social ties in the Japanese community (Toyama, 2016), it might be difficult for recent Japanese middle adults to develop their social relationships with various people. These cultural specificities in work–life environments and social relationships in communities might cause different normative trajectories of personality development in Japan compared with those in Western countries.

With respect to Extraversion and Openness, previous research in Western and non-Western countries suggested slight cultural differences. Given the possibility of decline in Extraversion, or at least the social vitality facet, and Openness in Western countries (e.g., Allemand et al., 2007; Donnellan & Lucas, 2008; Lucas & Donnellan, 2009; Specht et al., 2011; Terracciano et al., 2005), the present finding that the scores of Extraversion and Openness remain stable might support the notion of cultural differences in personality development. Despite its cross-sectional design, a previous study in Japan also showed there were no age differences in Extraversion and Openness (Kawamoto et al., 2015). This might be because Japanese young people recently tend to exhibit characteristics of associated with low levels of Extraversion and Openness, i.e. low ambition, inward-looking trend, low interest in going abroad, preference for low demanding jobs, and indecisive behaviors (Chen, 2012). The mean levels of Extraversion and Openness in Japanese people are relatively low from young age and remain stable rather than gradually decline across the life course.

The principal purpose of this study was to investigate the moderation effect of latent LH constructs. According to Figueredo et al. (2013), low-K people (susceptible people) tend to be more affected by positive and negative life events for better and for worse.

The present results showed some significant differences in life event effects between low-K and high-K individuals. For example, if low-K people experienced traffic- or job-related accident (item 5), they were more negatively affected, showing a decreased level of Extraversion and Openness; however, if high-K people experienced this event, they were less affected by it. Moreover, if low-K people engaged in sexual relations without emotional commitment (item 18), they were more affected, showing increases on the level of Extraversion and decreases on the level of Honesty–Humility; however, if high-K people experienced this event, they were less affected by it. These findings support the hypotheses of this study.

As for the effect of major deterioration in financial status (item 6) on the level of Honesty–Humility, high-K individuals were more affected. This outcome is not consistent with the hypothesis. When people experience deterioration in financial status, they should pull in their horns, work more, and become steady and reliable. These behaviors are future-oriented and applicable to high-K strategies. As high-K individuals have familiarity with these behaviors, their behavioral tendency became stronger in the face of deterioration in financial status. In contrast, low-K strategies were intrinsically adaptive to an unstable, unpredictable environment. Hence, a bad environment factor like deterioration in financial status might not have an influence on them.

As such, do LH constructs interact with any life events as expected by differential susceptibility theory? The answer to this question should be 'No'. For example, items 2 ('death of a person close to you') and 17 ('serious illness or injury of a person close to you'), which seem to be influential and impactful, did not interact with LH constructs. Presumably, it is important for interaction with LH constructs that they are directly related to the participants' fitness. LH constructs denote the tendencies that explain how organisms allocate their energy, time, and effort to somatic and reproductive effort depending on life circumstances. Hence, when the events straightforwardly affect the participants' circumstances, they modify their strategies that are the most adaptive to the alternative circumstances. In contrast, when the events do not strongly affect the participants' circumstances, they may not be influenced by the life events. Future research should consider the detailed characteristics of each environmental event.

Ellis et al. (2011) summarized the previous findings on the differential susceptibility model at genetic, epigenetic, neural, neuroendocrine, and behavioral levels. In those with adult samples, much research has mainly focused on the genetic or physiological markers like serotonin-related gene polymorphism (Cao et al., 2018) or amygdala reactivity (Gard et al., 2018). These factors are genetic or neuroendocrine levels. However, little research using adult samples has shown the differential susceptibility phenomenon at behavioral level. The LH constructs, which was dealt with as a moderating susceptible factor in this study, can be considered as a behavioral or psychological level marker. Previous research suggested that negative emotionality and/or highly-sensitive person are behavioral phenotypic markers of susceptibility (Belsky, 2005; Ellis et al. 2011). The LH constructs are considered to partly reflect those susceptible indicators (Figueredo et al., 2014). These findings, therefore, synthesize the two research lines of the differential susceptibility model and LH theory.

In addition, according to a meta-analytic study summarizing longitudinal studies with children up to 18 years (Slagt, Dubas, Deković, & van Aken, 2015), the differential susceptibility model was mainly supported in relatively early developmental stages. Slagt et al.

(2015) suggested two possible explanations for their findings. One is that although individuals with higher level of susceptibility remain susceptible over their lifetime, specific characteristics of their susceptibility might change depending on their developmental stage. Another explanation suggested that susceptibility might be observed during certain sensitive periods in life. The present findings do not support the latter possibility, but rather the former one. The results of this study showed that the LH constructs of middle adults could function as a moderating factor, susceptibility, and suggested that susceptible individuals remain susceptible at least until middle adulthood. Moreover, in the meta-analytic study by Slagt et al. (2015), it was shown that early children with high level of negative emotionality were likely to be influenced by both positive and negative environments for better and for worse. Although the LH constructs partly reflect negative emotionality (Figueredo et al., 2014), they are relatively different and independent. Putting things together, susceptible individuals remain susceptible, and notably, specific predispositions of their susceptibility might change from negative emotionality to related factors, such as LH constructs. Future research should examine the longitudinal associations between negative emotionality in early childhood and LH constructs in adulthood.

The strengths of this study include the relatively large sample size, the use of a relatively rare sample of Japanese adult population, and a unique viewpoint in focusing on latent LH constructs as individual susceptibility. Conversely, the following limitations should be taken into consideration. First, this study used a single, self-report questionnaire to measure participants' personality. Mono-rater measures of personality constructs are easily influenced by random and systematic error components (Campbell & Fiske, 1959). To avoid these biases, it is effective to administer concurrently additional measurement methods or independent ratings by well-informed observers (Hofstee, 1994). Future research should employ multiple-method or multiple-rater personality data to eliminate random and systematic error effects for investigating stability and change in personality. Especially, when focusing on middle adulthood, it must be useful to conduct an investigation at the couple level.

Second, the short assessment interval was also a limitation of this study. Many studies have examined stability and change in personality with relatively long assessment intervals, which could provide useful evidence regarding normative life-long trajectories of personality. Nonetheless, despite the short-term retest interval, this study also offered some mean-level changes in personality and examined individual differences in personality change with a focus on person-environmental interaction.

Third, this study missed the relatively small daily life experiences. Personality change may be induced by not only large high-impact life events but also many everyday experiences. Future research should examine this point.

Fourth, this study did not collect some information about demographic variables including household annual income, educational attainment, occupational level, and marital status. These important variables could interact with life events, which might cause complex developmental trajectories in personality.

Finally, this study did not directly measure the susceptibility concept, because its definition remains under discussion and a measurement scale has not been developed. For further investigation, the susceptibility concept should be clearly defined, and a measurement scale of it developed accordingly.

Acknowledgments

The author would like to thank Editage (www.editage.jp) for English language editing.

Funding

This research was supported by JSPS KAKENHI Grant Numbers JP14J12061 and JP17H01023.

ORCID

Tetsuya Kawamoto ⓘ http://orcid.org/0000-0003-4753-9225

References

Allemand, M., Zimprich, D., & Hertzog, C. (2007). Cross-sectional age differences and longitudinal age changes of personality in middle adulthood and old age. *Journal of Personality, 75*(2), 323–358. doi:10.1111/j.1467-6494.2006.00441.x

Antonucci, T. C., Akiyama, H., & Merline, A. (2001). Dynamics of social relationships in midlife. In M. E. Lachman (Ed.), *Handbook of midlife development* (pp. 571–598). New York: Wiley.

Ashton, M. C., & Lee, K. (2007). Empirical, theoretical, and practical advantages of the HEXACO model of personality structure. *Personality and Social Psychology Review, 11*(2), 150–166. doi: 10.1177/1088868306294907

Ashton, M. C., & Lee, K. (2009). The HEXACO-60: A short measure of the major dimensions of personality. *Journal of Personality Assessment, 91*(4), 340–345. doi:10.1080/00223890902935878

Ashton, M. C., Lee, K., & de Vries, R. E. (2014). The HEXACO honesty-humility, agreeableness, and emotionality factors. *Personality and Social Psychology Review, 18*(2), 139–152. doi:10. 1177/1088868314523838

Ashton, M. C., & Lee, K. (2016). Age trends in HEXACO-PI-R self-reports. *Journal of Research in Personality, 64*, 102–111. doi:10.1016/j.jrp.2016.08.008

Ardelt, M. (2000). Still stable after all these years? Personality stability theory revisited. *Social Psychology Quarterly, 63*(4), 392–405. doi:10.2307/2695848

Belsky, J. (1997). Variation in susceptibility to environmental influence: An evolutionary argument. *Psychological Inquiry, 8*(3), 182–186. doi:10.1207/s15327965pli0803_3

Belsky, J. (2005). Differential susceptibility to rearing influence: An evolutionary hypothesis and some evidence. In B. J. Ellis & D. F. Bjorklund (Eds.), *Origins of the social mind: Evolutionary psychology and child development*. New York, NY: Guilford Press.

Bentler, P. M. (1990). Comparative fit indexes in structural models. *Psychological Bulletin, 107*(2), 238–246. doi:10.1037/0033-2909.107.2.238

Bleidorn, W., Kandler, C., & Caspi, A. (2014). The behavioural genetics of personality development in adulthood: Classic, contemporary, and future trends. *European Journal of Personality, 28*(3), 244–255. doi:10.1002/per.1957

Brim, O. G., Ryff, C. D., & Kessler, R. C. (2004). *How healthy are we? A national study of well-being at midlife*. Chicago, IL: University of Chicago Press.

Campbell, D. T., & Fiske, D. W. (1959). Convergent and discriminant validation by the multi-trait-multimethod matrix. *Psychological Bulletin, 56*(2), 81–105. doi:10.1037/h0046016

Cao, Z., Wu, S., Wang, C., Wang, L., Soares, J. C., He, S.-C., & Zhang, X. Y. (2018). Serotonin transporter gene (5-HTT) rs6354 polymorphism, job-related stress, and their interaction in burnout in healthcare workers in a Chinese hospital. *Psychopharmacology, 235*(11), 3125–3135. doi:10.1007/s00213-018-5009-2

Chandra, V. (2012). Work–life balance: Eastern and western perspectives. *The International Journal of Human Resource Management, 23*, 1040–1056. doi:10.1080/09585192.2012.651339

Chen, S. (2012). The rise of (soushoukei danshi): Masculinity and consumption in contemporary Japan. In C. C. Otnes & L. T. Zayer (Eds.), *Gender, culture, and consumer behavior* (pp. 285–310). New York, NY: Routledge.

Donnellan, M. B., & Lucas, R. E. (2008). Age differences in the big five across the life span: Evidence from two national samples. *Psychology and Aging, 23*(3), 558–566. doi:10.1037/a0012897

Ellis, B. J., Boyce, W. T., Belsky, J., Bakermans-Kranenburg, M. J., & Van Ijzendoorn, M. H. (2011). Differential susceptibility to the environment: An evolutionary–neurodevelopmental theory. *Development and Psychopathology, 23*(1), 7–28. doi:10.1017/S0954579410000611

Ellis, B. J., Figueredo, A. J., Brumbach, B. H., & Schlomer, G. L. (2009). Fundamental dimensions of environmental risk: The impact of harsh versus unpredictable environments on the evolution and development of life history strategies. *Human Nature, 20*(2), 204–268. doi:10.1007/s12110-009-9063-7

Ferguson, C. J. (2010). A meta-analysis of normal and disordered personality across the life span. *Journal of Personality and Social Psychology, 98*(4), 659–667. doi:10.1037/a0018770

Figueredo, A., Vasquez, G., Brumbach, B., Schneider, S., Sefcek, J., Tal, I., ... Jacobs, W. (2006). Consilience and life history theory: From genes to brain to reproductive strategy. *Developmental Review, 26*(2), 243–275.

Figueredo, A. J., Vásquez, G., Brumbach, B. H., Sefcek, J. A., Kirsner, B. R., & Jacobs, W. J. (2005). The *K*-factor: Individual differences in life history strategy. *Personality and Individual Differences, 39*(8), 1349–1360.

Figueredo, A. J., Wolf, P. S. A., Olderbak, S. G., Gladden, P. R., Fernandes, H. B. F., Wenner, C., ... Rushton, J. P. (2014). The psychometric assessment of human life history strategy: A meta-analytic construct validation. *Evolutionary Behavioral Sciences, 8*(3), 148–185.

Figueredo, A. J., Woodley, M. A., Brown, S. D., & Ross, K. C. (2013). Multiple successful tests of the strategic differentiation-integration effort (*SD-IE*) hypothesis. *Journal of Social, Evolutionary, and Cultural Psychology, 7*(4), 361–383.

Gard, A. M., Shaw, D. S., Forbes, E. E., & Hyde, L. W. (2018). Amygdala reactivity as a marker of differential susceptibility to socioeconomic resources during early adulthood. *Developmental Psychology, 54*(12), 2341–2355. doi:10.1037/dev0000600

Goldberg, L. R. (1993). The structure of phenotypic personality traits. *American Psychologist, 48*(1), 26–34. doi:10.1037/0003-066X.48.1.26

Helson, R., Jones, C., & Kwan, V. S. Y. (2002). Personality change over 40 years of adulthood: Hierarchical linear modeling analyses of two longitudinal samples. *Journal of Personality and Social Psychology, 83*(3), 752–766. doi:10.1037//0022-3514.83.3.752

Helson, R., & Soto, C. J. (2005). Up and down in middle age: Monotonic and nonmonotonic changes in roles, status, and personality. *Journal of Personality and Social Psychology, 89*(2), 194–204. doi:10.1037/0022-3514.89.2.194

Hobson, B. (Ed.) (2013). *Rklife balance: The agency and capabilities gap.* Oxford, UK: Oxford University Press.

Hofstee, W. T. (1994). Who should own the definition of personality?. *European Journal of Personality, 8*(3), 149–162. doi:10.1002/per.2410080302

Hopwood, C. J., Donnellan, M. B., Blonigen, D. M., Krueger, R. F., McGue, M., Iacono, W. G., & Burt, S. A. (2011). Genetic and environmental influences on personality trait stability and growth during the transistion to adulthood: A three-wave longitudinal study. *Journal of Personality and Social Psychology, 100*(3), 545–556. doi:10.1037/a0022409

Hu, L., & Bentler, P. M. (1999). Cutoff criteria for fit indexes in covariance structure analysis: Conventional criteria versus new alternatives. *Structural Equation Modeling, 6*(1), 1–55. doi:10.1080/10705519909540118

Hudson, N. W., Roberts, B. W., & Lodi-Smith, J. (2012). Personality trait development and social investment in work. *Journal of Research in Personality, 46*(3), 334–344. doi:10.1016/j.jrp.2012.03.002

Jessee, A., Mangelsdorf, S. C., Brown, G. L., Schoppe-Sullivan, S. J., Shigeto, A., & Wong, M. S. (2010). Parents' differential susceptibility to the effects of marital quality on sensitivity across the first year. *Infant Behavior and Development, 33*(4), 442–452. doi:10.1016/j.infbeh.2010.04.010

Kandler, C., Bleidorn, W., Riemann, R., Angleitner, A., & Spinath, F. M. (2012). Life events as environmental states and genetic traits and the role of personality: A longitudinal twin study. *Behavior Genetics, 42*(1), 57–72. doi:10.1007/s10519-011-9491-0

Kandler, C., Bleidorn, W., Riemann, R., Spinath, F. M., Thiel, W., & Angleitner, A. (2010). Sources of cumulative continuity in personality: A longitudinal multiple-rater twin study. *Journal of Personality and Social Psychology, 98*(6), 995–1008. doi:10.1037/a0019558

Kawamoto, T. (2015). The translation and validation of the Mini-K scale in Japanese. *Japanese Psychological Research, 57*(3), 254–267. doi:10.1111/jpr.12083

Kawamoto, T. (2016). Personality change from life experiences: Moderation effect of attachment security. *Japanese Psychological Research, 58*(2), 218–231. doi:10.1111/jpr.12110

Kawamoto, T., & Endo, T. (2019). Sources of variances in personality change during adolescence. *Personality and Individual Differences, 141*, 182–187. doi:10.1016/j.paid.2019.01.018

Kawamoto, T., Oshio, A., Abe, S., Tsubota, Y., Hirashima, T., Ito, H., & Tani, I. (2015). Age and gender differences of Big Five personality traits in a cross-sectional Japanese sample. *The Japanese Journal of Developmental Psychology, 26*, 107–122.

Le, K., Donnellan, M. B., & Conger, R. (2014). Personality development at work: Workplace conditions, personality changes, and the correspondive principle. *Journal of Personality, 82*(1), 44–56. doi:10.1111/jopy.12032

Lewis, D. M. G. (2015). Evolved individual differences: Advancing a condition-dependent model of personality. *Personality and Individual Differences, 84*, 63–72. doi:10.1016/j.paid.2014.10.013

Lucas, R. E., & Donnellan, M. B. (2009). Age differences in personality: Evidence from a nationally representative Australian sample. *Developmental Psychology, 45*(5), 1353–1363. doi:10.1037/a0013914

Lüdtke, O., Roberts, B. W., Trautwein, U., & Nagy, G. (2011). A random walk down university avenue: Life paths, life events, and personality trait change at the transition to university life. *Journal of Personality and Social Psychology, 101*(3), 620–637. doi:10.1037/a0023743

MacDermid, S. M., Franz, C. E., & De Reus, L. A. (1998). Generativity: At the crossroads of social roles and personality. In D. P. McAdams & E. de St. Aubin (Eds.), *Generativity and adult development: How and why we care for the next generation* (pp. 181–226). Washington, DC: American Psychological Association.

McArdle, J. J. (2009). Latent variable modeling of differences and changes with longitudinal data. *Annual Review of Psychology, 60*, 577–605. doi:10.1146/annurev.psych.60.110707.163612

McCrae, R. R., Costa, P. T., de Lima, M. P., Simões, A., Ostendorf, F., Angleitner, A., … Piedmont, R. L. (1999). Age differences in personality across the adult life span: Parallels in five cultures. *Developmental Psychology, 35*(2), 466–477. doi:10.1037/0012-1649.35.2.466

Mroczek, D. K., & Spiro, A. III (2003). Modeling intraindividual change in personality traits: Findings from the Normative Aging Study. *The Journals of Gerontology: Series B: Psychological Sciences and Social Sciences, 58*, 153–165.

Muthén, L. K., & Muthén, B. (2012). *Mplus user's guide*, 7th ed. Los Angeles, CA: Muthén & Muthén.

Plomin, R., Lichtenstein, P., Pedersen, N. L., McClearn, G. E., & Nesselroade, J. R. (1990). Genetic influence on life events during the last half of the life span. *Psychology and Aging, 5*(1), 25–30.

Roberts, B. W., Caspi, A., & Moffitt, T. E. (2003). Work experiences and personality development in young adulthood. *Journal of Personality and Social Psychology*, *84*(3), 582–593. doi:10.1037//0022-3514.84.3.582

Roberts, B. W., & DelVecchio, W. F. (2000). The rank-order consistency of personality traits from childhood to old age: A quantitative review of longitudinal studies. *Psychological Bulletin*, *126*(1), 3–25. doi:10.1037//0033-2909.126.1.3

Roberts, B. W., Walton, K. E., & Viechtbauer, W. (2006). Patterns of mean-level change in personality traits across the life course: A meta-analysis of longitudinal studies. *Psychological Bulletin*, *132*(1), 1–25. doi:10.1037/0033-2909.132.1.1

Roberts, B. W., & Wood, D. (2006). Personality development in the context of the neo-socioanalytic model of personality. In D. K. Mroczek., & T. D. Little (Eds.), *Handbook of personality development* (pp. 11–39). Mahwah, NJ: Lawrence Erlbaum Associates Publishers.

Roberts, B. W., Wood, D., & Caspi, A. (2008). The development of personality traits in adulthood. In O. P. John, R. W. Robins, & L. A. Pervin (Eds.), *Handbook of personality: Theory and research* (pp. 375–398). New York, NY: Guilford Press.

Slagt, M., Dubas, J. S., Denissen, J. J., Deković, M., & van Aken, M. A. (2015). Personality traits as potential susceptibility markers: Differential susceptibility to support among parents. *Journal of Personality*, *83*(2), 155–166. doi:10.1111/jopy.12091

Soto, C. J., John, O. P., Gosling, S. D., & Potter, J. (2011). Age differences in personality traits from 10 to 65: Big Five domains and facets in a large cross-sectional sample. *Journal of Personality and Social Psychology*, *100*(2), 330–348. doi:10.1037/a0021717

Specht, J., Egloff, B., & Schmukle, S. C. (2011). Stability and change of personality across the life course: The impact of age and major life events on mean-level and rank-order stability of the Big Five. *Journal of Personality and Social Psychology*, *101*(4), 862–882. doi:10.1037/a0024950

Steiger, J. H. (1990). Structural model evaluation and modification: An interval estimation approach. *Multivariate Behavioral Research*, *25*(2), 173–180. doi:10.1207/s15327906mbr2502_4

Terracciano, A., McCrae, R. R., Brant, L. J., & Costa, P. T. Jr. (2005). Hierarchical linear modeling analyses of the NEO-PI-R Scales in the Baltimore Longitudinal Study of Aging. *Psychology and Aging*, *20*(3), 493–506. doi:10.1037/0882-7974.20.3.493

Toyama, K. (2016). The isolation of child-rearing families in urban area: From the analysis of trust in local communities using SSP2015. *Research Journal of Graduate Students of Letters*, *16*, 209–230.

Tucker, L. R., & Lewis, C. (1973). A reliability coefficient for maximum likelihood factor analysis. *Psychometrika*, *38*(1), 1–10. doi:10.1007/BF02291170

Vaidya, J. G., Gray, E. K., Haig, J., & Watson, D. (2002). On the temporal stability of personality: Evidence for differential stability and the role of life experiences. *Journal of Personality and Social Psychology*, *83*(6), 1469–1484. doi:10.1037//0022-3514.83.6.1469

van Aken, M. A. G., Denissen, J. J. A., Branje, S. J. T., Dubas, J. S., & Goossens, L. (2006). Midlife concerns and short-term personality change in middle adulthood. *European Journal of Personality*, *20*(6), 497–513. doi:10.1002/per.603

Wakabayashi, A. (2014). A sixth personality domain that is independent of the Big Five domains: The psychometric properties of the HEXACO Personality Inventory in a Japanese sample. *Japanese Psychological Research*, *56*, 211–223.

Walton, K. E., Huyen, B. T. T., Thorpe, K., Doherty, E. R., Juarez, B., D'Accordo, C., & Reina, M. T. (2013). Cross-sectional personality differences from age 16–90 in a Vietnamese sample. *Journal of Research in Personality*, *47*(1), 36–40. doi:10.1016/j.jrp.2012.10.011

Wilson, E. O. (1975). *Sociobiology: The new synthesis*. Cambridge, MA: Harvard University.

Wood, D., & Denissen, J. J. A. (2015). A functional perspective on personality trait development. In K. J. Reynolds., & N. R. Branscombe (Eds.), *Psychology of change: Life contexts, experiences, and identities* (pp. 97–115). New York, NY: Psychology Press.

Effect of Depressive Symptoms and Sex on the Relationship Between Loneliness and Cigarette Dependence: A Moderated Mediation

Carmela Martínez-Vispo (iD), Ana López-Durán (iD), Rubén Rodríguez-Cano (iD), Elena Fernández del Río (iD), Carmen Senra (iD), and Elisardo Becoña (iD)

ABSTRACT
Loneliness is a subjective and emotionally unpleasant experience of perceiving insufficient social relationships. Previous research has revealed that loneliness constitutes a psychosocial risk factor for depression, and is also related to unhealthy behaviors such as smoking. This study aims to examine the relation between loneliness, depression, and cigarette dependence, and to explore the role of sex in this relationship. A total sample of 275 adult treatment-seeking daily smokers ($Mage = 45.3$; 61.5% females) was used. Our results showed a significant correlation between higher scores of loneliness, depressive symptoms, and cigarette dependence. In addition, mediation analysis showed a significant indirect effect of loneliness on cigarette dependence, via depressive symptoms. Regarding the effect of sex, we found that this variable significantly moderated the relationship between depressive symptoms and cigarette dependence. Results of this study extend previous literature by showing that, in treatment seeking smokers, loneliness is a significant predictor of depressive symptoms, and through this relation, it predicts cigarette dependence. Additionally, sex was a significant moderator of this relation. These findings have several clinical implications, and also contribute to the understanding of cigarette dependence, which is a well-known barrier for smoking cessation.

Loneliness can be defined as an emotionally unpleasant experience of perceiving insufficient social relationships in terms of type, quality, or quantity relative to the perceived need (Hawkley & Cacioppo, 2010; Peplau & Perlman, 1982). Loneliness is a subjective experience clearly distinct from social isolation, which can be measured objectively (e.g. living alone, marital status, network size, frequency of social contact, time alone). In fact, research has shown that loneliness can be experienced independently of social contact (Russell, Cutrona, McRae, & Gomez, 2012), and that lonely and nonlonely people engage in similar activities and spend equivalent time alone during the day (Hawkley, Burleson, Berntson, & Cacioppo, 2003). Studies have suggested that some cognitive-emotional processes might underline such observations, highlighting the relevance of self-regulatory processes, hyper-vigilance of social clues (which could introduce attentional, and memory biases), emotional functioning, negative repetitive thinking, and other variables as the presence of anxiety and stress (Cacioppo et al., 2000; Cacioppo, Grippo, London, Goossens, & Cacioppo, 2015; Sadeghi Bahmani et al., 2018; Zawadzki, Graham, & Gerin, 2013).

Loneliness has emerged as a psychosocial risk factor that is related to a higher probability of mortality, as revealed in a recent meta-analytic review that found that, after accounting for multiple covariates, loneliness increased the likelihood of death by 26% when compared with nonloneliness (Holt-Lunstad, Smith, Baker, Harris, & Stephenson, 2015). Moreover, recent research has revealed that loneliness has an impact on physical and mental health (Shankar, McMunn, Banks, & Steptoe, 2011; Steptoe, Shankar, Demakakos, & Wardle, 2013; Valtorta, Kanaan, Gilbody, Ronzi, & Hanratty, 2016). For instance, in a large cross-sectional study, Richard et al. (2017) found that lonely individuals more frequently reported chronic diseases (odds ratio [OR] 1.41), and psychological distress (OR 3.74) that those not experiencing loneliness. Regarding the relation between loneliness and mental health, some studies have found a consistent and strong association with depressive symptomatology (Cacioppo, Hughes, Waite, Hawkley, & Thisted, 2006). Longitudinal studies have even reported that loneliness could be considered as a risk factor for depressive symptoms (Hawkley & Cacioppo, 2010; Luo, Hawkley, Waite, & Cacioppo, 2012).

It has also been documented that loneliness is related to unhealthy behaviors such as, alcohol and substance use (Beutel et al., 2017; Lauder, Mummery, Jones, & Caperchione, 2006), including cigarette smoking (Habibi et al., 2018; Richard et al., 2017; Shankar et al., 2011). Research conducted in the general population has shown that higher loneliness was associated with an increased rate of current smoking status (Beutel et al., 2017). In addition, in a 10-year longitudinal study carried out with a population-representative sample of older English adults, it was found that loneliness was negatively related to successful smoking cessation (Kobayashi & Steptoe, 2018). In the context of smoking cessation interventions, previous studies have shown that loneliness is a significant predictor of lower smoking cessation self-efficacy (Shuter, Moadel, Kim, Weinberger, & Stanton, 2014), and that it is positively related to smoking status after receiving an intervention to quit smoking (Moadel et al., 2012). Despite the existing literature establishing a relation between loneliness and smoking, some studies have not found such an association. In fact, in a recent systematic review examining the association between loneliness and smoking a positive association was found, but only in half of the 23 studies reviewed (Dyal & Valente, 2015). The authors highlight the need to consider depression when investigating this association, as it could be impacting this relationship. Actually, depressive symptoms are related not only to loneliness, as mentioned, but also to smoking and cigarette dependence (Breslau, Johnson, Hiripi, & Kessler, 2001; Goodwin et al., 2017). Concretely, research has shown that smokers with depressive symptoms report a greater probability of being cigarette dependent, and experience a stronger withdrawal syndrome when compared to non-depressed smokers (Jamal, Willem Van der Does, Cuijpers, & Penninx, 2012; Weinberger et al., 2017).

Furthermore, it is necessary to clarify the impact that sex may have on such a relationship, as some differences have been found between females and males with respect to loneliness, depressive symptoms, and smoking-related variables. For instance, most studies show that females tend to report loneliness and depressive symptoms more frequently than males (De Jong Gierveld & Van Tilburg, 2010; Dong & Chen, 2017; Whiteford, Ferrari, Degenhardt, Feigin, & Vos, 2015), whereas it has been suggested that males tend to experience greater cigarette dependence (Okita et al., 2016; Perkins et al., 2006).

Previous research highlights the relevance of cigarette dependence on smoking persistence and relapse during and after smoking cessation treatment (Fagerstrom, Russ, Yu, Yunis, & Foulds, 2012; Kenford et al., 2002). To date, however, very few studies have examined loneliness in smokers, and its relation to depression and cigarette dependence. The analysis of the relation among these variables would inform of the impact of psychosocial variables on cigarette dependence, and consequently, would help to improve smoking cessation interventions.

Thus, the current study investigates for the first time: (a) the possible relationship between loneliness, depression, and cigarette dependence; (b) the possible mediation of depressive symptoms in the relationship between loneliness and cigarette dependence; and (c) the possible moderation of sex in that relationship. Therefore, based on the aforementioned literature, we formulated three hypotheses: (1) we expected that higher loneliness scores correlated with higher depression and cigarette dependence scores; (2) we expected that depression scores mediated in the relation between loneliness and cigarette dependence scores; and (3) we expected that sex would be a significant moderator in the relation between loneliness, depression, and cigarette dependence.

Methods

Participants

The sample included 275 treatment-seeking daily adult smokers recruited from the community to participate in a smoking cessation randomized controlled trial (conducted in Spain), based in a cognitive-behavioral intervention without pharmacotherapy (clinicialtrials.gov# NCT02844595). Individuals were eligible if they were at least 18-years-old, wished to participate in the smoking cessation treatment, provided written informed consent, and smoked at least eight cigarettes per day. Exclusion criteria were: a diagnosis of severe mental disorder (bipolar disorder and/or psychotic disorder); other substance use disorders (alcohol, cannabis, stimulants, hallucinogens and/or opioids); having participated in the same or similar treatment over the previous year or having received pharmacological treatment to quit smoking over the previous year; presence of a high life-risk pathology (i.e. recent myocardial infarction); and/or using tobacco products other than cigarettes.

Measures

Assessment examined demographics, cigarette dependence, loneliness, and current depression symptoms. We used the validated Spanish version of the following instruments.

- Smoking Habit Questionnaire (Elisardo Becoña, 1994), designed to gather information on sociodemographic variables (e.g. sex, age, marital status, educational level) and tobacco use (e.g., number of cigarettes smoked per day, use of other tobacco products different from cigarettes, quit attempts).

- Los Angeles Loneliness Scale (UCLA-3; Russell, 1996; Spanish version by Vázquez & García-Bóveda, 1994). This self-report measure consists of 20 items, with four response options corresponding to the frequency of the item (e.g. "How often do you feel that you lack companionship?" "How often do you feel close to people?") Higher scores indicate a higher level of loneliness perception. In this sample, the Cronbach's alpha of this instrument was .89.

- Beck Depression Inventory-II (BDI-II; Beck, Steer, & Brown, 1996; Spanish version by Sanz & Vazquez, 2011). This 21-item self-report scale measures current depressive symptoms. Each item has four response options, from 0 to 3, referring to how the participant has felt over the last two weeks (e.g., "feeling sad", "feeling discouraged about the future"). The total score can range from 0 to 63, with higher scores indicating a higher level of depressive symptoms. In this sample, the Cronbach's alpha of this instrument was .90.

- Fagerström Test of Cigarette Dependence (FTCD; Heatherton, Kozlowski, Frecker, & Fagerström, 1991; Spanish version by Becoña & Vázquez, 1998). This six-item instrument assesses cigarette dependence (e.g. "which cigarette would you hate to give up?"; "how many cigarettes/day do you smoke?"). Scores ≥ 6 are considered to be indicative of dependence. In this sample, the Cronbach's alpha of this instrument was .65.

Procedure

The current study is based on the secondary analysis of baseline data from the mentioned above randomized controlled trial. A more detailed description of the study procedures can be found in Becoña et al. (2017), and Martínez-Vispo et al. (in press). Participants were recruited between January 2016 and April 2017 through advertisements, by word of mouth, and referral from the services of the healthcare system. The study was approved by the Bioethics Committee of the University of Santiago de Compostela (Spain). All participants provided written informed consent before entering the study.

Data Analytic Strategy

Descriptive data and frequency analyses of the studied variables were conducted and are reported as means with standard deviations or frequencies with the corresponding percentages (Table 1). Correlations among study variables were also examined.

Two simple mediation models (Figure 1) were performed to test whether depressive symptoms (mediator variable = M) have an indirect effect on the relation between loneliness (independent variable = X) and cigarette dependence (dependent variable = Y), with and without covariates (sex, age, marital status, education, working status).

Two moderated mediation models (Figure 1) were constructed to test the role of sex in moderating the hypothesized mediation effect, following the approach of Preacher and Hayes (2008). Firstly, we tested the first stage of moderated mediation for proposed model using PROCESS "Model 7"; and then, we tested the second stage of moderated mediation using PROCESS "Model 14". We used the PROCESS macro V3.1. for SPSS, version 24.0, developed by Hayes and Little (2018) to examine mediation and

Table 1. Descriptive Data of the Total Sample ($N = 275$).

	Mean (SD) % (N)
Sex (female)	61.5 (169)
Age	45.3 (10.9)
Marital status (married or living with a partner)	50.9 (140)
Education	
<HS diploma	21.4 (59)
HS diploma or GED	38.2 (105)
College or technical school	40.4 (111)
Current work situation (working)	58.9 (162)
UCLA-3	35.1 (9.2)
BDI-II	10.5 (9.1)
FTCD (dependent $\geq$ 6 score)	42.5 (117)

BDI-II: Beck Depression Inventory-II; GED: general education; HS: high school; FCTC: Fagerström Test for Cigarette Dependence (1 = FTCD scores $\geq$ 6; 0 = FTCD scores < 6); UCLA-3: loneliness scale.

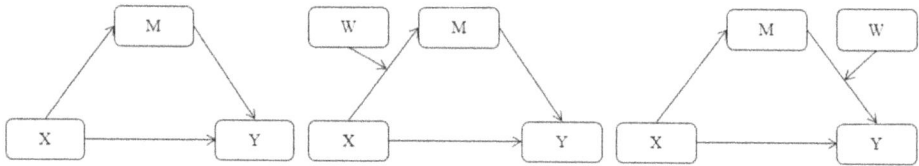

Figure 1. Conceptual mediation and moderated mediation models (4, 7, and 14). Note: X: independent variable; Y: dependent variable; M: mediator variable; W: moderator variable. Model 4: left; Model 7 centered, and Model 14: right.

moderated mediation models. Bootstrap resampling techniques were performed (with 20.000 re-samples), and a 95% bias-corrected confidence interval (BootCI) was used to evaluate indirect effects (Preacher & Hayes, 2008). Results are presumed to be significant if the CIs do not include zero. Significance of moderated mediation was tested with Hayes' index of moderated mediation (Hayes, 2018).

Results

Descriptive Results

Descriptive data and self-report measures are presented in Table 1. The bivariate correlations showed that loneliness was significantly related to depressive symptoms ($r = 0.51$, $p = \leq .01$) and to cigarette dependence ($r = 0.12$, $p = \leq 0.05$). Moreover, depressive symptoms correlated positively with cigarette dependence ($r = 0.26$, $p = \leq 0.01$).

Mediation Models

Simple mediation analysis (Model 4) examined the relations between the independent variable (X = loneliness), the dependent variable (Y = cigarette dependence), and the mediator variable (M = depressive symptoms). In the model without covariates (Table 2), loneliness had a significant indirect effect on cigarette dependence via depressive symptoms ($B = 0.035$; SE = 0.010, 95% BootCI [0.017, 0.058]) as the 95% confidence interval of the point estimate did not cross zero, whereas the direct was nonsignificant ($B = -0.007$; SE = 0.016, 95% BootCI [−0.039, 0.023]). When including the covariates in the model (Table

Table 2. Mediation Analysis Results.

Predictor (X)	Path	B	SE	t	p	LLCI	ULCI	Path	B	SE	z	p	LLCI	ULCI
		Mediator (M) Depressive symptoms						Outcome (Y) Cigarette dependence						
Loneliness	a	0.50	0.05	9.88	0.001	0.408	0.611	c′	−0.00	0.01	−0.48	0.627	−0.039	0.023
Depressive symptoms	—	—	—	—	—	—	—	b	0.06	0.01	3.95	0.001	0.034	0.103
		Mediator (M) Depressive symptoms						Outcome (Y) Cigarette dependence						
Predictor (X)	Path	B	SE	t	p	LLCI	ULCI	Path	B	SE	z	p	LLCI	ULCI
Loneliness	a	0.49	0.05	9.75	0.001	0.393	0.591	c′	−0.00	0.01	−0.46	0.644	−0.039	0.024
Depressive symptoms	—	—	—	—	—	—	—	b	0.07	0.01	3.91	0.001	0.036	0.108
Sex		0.34	0.94	0.36	0.718	−1.523	2.207		−0.42	0.26	−1.60	0.109	−0.940	0.094
Age		−0.07	0.04	−1.81	0.071	−0.161	0.006		0.00	.01	0.82	0.409	−0.013	0.033
Marital status		−0.45	0.94	−0.48	0.630	−2.320	1.408		−0.52	0.26	−1.98	0.047	−1.053	−0.005
Education		−3.33	0.99	−3.33	0.001	−5.297	−1.362		−0.30	0.28	−1.05	0.292	−0.859	0.259
Working status		−1.93	0.98	−1.96	0.050	−3.874	0.006		0.40	0.28	1.41	0.157	−0.154	0.954

LLCI: lower limit confidence interval; SE: standard error; ULCI: upper limit confidence interval.

2), a similar result was found, showing that the indirect effect of depression remained significant ($B = 0.035$; SE $= 0.010$, 95% BootCI [0.017, 0.060]), whereas the direct effect was nonsignificant ($B = -0.007$; SE $= 0.016$, 95% BootCI [−0.039, 0.024]).

A reverse model was conducted examining whether loneliness could mediate in the relation between depressive symptoms (X) and cigarette dependence (Y). This model showed a nonsignificant indirect effect of loneliness in this relation ($B = -0.001$, 95% BootCI [−0.01, 0.008].

Moderated Mediation Models

Two models were used to analyze whether sex moderated the mediation effect of depressive symptoms in the relation between loneliness on cigarette dependence.

To test the first stage of moderated mediation, we used PROCESS Model 7 (Figure 1) with loneliness as the independent variable (X) and cigarette dependence as the dependent variable (Y). Depressive symptoms were entered as the mediator variable (M), and we also included age, marital status, education, and working status as covariates. Sex was entered as moderator (W). The direct effect (c' path) of loneliness on cigarette dependence after controlling for depressive symptoms (M), sex (W), and the interaction of loneliness and sex (X*W) was nonsignificant ($B = -0.010$; SE $= 0.016$, 95% BootCI [−0.041, 0.021]). There was a significant conditional indirect effect for both sexes (Table 3), but the moderated mediation effect was nonsignificant ($B = 0.004$; SE $= 0.009$, 95% BootCI [−0.015, 0.023]).

To test the second stage of moderated mediation, we used the PROCESS Model 14 (Figure 1). The interaction between depressive symptoms and sex (M*V) was significant (Table 3). As in the previous analysis, the direct effect (c' path) was nonsignificant (B $= -0.008$; SE $= 0.016$, 95% BootCI [−0.040, 0.024]). There was a significant conditional indirect effect of loneliness on cigarette dependence through depressive symptoms for both sexes. The index of moderated mediation was significant ($B = -0.042$; SE $= 0.019$, 95% BootCI [−0.085, −0.010]), indicating that the strength of the indirect effect of loneliness on cigarette dependence through depressive symptoms was significant and dependent on sex. This effect was significant for both sexes, although it was higher for

Table 3. Moderated Mediation Analysis Results.

Model 7	B	SE	p	LLCI	ULCI
X→M (a)	0.443	0.091	0.001	0.263	0.623
M→Y (b)	0.074	0.018	0.001	0.038	0.111
X→Y (c′)	−0.010	0.016	0.539	−0.041	0.021
X*W→M	0.053	0.109	0.624	−0.162	0.026
Conditional mediation for males	0.033	0.011		0.015	0.058
Conditional mediation for females	0.037	0.011		0.018	0.063
Index of moderated mediation	0.004	0.0096		−0.015	0.023
Model 14	**B**	**SE**	**p**	**LLCI**	**ULCI**
X→M (a)	0.481	0.50 3	0.001	0.383	0.580
M→Y (b)	0.137	0.034	0.001	0.070	0.204
X→Y (c′)	−0.008	0.016	0.627	−0.040	0.024
M*V→Y	−0.087	0.037	0.020	−0.161	−0.013
Conditional mediation for males	0.066	0.018		0.038	0.111
Conditional mediation for females	0.024	0.011		0.005	0.049
Index of moderated mediation	−0.042	0.019		−0.085	−0.010

Covariates included in the analysis: age, marital status, education, working status. X: loneliness; Y: cigarette dependence (0 = nondependent; 1 = dependent); M: depressive symptoms; W: sex (0 = male; 1 = female; path a); V = sex (0 = male; 1 = female; path b). LLCI: lower limit confidence interval; SE: standard error; ULCI: upper limit confidence interval.

males ($B = 0.066$; SE $= 0.018$, 95% BootCI [0.038, 0.111]) than for females ($B = 0.024$; SE $= 0.011$, 95% BootCI [0.005, 0.049]).

Discussion

To our knowledge, the current investigation is the first study to examine the relation between loneliness, depressive symptoms, and cigarette dependence in a sample of treatment-seeking smokers. Our findings showed that the study variables correlated positively, confirming our first hypothesis. This is consistent with previous research showing that loneliness is associated with higher levels of depressive symptoms (Erzen & Çikrikci, 2018). Regarding the relation between loneliness and cigarette dependence, we found a positive and significant correlation, with greater scores in loneliness associated with being cigarette dependent. This finding extends previous studies reporting that loneliness is related to a greater probability of smoking cigarettes (DeWall & Pond, 2011; Dyal & Valente, 2015; Matthews et al., 2019), as to date, the relation with cigarette dependence has not been studied.

Regarding our second hypothesis, mediation-related results of this study showed that loneliness has no direct effect on cigarette dependence, but it has significant indirect effects via depressive symptoms in this sample of smokers seeking smoking-cessation treatment. Furthermore, this indirect effect remained significant after accounting for age, sex, marital status, education level, and working status. When examining the effect of sex, we found that it was a significant moderator of the indirect effect of loneliness on cigarette dependence through depressive symptoms, which support our third hypothesis. Concretely, moderated mediation analyses showed that this conditional effect was only significant within the path between depressive symptoms and cigarette dependence, with males showing greater levels of risk of dependence. In contrast, the pathway from loneliness to depressive symptoms did not differ as a function of sex, which implies that loneliness predicts depression equally for males and females.

The main finding of this study suggests that, in treatment-seeking smokers, higher loneliness predicts cigarette dependence through depressive symptoms. Different explanations for this relation can be drawn, as cigarette dependence is a complex and multidimensional phenomenon that involves a broad range of psychological, social, and physiological variables (Fagerstrom, 2012; Piper et al., 2004). In this sense, mood management has been suggested as a relevant factor for cigarette dependence (Baker, Piper, McCarthy, Majeskie, & Fiore, 2004). Previous research has shown that dependent smokers tend to use smoking not only as a coping strategy to deal with psychological distress and negative affect, but also as a way of increasing positive affect (Audrain-McGovern, Wileyto, Ashare, Cuevas, & Strasser, 2014; Spring, Pingitore, & McChargue, 2003). Thus, considering our results, lonely smokers with higher levels of depressive symptoms may have a higher probability of cigarette dependence because of their expectation that smoking will alleviate this negative emotional state. Additionally, social-related motivational factors, such as the desire for increased acceptance and social belonging, may influence the value of cigarette smoking for lonely smokers, as suggested by DeWall and Pond (2011). It has also been proposed that smoking may be considered as a facilitator for social behavior, functioning as a way to contact with others (Baker, Brandon, & Chassin, 2004). In addition, the cigarette is sometimes considered as a "friend" when an individual feels lonely (Fagerstrom, 2012), which can have special relevance when depressive symptoms are present. Regarding physiological factors related to cigarette dependence, previous studies have reported the existence of sex differences. In accordance, the moderator role of sex found in the path between depressive symptoms and cigarette dependence is consistent with previous research suggesting that males may be more sensitive to nicotine effects than females (Perkins, 2008), and also that males experiences greater relief of negative affective responses after smoking (Perkins & Karelitz, 2015).

Some limitations of the current investigation should be noted. First, due to the cross-sectional nature of our data, causal and temporal interpretations could not be established. Future research should examine longitudinal associations between loneliness, depressive symptoms, and cigarette dependence, and also the interaction and impact of these variables on smoking cessation outcomes. Secondly, we used a sample of treatment-seeking smokers from Spain; thus, it remains unclear whether our results could be generalized to smokers from the general population or from other cultural backgrounds. Studies conducted in nonclinical samples and cross-cultural research are needed in order to determine to what extend the relation among the variables found in this study can be generalized. Third, the study measures were self-report instruments, and can therefore be affected by response bias.

Despite these limitations, the present study has several strengths and extends previous literature by showing that, in treatment-seeking smokers, loneliness is not only a significant predictor of depressive symptoms, but also, through this relation, it has an effect on cigarette dependence that is greater for males. Previous studies examining loneliness in the context of smoking-cessation interventions have shown that this psychosocial variable is a significant predictor of lower smoking-cessation self-efficacy (Shuter et al., 2014), and that it is related to smoking status (Moadel et al., 2012). To our knowledge, this is the first study that examines the relation between loneliness, depressive symptoms, and cigarette dependence in a sample of treatment-seeking smokers, considering sex as a possible moderator. Examination of this relationship contributes to the understanding of cigarette dependence, which constitutes a well-known barrier to abstinence. Thus, our results are also helpful, as they may guide the development of targeted smoking-cessation interventions, which should consider loneliness, its relation to depressive symptoms, and sex differences. For instance, some authors have suggested that introduce strategies aimed to enhance social support, to identify automatic negative thoughts related to social interactions, and to change maladaptive social perception and cognition could be adequate intervention approaches (Cacioppo et al., 2015; Masi, Chen, Hawkley, & Cacioppo, 2011; Qualter et al., 2015). Additional research is needed to assess whether the inclusion of such strategies in smoking cessation treatments would increase abstinence outcomes.

Overall, these findings provide support for the role of loneliness in cigarette dependence, considering depressive symptoms as a relevant variable in such a relation among treatment-seeking smokers.

Funding

This research was supported by the Spanish Ministry of Economy and Competiveness and by ERDF (European Regional Development Fund) (Project reference: PSI2015-66755-R).

ORCID

Carmela Martínez-Vispo ⓘ http://orcid.org/0000-0002-8503-1791
Ana López-Durán ⓘ http://orcid.org/0000-0001-7661-8972
Rubén Rodríguez-Cano ⓘ http://orcid.org/0000-0001-6934-2939
Elena Fernández del Río ⓘ http://orcid.org/0000-0002-9645-8109
Carmen Senra ⓘ http://orcid.org/0000-0001-5980-6680
Elisardo Becoña ⓘ http://orcid.org/0000-0002-6639-3834

References

Audrain-McGovern, J., Wileyto, E. P., Ashare, R., Cuevas, J., & Strasser, A. A. (2014). Reward and affective regulation in depression-prone smokers. *Biological Psychiatry*, 76(9), 689–697. doi:10.1016/j.biopsych.2014.04.018

Baker, T. B., Brandon, T. H., & Chassin, L. (2004). Motivational influences on cigarette smoking. *Annual Review of Psychology*, 55(1), 463–491. doi:10.1146/annurev.psych.55.090902.142054

Baker, T. B., Piper, M. E., McCarthy, D. E., Majeskie, M. R., & Fiore, M. C. (2004). Addiction motivation reformulated: An affective processing model of negative reinforcement. *Psychological Review*, 111(1), 33–51. doi:10.1037/0033-295X.111.1.33

Beck, A., Steer, R., & Brown, G. (1996). Beck depression inventory (2nd ed). Manual. San Antonio, TX: The Psychological Corporation.

Becoña, E. (1994). Evaluación de la conducta de fumar [Assessment of smoking behavior]. In L. J. Graña (Ed.), *Conductas adictivas: teoría, evaluación y tratamiento.* (pp. 403–454). Madrid, Spain: Debate.

Becoña, E., Martínez-Vispo, C., Senra, C., López-Durán, A., Rodríguez-Cano, R., & Fernández del Río, E. (2017). Cognitive-behavioral treatment with behavioral activation for smokers with depressive symptomatology: Study protocol of a randomized controlled trial. *BMC Psychiatry*, 17(1), 134. doi:10.1186/s12888-017-1301-7

Becoña, E., & Vázquez, F. L. (1998). The Fagerström Test for Nicotine Dependence in a Spanish sample. *Psychological Reports*, 83(3_suppl), 1455–1458. doi:10.2466/pr0.1998.83.3f.1455

Beutel, M. E., Klein, E. M., Brähler, E., Reiner, I., Jünger, C., Michal, M., … Tibubos, A. N. (2017). Loneliness in the general population: Prevalence, determinants and relations to mental health. *BMC Psychiatry*, 17(1), 97. doi:10.1186/s12888-017-1262-x

Breslau, N., Johnson, E. O., Hiripi, E., & Kessler, R. (2001). Nicotine dependence in the United States. *Archives of General Psychiatry*, 58(9), 810. doi:10.1001/archpsyc.58.9.810

Cacioppo, J. T., Ernst, J. M., Burleson, M. H., McClintock, M. K., Malarkey, W. B., Hawkley, L. C., … Berntson, G. G. (2000). Lonely traits and concomitant physiological processes: The MacArthur social neuroscience studies. *International Journal of Psychophysiology*, 35(2-3), 143–154. doi:10.1016/S0167-8760(99)00049-5

Cacioppo, J. T., Hughes, M. E., Waite, L. J., Hawkley, L. C., & Thisted, R. A. (2006). Loneliness as a specific risk factor for depressive symptoms: Cross-sectional and longitudinal analyses. *Psychology and Aging*, 21(1), 140–151. doi:10.1037/0882-7974.21.1.140

Cacioppo, S., Grippo, A. J., London, S., Goossens, L., & Cacioppo, J. T. (2015). Loneliness: Clinical import and interventions. *Perspectives on Psychological Science*, 10(2), 238–249. doi: 10.1177/1745691615570616

De Jong Gierveld, J., & Van Tilburg, T. (2010). The De Jong Gierveld short scales for emotional and social loneliness: Tested on data from 7 countries in the UN generations and gender surveys. *European Journal of Ageing*, 7(2), 121–130. doi:10.1007/s10433-010-0144-6

DeWall, C. N., & Pond, R. S. (2011). Loneliness and smoking: The costs of the desire to reconnect. *Self and Identity*, 10(3), 375–385. doi:10.1080/15298868.2010.524404

Dong, X., & Chen, R. (2017). Gender differences in the experience of loneliness in U.S. Chinese older adults. *Journal of Women & Aging*, 29(2), 115–125. doi:10.1080/08952841.2015.1080534

Dyal, S. R., & Valente, T. W. (2015). A systematic review of loneliness and smoking: Small effects, big implications. *Substance Use & Misuse*, *50*(13), 1697–1716. doi:10.3109/10826084.2015.1027933

Erzen, E., & Çikrikci, Ö. (2018). The effect of loneliness on depression: A meta-analysis. *International Journal of Social Psychiatry*, *64*(5), 427–435. doi:10.1177/0020764018776349

Fagerstrom, K. (2012). Determinants of tobacco use and renaming the FTND to the Fagerstrom test for cigarette dependence. *Nicotine & Tobacco Research*, *14*(1), 75–78. doi:10.1093/ntr/ntr137

Fagerstrom, K., Russ, C., Yu, C.-R., Yunis, C., & Foulds, J. (2012). The Fagerstrom test for nicotine dependence as a predictor of smoking abstinence: A pooled analysis of varenicline clinical trial data. *Nicotine & Tobacco Research*, *14*(12), 1467–1473. doi:10.1093/ntr/nts018

Goodwin, R. D., Wall, M. M., Garey, L., Zvolensky, M. J., Dierker, L., Galea, S., ... Hasin, D. S. (2017). Depression among current, former, and never smokers from 2005 to 2013: The hidden role of disparities in depression in the ongoing tobacco epidemic. *Drug and Alcohol Dependence*, *173*, 191–199. doi:10.1016/j.drugalcdep.2016.11.038

Habibi, M., Hosseini, F., Darharaj, M., Moghadamzadeh, A., Radfar, F., & Ghaffari, Y. (2018). Attachment style, perceived loneliness, and psychological well-being in smoking and non-smoking university students. *Journal of Psychology: Interdisciplinary and Applied*, *152*(4), 226–236. doi:10.1080/00223980.2018.1446894

Hawkley, L. C., Burleson, M. H., Berntson, G. G., & Cacioppo, J. T. (2003). Loneliness in everyday life: Cardiovascular activity, psychosocial context, and health behaviors. *Journal of Personality and Social Psychology*, *85*(1), 105–120. doi:10.1037/0022-3514.85.1.105

Hawkley, L. C., & Cacioppo, J. T. (2010). Loneliness matters: A theoretical and empirical review of consequences and mechanisms. *Annals of Behavioral Medicine*, *40*(2), 218–227. doi:10.1007/s12160-010-9210-8

Hayes, A. F. (2018). Partial, conditional, and moderated moderated mediation: Quantification, inference, and interpretation. *Communication Monographs*, *85*(1), 4–40. doi: 10.1080/03637751.2017.1352100

Hayes, A. F., & Little, T. D. (2018). Introduction to mediation, moderation, and conditional process analysis: A regression-based approach (2nd ed). New York, NY: Guilford Press.

Heatherton, T. F., Kozlowski, L. T., Frecker, R. C., & Fagerström, K. O. (1991). The Fagerström test for nicotine dependence: A revision of the Fagerström tolerance questionnaire. *British Journal of Addiction*, *86*(9), 1119–1127. doi:10.1111/j.1360-0443.1991.tb01879.x

Holt-Lunstad, J., Smith, T. B., Baker, M., Harris, T., & Stephenson, D. (2015). Loneliness and social isolation as risk factors for mortality. *Perspectives on Psychological Science*, *10*(2), 227–237. doi:10.1177/1745691614568352

Jamal, M., Willem Van der Does, A. J., Cuijpers, P., & Penninx, B. W. J. H. (2012). Association of smoking and nicotine dependence with severity and course of symptoms in patients with depressive or anxiety disorder. *Drug and Alcohol Dependence*, *126*(1-2), 138–146. doi:10.1016/j.drugalcdep.2012.05.001

Kenford, S. L., Smith, S. S., Wetter, D. W., Jorenby, D. E., Fiore, M. C., & Baker, T. B. (2002). Predicting relapse back to smoking: Contrasting affective and physical models of dependence. *Journal of Consulting and Clinical Psychology*, *70*(1), 216–227. doi:10.1037//0022-006X.70.1.216

Kobayashi, L. C., & Steptoe, A. (2018). Social isolation, loneliness, and health behaviors at older ages: Longitudinal cohort study. *Annals of Behavioral Medicine*, *52*(7), 582–593. doi:10.1093/abm/kax033

Lauder, W., Mummery, K., Jones, M., & Caperchione, C. (2006). A comparison of health behaviours in lonely and non-lonely populations. *Psychology, Health & Medicine*, *11*(2), 233–245. doi:10.1080/13548500500266607

Luo, Y., Hawkley, L. C., Waite, L. J., & Cacioppo, J. T. (2012). Loneliness, health, and mortality in old age: A national longitudinal study. *Social Science & Medicine*, *74*(6), 907–914. doi: 10.1016/j.socscimed.2011.11.028

Martínez-Vispo, C., Rodríguez-Cano, R. A., López-Durán, A., Senra, C., Fernández del Río, E., & Becoña, E. (in press). Cognitive-behavioral treatment with behavioral activation for smoking cessation: Randomized controlled trial. PlosOne.

Masi, C. M., Chen, H.-Y., Hawkley, L. C., & Cacioppo, J. T. (2011). A meta-analysis of interventions to reduce loneliness. *Personality and Social Psychology Review*, *15*(3), 219–266. doi: 10.1177/1088868310377394

Matthews, T., Danese, A., Caspi, A., Fisher, H. L., Goldman-Mellor, S., Kepa, A., … Arseneault, L. (2019). Lonely young adults in modern Britain: Findings from an epidemiological cohort study. *Psychological Medicine*, *49*(02), 268–277. doi:10.1017/S0033291718000788

Moadel, A. B., Bernstein, S. L., Mermelstein, R. J., Arnsten, J. H., Dolce, E. H., & Shuter, J. (2012). A randomized controlled trial of a tailored group smoking cessation intervention for HIV-infected smokers. *JAIDS Journal of Acquired Immune Deficiency Syndromes*, *61*(2), 208–215. doi:10.1097/QAI.0b013e3182645679

Okita, K., Petersen, N., Robertson, C. L., Dean, A. C., Mandelkern, M. A., & London, E. D. (2016). Sex differences in midbrain dopamine D2-type receptor availability and association with nicotine dependence. *Neuropsychopharmacology*, *41*(12), 2913–2919. doi:10.1038/npp.2016.105

Peplau, L. A., & Perlman, D. (1982). Perspectives on loneliness. In L. A. Peplau & D. Perlman (Eds.), *Loneliness: A sourcebook of current theory, research and therapy* (pp. 1–18). New York, NY: John Wiley & Sons.

Perkins, K. A. (2008). *Sex differences in nicotine reinforcement and reward: Influences on the persistence of tobacco smoking* (pp. 143–169). New York, NY: Springer.

Perkins, K. A., Doyle, T., Ciccocioppo, M., Conklin, C., Sayette, M., & Caggiula, A. (2006). Sex differences in the influence of nicotine dose instructions on the reinforcing and self-reported rewarding effects of smoking. *Psychopharmacology*, *184*(3-4), 600–607. doi:10.1007/s00213-005-0103-7 doi:10.1007/s00213-005-0103-7

Perkins, K. A., & Karelitz, J. L. (2015). Sex differences in acute relief of abstinence-induced withdrawal and negative affect due to nicotine content in cigarettes. *Nicotine & Tobacco Research*, *17*(4), 443–448. doi:10.1093/ntr/ntu150

Piper, M. E., Piasecki, T. M., Federman, E. B., Bolt, D. M., Smith, S. S., Fiore, M. C., & Baker, T. B. (2004). A multiple motives approach to tobacco dependence: The Wisconsin Inventory of Smoking Dependence Motives (WISDM-68). *Journal of Consulting and Clinical Psychology*, *72*(2), 139–154. doi:10.1037/0022-006X.72.2.139

Preacher, K. J., & Hayes, A. F. (2008). Asymptotic and resampling strategies for assessing and comparing indirect effects in multiple mediator models. *Behavior Research Methods*, *40*(3), 879–891. doi:10.3758/BRM.40.3.879

Qualter, P., Vanhalst, J., Harris, R., Van Roekel, E., Lodder, G., Bangee, M., … Verhagen, M. (2015). Loneliness across the life span. *Perspectives on Psychological Science*, *10*(2), 250–264. doi:10.1177/1745691615568999

Richard, A., Rohrmann, S., Vandeleur, C. L., Schmid, M., Barth, J., & Eichholzer, M. (2017). Loneliness is adversely associated with physical and mental health and lifestyle factors: Results from a Swiss national survey. *Plos One*, *12*(7), e0181442. doi:10.1371/journal.pone.0181442

Russell, D. W. (1996). UCLA loneliness scale (Version 3): Reliability, validity, and factor structure. *Journal of Personality Assessment*, *66*(1), 20–40. doi:10.1207/s15327752jpa6601_2

Russell, D. W., Cutrona, C. E., McRae, C., & Gomez, M. (2012). Is loneliness the same as being alone?. *Journal of Psychology: Interdisciplinary and Applied*, *146*(1-2), 7–22. doi:10.1080/00223980.2011.589414

Sadeghi Bahmani, D., Faraji, P., Faraji, R., Lang, U. E., Holsboer-Trachsler, E., Brand, S., … Brand, S. (2018). Is emotional functioning related to academic achievement among university students? Results from a cross-sectional Iranian sample. *Revista Brasileira de Psiquiatria*, *40*(3), 290–295. doi:10.1590/1516-4446-2017-2434

Sanz, J., & Vazquez, C. (2011). Adaptación española del Inventario para Depresión de Beck-II (BDI-II) [Spanish adaptation of the Beck Depression Inventory—II (BDI-II)]. Manual. Madrid, Spain: Pearson.

Shankar, A., McMunn, A., Banks, J., & Steptoe, A. (2011). Loneliness, social isolation, and behavioral and biological health indicators in older adults. *Health Psychology*, *30*(4), 377–385. doi: 10.1037/a0022826

Shuter, J., Moadel, A. B., Kim, R. S., Weinberger, A. H., & Stanton, C. A. (2014). Self-efficacy to quit in HIV-infected smokers. *Nicotine & Tobacco Research, 16*(11), 1527–1531. doi:10.1093/ntr/ntu136

Spring, B., Pingitore, R., & McChargue, D. E. (2003). Reward value of cigarette smoking for comparably heavy smoking schizophrenic, depressed, and nonpatient smokers. *American Journal of Psychiatry, 160*(2), 316–322. doi:10.1176/appi.ajp.160.2.316

Steptoe, A., Shankar, A., Demakakos, P., & Wardle, J. (2013). Social isolation, loneliness, and all-cause mortality in older men and women. *Proceedings of the National Academy of Sciences, 110*(15), 5797–5801. doi:10.1073/pnas.1219686110

Valtorta, N. K., Kanaan, M., Gilbody, S., Ronzi, S., & Hanratty, B. (2016). Loneliness and social isolation as risk factors for coronary heart disease and stroke: Systematic review and meta-analysis of longitudinal observational studies. *Heart, 102*(13), 1009–1016. doi:10.1136/heartjnl-2015-308790

Vázquez, A. J., & García-Bóveda, J. (1994). RULS: Escala de soledad UCLA revisada. *Fiabilidad y Validez de Una Versión Española. Revista de Psicología de La Salud, 6*(1), 46–54. doi:10.21134/PSSA.V6I1.1224

Weinberger, A. H., Kashan, R. S., Shpigel, D. M., Esan, H., Taha, F., Lee, C. J., … Goodwin, R. D. (2017). Depression and cigarette smoking behavior: A critical review of population-based studies. *The American Journal of Drug and Alcohol Abuse, 43*(4), 416–431. doi:10.3109/00952990.2016.1171327

Whiteford, H. A., Ferrari, A. J., Degenhardt, L., Feigin, V., & Vos, T. (2015). The global burden of mental, neurological and substance use disorders: An analysis from the Global Burden of Disease Study 2010. *Plos One, 10*(2), e0116820. doi:10.1371/journal.pone.0116820

Zawadzki, M. J., Graham, J. E., & Gerin, W. (2013). Rumination and anxiety mediate the effect of loneliness on depressed mood and sleep quality in college students. *Health Psychology, 32*(2), 212–222. doi:10.1037/a0029007

Body Dysmorphic Symptoms, Functional Impairment, and Depression: The Role of Appearance-Based Teasing

Hilary Weingarden and Keith D. Renshaw

ABSTRACT

Body dysmorphic disorder is associated with elevated social and occupational impairment and comorbid depression, but research on risk factors for body dysmorphic symptoms and associated outcomes is limited. Appearance-based teasing may be a potential risk factor. To examine the specificity of this factor, the authors assessed self-reported appearance-based teasing, body dysmorphic, and obsessive-compulsive symptom severity, functional impairment (i.e., social, occupational, family impairment), and depression in a nonclinical sample of undergraduates. As hypothesized, appearance-based teasing was positively correlated with body dysmorphic symptoms. The correlation between teasing and body dysmorphic symptoms was stronger than that between teasing and obsessive-compulsive symptom severity. Last, body dysmorphic symptom severity and appearance-based teasing interacted in predicting functional impairment and depression. Specifically, appearance-based teasing was positively associated with depression and functional impairment only in those with elevated body dysmorphic symptoms. When a similar moderation was tested with obsessive-compulsive, in place of body dysmorphic, symptom severity, the interaction was nonsignificant. Findings support theory that appearance-based teasing is a specific risk factor for body dysmorphic symptoms and associated functional impairment.

Body dysmorphic disorder (BDD) is a severe and understudied psychological disorder, characterized by distressing preoccupations with imagined defects in one's physical appearance (American Psychiatric Association [APA], 2013). In most cases of BDD, an actual physical flaw in one's appearance does not exist and is imagined by the sufferer. However, in cases where a physical flaw is present, the individual's concern and preoccupation must be greatly out of proportion to the flaw itself (APA, 2013). In response to obsessive preoccupations about an imagined flaw(s), individuals suffering from BDD typically engage in impairing and time-consuming compulsive rituals, such as repetitive mirror-checking, camouflaging body parts of concern, and repetitive grooming.

As BDD is characterized by these obsessive preoccupations and repetitive, compulsive behaviors, it shares many phenomenological similarities with obsessive-compulsive disorder (OCD). In addition, comorbidity rates between BDD and OCD are elevated (Phillips, Menard, Fay, & Weisberg, 2005), and OCD may be the most frequent psychiatric diagnosis among relatives of people with BDD (Hollander, 1993). Consequently, BDD is classified as an obsessive-compulsive related disorder in the DSM-5 (APA, 2013). Although it is not frequently studied, BDD is not an uncommon disorder, with point-prevalence estimates between 1.7–2.4% (Buhlmann et al., 2010; Koran, Abujaoude, Large, & Serpe, 2008; Rief, Buhlmann, Wilhelm, Borkenhagen, & Brahler, 2006) and prevalence in a general adult psychiatric inpatient unit documented to be as high as 16% (Conroy et al., 2008).

Despite the relatively lower level of attention devoted to BDD in the empirical literature, BDD is associated with marked functional impairment across a wide range of domains. For instance, occupational impairment in BDD exceeds that found in both the general population and in related disorders, like OCD (Chosak et al., 2008; Frare, Perugi, Ruffolo, & Toni, 2004). Rates of unemployment in BDD samples are documented between 39–53% (Didie, Menard, Stern, & Phillips, 2008; Frare et al.; Perugi et al., 1997; Veale, Boocock, Gournay, & Dryden, 1996), and 30% of individuals with BDD report being housebound due to the disorder (Phillips, 1996; Phillips et al., 2006; Rief et al., 2006). Among those with BDD who are able to maintain jobs, work impairment is nearly universal (Phillips et al., 2006; Phillips, McElroy, Keck, Pope, & Hudson, 1993). As with occupational impairment, individuals with BDD also generally experience more severe social impairment than in related disorders like OCD (Frare et al., 2004). Almost all participants (96–100%) in two BDD samples reported moderate to extreme social dysfunction (Phillips & Diaz, 1997; Phillips et al., 2006), and 90% of another sample was either single or divorced (Fontenelle et al., 2006). Last, the rate of comorbid major depressive disorder in BDD is documented between 75–81% (Phillips et al., 2005, 2006), higher than that typically documented in related disorders, such as OCD (Phillips, Gunderson, Mallya, McElroy, & Carter, 1998).

Elevated functional impairment (i.e., occupational, social, family) and depression in the BDD population contribute to substantial suffering and costs, at both individual and societal levels. Therefore, it is important to focus research attention on identifying risk factors both for BDD symptoms and for the elevated levels of functional impairment and depression that may accompany such symptoms. Although empirical research on risk factors for functional impairment and depression in relation to BDD and body dysmorphic symptoms is in its infancy, recent theoretical models of BDD and body dissatisfaction propose factors that warrant investigation. In particular, appearance-based teasing during youth has been posited as an important social-developmental risk factor in the etiology of body dysmorphic symptoms (Feusner, Neziroglu, Wilhelm, Mancusi, & Bohon, 2010). Indeed, two previous studies demonstrated that individuals with BDD retrospectively reported greater appearance-based teasing during childhood than a healthy control group and a matched non-BDD group from a community sample (Buhlmann, Cook, Fama, & Wilhelm, 2007; Buhlmann et al., 2011). Similarly, retrospective reports of childhood bullying were significantly associated with symptoms of muscle dysmorphia (a variant of BDD) in a sample of adult male bodybuilders (Boyda & Shevlin, 2011), and a separate study showed that muscle dysmorphia symptoms and childhood bullying each significantly predicted functional impairment (e.g., low self-esteem, global psychopathology) in a sample of 100 male bodybuilders (Wolke & Sapouna, 2008).

These studies provide preliminary evidence that appearance-based teasing may be related to BDD and body dysmorphic symptoms. However, research remains in its early stages. Thus, the present study addresses several novel next steps in researching the role of appearance-based teasing in body dysmorphic symptom severity, functional impairment (i.e., social, occupational, family), and depression. Appearance preoccupations are a phenomenon that occurs on a wide spectrum of severity within the general population. Given the highly preliminary state of current research on appearance-based teasing in BDD and the need for further research, the present study uses a nonclinical sample in order to test the next research questions.

The present study addresses a number of important gaps in the literature to date. First, prior studies do not establish whether appearance-based teasing is a specific risk factor for body dysmorphic symptoms, or a general risk factor for broader psychopathology. The specificity of appearance-based teasing as a risk factor is an important distinction, as it would provide information about whether, as is theoretically posited, appearance-based teasing is specifically implicated as a risk factor to the development of BDD over other forms of psychological distress. Thus, the first aim of the present study was to extend previous findings by comparing the association of recalled history of appearance-based teasing with body dysmorphic symptom severity to the association between appearance-based teasing and related obsessive-compulsive symptom severity (Aim 1). Obsessive-compulsive symptoms were chosen as a stringent comparison, due to their phenomenological similarity (i.e., presence of obsessions and compulsions) to body dysmorphic symptoms. We hypothesized that self-reported appearance-based teasing would be more strongly associated with body dysmorphic symptom severity than with obsessive-compulsive symptom severity.

In addition, while some studies have shown a link between BDD symptoms and appearance-based teasing, theoretical conceptualizations of BDD also posit that appearance-based teasing may be a risk factor to the elevated functional impairment and depression documented in those with BDD (e.g., Buhlmann et al., 2007). However, only one prior study tests the association between appearance-based teasing, self-esteem, and global psychopathology with symptoms of muscle dysmorphia (Wolke & Sapouna, 2008). Thus, to address this gap in the literature, we next examined appearance-based teasing and BDD symptoms as concomitant risk factors for functional impairment (i.e., social, occupational, family) and depression (Aim 2). Given the research reviewed above, we expected that body dysmorphic symptom severity would predict functional impairment and depression. Building on prior research, we also hypothesized that a history of appearance-based teasing would predict functional impairment and depression, even when accounting for body dysmorphic symptom severity.

Moreover, theoretical conceptualizations of BDD suggest that appearance-based teasing is a particularly relevant risk factor for functional impairment among those with elevated body dysmorphic symptoms. For instance, individuals with BDD typically possess severely negative cognitions about themselves and their appearance, and they also possess distorted beliefs about the importance of one's physical appearance in general (Cororve & Gleaves, 2001). Thus, appearance-based teasing may be more likely to be internalized and interpreted negatively among individuals suffering from elevated body dysmorphic symptoms. As a result, appearance-based teasing may be a greater risk factor for functional impairment and depression among those with elevated BDD symptoms, compared to those with low BDD symptoms. We thus hypothesized that there would be an interactive effect of appearance-based teasing and body dysmorphic symptom severity, such that appearance-based teasing would be more strongly associated with depression and functional impairment in those with more severe body dysmorphic symptoms compared to those with less severe body dysmorphic symptoms.

Moreover, to build on our initial aim to test whether appearance-based teasing is a risk factor specific to BDD (as opposed to a risk factor for psychopathology more broadly), we also ran a parallel set of moderation analyses, with obsessive-compulsive symptom severity in place of body dysmorphic symptom severity. We hypothesized that obsessive-compulsive symptom severity would *not* significantly moderate the association of appearance-based teasing with either functional impairment or depression. Such a finding would lend further evidence that appearance-based teasing is a more specific risk factor for those with elevated BDD symptoms, as opposed to those with elevated symptoms of broader, related types of psychopathology.

Method

Participants

Participants consisted of 435 college students from George Mason University, a highly diverse university in Northern Virginia. Participants completed measures online, in return for credit in an introductory psychology course or a handful of more advanced courses. Inclusion criteria required that participants be at least 18 years of age. To ensure data integrity, we excluded participants who either spent too little time completing the survey (approximately 25 minutes or fewer), or did not appropriately answer two questions embedded in the survey as quality checks. These checks resulted in exclusion of 38 individuals, leaving a final sample of 397 participants. These participants ranged in age from 18 to 45 years ($M = 21.27$, $SD = 3.87$). The majority of participants were female (81%) and unmarried (87%). In addition, 52% of participants identified as White; 10% identified as African American; 24% identified as East Asian, Southeast Asian, or Middle Eastern; 9% identified as "other"; and the remainder of participants did not report their race.

Procedures

All procedures were approved by the university's Institutional Review Board. Participants completed the study online via Qualtrics, a secure Internet survey provider. They were first directed to an Informed Consent page, which required that they read and indicate agreement (by choosing an "I agree" option) before beginning the study. Participants were then able to proceed through study questionnaires, which took approximately 40 to 90 minutes to complete. Participants were awarded course credit as compensation for their time. Of note, list-wise deletion was used to handle missing data (which ranged from 8.3–13.6% in the present study analyses), as recommendations in the literature suggest that list-wise deletion is an appropriate strategy for up to 20% missing data (Peng, Harwell, Liou, & Ehman, 2006).

Measures

Yale-Brown Obsessive Compulsive Scale Modified for BDD (BDD Y-BOCS; Phillips, Hollander, Rasmussen, & Aronowitz, 1997)

The self-report BDD Y-BOCS, an adaptation from the clinician-administered BDD Y-BOCS (Phillips et al., 1997), was used to assess BDD symptom severity. For example, item 1 asks, "How much of your time is occupied by THOUGHTS about a defect or flaw in your appearance?" Following procedures used in prior studies (e.g., Marques, Weingarden, LeBlanc, & Wilhelm, 2011), we used a 10-item, self-report version of the measure, which omits two items from the clinician-administered BDD Y-BOCS (these two items measure insight and avoidance, which are difficult to assess accurately via self-report). The items use a 5-point Likert scale, with total scores on the measure ranging from 0 to 40, and higher scores indicating more severe BDD symptoms. A score of 16 or greater has been used as a clinical cutoff with the 10-item self-report adaptation of the BDD Y-BOCS (e.g., Marques, Weingarden, et al., 2011; Marques, LeBlanc, et al., 2011). The 12-item version demonstrates strong test-retest reliability, internal consistency ($\alpha =.80$), and sensitivity to change with treatment (Phillips et al., 1997). Likewise, psychometric properties of the 10-item version are comparably strong for reliability, convergent and discriminant validity, sensitivity to change, and factor structure, (Phillips et al., 1997). Internal consistency in the present study was also strong ($\alpha =.88$).

Obsessive-Compulsive Inventory-Revised (OCI-R; Foa et al., 2002)

The OCI-R is an 18-item, self-report scale that assesses severity of OCD symptoms. Questions are rated on a Likert scale ranging from 0 (*not at all*) to 4 (*extremely*), with total scores ranging from 0–72. The recommended cutoff score for detecting OCD is 21 (Foa et al.), and the mean for individuals with OCD is 28 (Foa et al.). The total scale has strong internal consistency within a clinical population ($\alpha =.81$), test-retest reliability assessed over a 2-week period, and convergent validity with the Yale-Brown Obsessive Compulsive Scale (Y-BOCS; Foa et al.). In the present study, the OCI-R also demonstrated strong internal consistency ($\alpha =.91$).

Depression Anxiety Stress Scale – Short Form (DASS-21; Lovibond & Lovibond, 1995)

Depression was measured using the 7-item depression subscale of the Depression Anxiety Stress Scale – Short Form. Items are scored from 0 (*did not apply to me at all*) to 3 (*applied to me very much or most of the time*), and depression items are summed and multiplied by two to achieve the final subscale score that is equivalent to the full 14-item DASS subscale. Higher scores indicate greater depressive severity. Scores on the depression subscale can be classified as *normal* (0–9), *mild* (10–13), *moderate* (14–20), *severe* (21–27), and *extremely severe* (28+). The DASS-depression subscale demonstrates strong internal consistency in both non-clinical ($\alpha =.88$; Henry & Crawford, 2005) and clinical samples ($\alpha =.96$; Brown, Chorpita, Korotitsch, & Barlow, 1997). The scale has strong concurrent validity with the Beck Depression Inventory (Beck, Rush, Shaw, & Emery, 1979), *rs* $=.74$ and .79 (Antony, Bieling, Cox, Enns, & Swinson, 1998; Lovibond & Lovibond), and it demonstrates discriminant validity with measures of anxiety (Antony et al.; Lovibond & Lovibond). Internal consistency in the present study was also strong ($\alpha =.91$).

Sheehan Disability Scale (SDS; Sheehan, Harnett-Sheehan, & Raj, 1996)

The SDS was used in the present study to assess functional impairment due to mental health symptoms. The SDS assesses functional impairment across three major life domains: social, school/occupational, and family/home. A single question is used to assess each domain, with the summed total score representing global functional impairment due to symptoms. Items are scored on a 10-point Likert scale, with higher scores representing greater functional impairment. The SDS does not have recommended cutoff scores, although it has been recommended that scores of five or greater on any individual item should flag clinician's attention (Sheehan et al.). The SDS has strong internal consistency ($\alpha = .89$; Sheehan et al.), and it showed similarly strong internal consistency in the present sample ($\alpha = .89$), as well.

Perception of Teasing Scale (POTS; Thompson, Cattarin, Fowler, & Fisher, 1995)

The POTS assesses recalled frequency of bullying and teasing from ages 5–6. The measure uses a 5-point Likert scale, with lower scores indicating less frequent bullying. There are no recommended cutoff scores for the measure. In the present study, the 6-item appearance-based teasing and bullying subscale was used, and the wording was slightly modified to assess general appearance bullying, rather than weight-based bullying (e.g., changing "People made fun of you because you were heavy" to "People made fun of you because of your appearance"). Prior research has shown that this subscale demonstrates convergent validity with measures of body image anxiety and body dissatisfaction, as well as strong internal consistency ($\alpha = .88$; Thompson et al.). In the present sample, the POTS also had strong internal consistency ($\alpha = .89$).

Results

Aim 1

Means, standard deviations, and intercorrelations for study variables are reported in Table 1. In the present sample, 69 participants (15.9%) scored in the range of elevated body dysmorphic symptoms (16 or greater) on the BDD Y-BOCS. Our first aim was to evaluate the association of appearance-based teasing with body dysmorphic symptom severity and compare this to the association of appearance-based teasing with obsessive-compulsive symptom severity. Consistent with our hypotheses and prior research, self-reported history of childhood appearance-based teasing was positively associated with body dysmorphic symptom

Table 1. Means, standard deviations and intercorrelations for study variables.

	1	2	3	4	5
1. BDD Y-BOCS					
2. OCI-R	.33*				
3. POTS	.33*	.20*			
4. SDS Total	.47*	.37*	.31*		
5. DASS depression	.45*	.40*	.24*	.65*	
Mean	9.72	12.70	11.92	6.22	8.61
SD	6.32	11.13	5.41	7.03	9.56

Note. BDD Y-BOCS = Body Dysmorphic Disorder Yale-Brown Obsessive Compulsive Scale; OCI-R = Obsessive Compulsive Inventory-Revised; POTS = Perception of Teasing Scale; SDS = Sheehan Disability Scale; DASS = Depression Anxiety Stress Scale 21-Item Version.*$p < .001$.

severity, with a medium effect (see Table 1). Also consistent with our hypotheses, the association between appearance-based teasing and obsessive-compulsive symptom severity was less strong (small to medium effect, see Table 1). A statistical comparison of the strengths of these correlations (see Steiger, 1980) indicated that they were significantly different, $t(363)$ = 2.26, $p < .05$.

Aim 2

Our second aim was to examine the roles of appearance-based teasing, body dysmorphic symptom severity, and their interaction as risk factors for functional impairment and depression. Using hierarchical moderated regression, we first regressed our outcome variables (total functional impairment in one regression and depression in a second regression) onto a centered version of appearance-based teasing and a centered body dysmorphic symptom severity variable (step 1), and their interaction (step 2). The overall regression of functional impairment was significant, $F(3, 360) = 44.72$, $p < .001$, $R^2 = .27$. Coefficients are shown in Table 2. Both main effects were significant, with more severe reports of appearance-based teasing and more severe body dysmorphic symptoms both predicting greater functional impairment, with small and medium-to-large effects, respectively. In addition, as hypothesized, the moderation effect was significant, $\delta R^2 = .02$. A simple slope test showed that the positive association between appearance-based teasing and total functional impairment was moderately strong and significant for those with high ($+1$ SD above mean) body dysmorphic symptom severity ($\beta = .28$, $p < .001$), but weak and non-significant for those with low (-1 SD below mean) body dysmorphic symptom severity ($\beta = .04$, $p = .59$) (see Figure 1).

In the hierarchical moderated regression of depression severity, the overall model was again significant, $F(3, 355) = 35.74$, $p < .001$, $R^2 = .23$. Coefficients are again shown in Table 2. Although there was no significant effect of appearance-based teasing on depression, body dysmorphic symptom severity once again predicted significantly greater depression, with a small-to-medium effect. In addition, as hypothesized, body dysmorphic symptom severity again moderated the effect of appearance-based teasing on depression, $\delta R^2 = .02$. The simple slope test demonstrated that the association between appearance-based teasing and depression was small-to-moderate and significantly positive ($\beta = .22$, $p < .001$) for those with high ($+1$ SD above mean) body dysmorphic symptom severity but weak and non-significantly negative ($\beta = -.06$, $p = .41$) for those with low (-1 SD below mean) body

Table 2. Standardized coefficients from regressions of functional impairment and depression onto teasing, body dysmorphic or obsessive compulsive symptom severity, and the interaction of teasing with symptom severity.

	BDD		OCD	
	Functional Impairment	Depression	Functional Impairment	Depression
	β	β	β	β
Appearance-Teasing	.16**	.08	.26***	.19***
BDD/OCD Symptom Severity	.40***	.39***	.33***	.40***
Teasing × BDD/OCD Severity	.13**	.15**	.08	−.04

Note. OCD = obsessive compulsive disorder; BDD = body dysmorphic disorder. *p < .001.

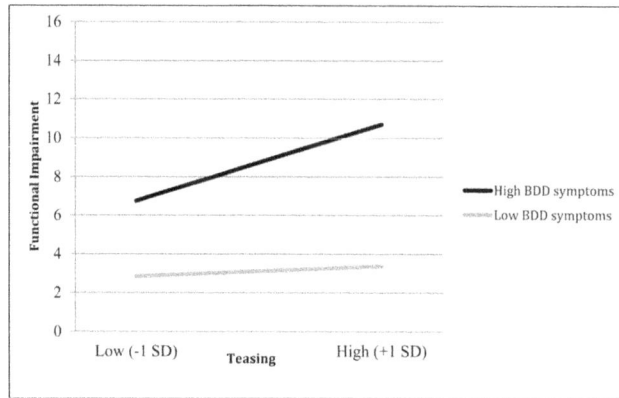

Figure 1. Body dysmorphic symptoms as a moderator of appearance-based teasing on functional impairment.

dysmorphic symptom severity (see Figure 2). Thus, for those with elevated body dysmorphic symptoms, appearance-based teasing predicted greater functional impairment and depression.

Last, to examine the specificity of these interaction effects to body dysmorphic symptoms, we ran a parallel set of hierarchical moderated linear regression analyses, with obsessive-compulsive symptom severity in place of body dysmorphic symptom severity. The overall regression of functional impairment was significant, $F(3, 342) = 33.61$, $p < .001$, $R^2 = .23$. As expected, although both appearance-based teasing and obsessive-compulsive symptom severity significantly predicted functional impairment with moderate effects, obsessive-compulsive symptom severity was not a significant moderator of the association of appearance-based teasing with functional impairment $\delta R^2 = .01$ (see Table 2). As with functional impairment, the overall regression of depression was significant, $F(3, 339) = 28.54$, $p < .001$, $R^2 = .20$. Again, as expected, although both appearance-based teasing and obsessive-compulsive symptom severity significantly predicted depression, with small and medium-to-large effects, respectively, obsessive-compulsive symptom severity was not a significant moderator of the association of appearance-based teasing with depression, $\delta R^2 = .00$. Thus, moderation

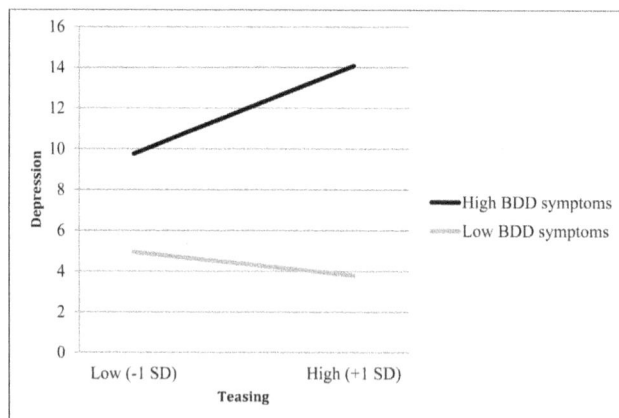

Figure 2. Body dysmorphic symptoms as a moderator of appearance-based teasing on depression.

of the association of appearance-based teasing with negative outcomes was limited to body dysmorphic symptom severity.

Discussion

Given the severity of BDD and its associated outcomes, it is important to focus research attention on identifying potential risk factors to BDD symptoms and associated problems. Clinical models of BDD posit that appearance-based teasing may play an important role in the development of BDD, and in the relationship between BDD and negative outcomes such as functional impairment (i.e., social, occupational, family) and depression. However, to date limited research has studied appearance-based teasing in conjunction with BDD or sub-clinical body dysmorphic symptoms as related to negative outcomes. Moreover, to the best of our knowledge, no research has examined the specificity of appearance-based teasing as a risk factor to poor outcomes in body dysmorphic symptoms, as compared to symptoms of related disorders, such as OCD. Information about the specificity of appearance-based teasing to BDD, in particular, would bolster the theoretical stance that appearance-based teasing is especially important as a risk factor among those with BDD, as opposed to being a risk factor for more generalized psychological distress. Thus, this information would contribute to our current understanding of BDD. The present study aimed to address these issues in a preliminary study to lay the groundwork for potential future investigations in clinical samples.

Consistent with prior research (Boyda & Shevlin, 2011) and our expectations, higher rates of self-reported appearance-based teasing were associated with more severe body dysmorphic symptoms. Moreover, this association was significantly stronger than that between appearance-based teasing and obsessive-compulsive symptom severity. These results contribute preliminary, novel empirical data to the yet unstudied theoretical conceptualization that appearance-based teasing during childhood is a *specific* risk factor for the development of body dysmorphic symptoms (e.g., Feusner et al., 2010), compared to symptoms of other types of psychopathology. These results suggest that future research on this issue in clinical samples is warranted. More specifically, future longitudinal research that follows the influence of appearance-based teasing on body image and BDD symptoms from an early age over time would help address whether such findings are truly reflective of developmental trajectories toward BDD or possibly influenced by recall bias of those with BDD.

Furthermore, only one prior study has tested the theorized link between appearance-based teasing and functional impairment within a sample of individuals with body dysmorphic symptoms, finding that appearance-based teasing accounted for variance in functional impairment within a sample of individuals with symptoms of muscle dysmorphia (Wolke & Sapouna, 2008). Such information can contribute not only to our understanding of risk for negative outcomes among BDD sufferers, but also to our understanding of the negative effects of appearance-based teasing on subsequent mental health problems. Thus, to extend this literature, the present study examined the role of recalled appearance-based teasing as a risk factor for elevated functional impairment and depression associated with body dysmorphic symptoms. Both appearance-based teasing and body dysmorphic symptom severity were associated with worse functional impairment in our sample, and body dysmorphic symptom severity also predicted worse depression among the sample. Moreover, appearance-based teasing was more strongly associated with both functional impairment and depression among those with elevated body dysmorphic symptoms, compared to those with low body dysmorphic symptoms. This suggests that appearance-based teasing may not be an equal risk factor for all individuals. Rather, it may be an especially relevant risk factor to functional impairment and depression for those with elevated concerns about the appearance of their body. Of note, this pattern was specific to symptoms related to bodily appearance concerns, as the same pattern was not obtained when examining obsessive-compulsive symptom severity. It is possible that inflated beliefs regarding the importance of physical appearance that accompany body dysmorphic symptoms lead individuals to be more affected by history of appearance-based teasing during childhood. At the same time, given the cross-sectional nature of our data, it is also possible that elevated body dysmorphic symptoms contribute to enhanced recall of appearance-based teasing and more negative outcomes, potentially inflating their association.

The present findings are consistent with existing, yet highly under-tested, theoretical models of appearance-based teasing as an important social-developmental risk factor for BDD symptoms, specifically (e.g., Feusner et al., 2010). If the findings regarding associations of recalled teasing with functional impairment and depression among those with elevated body dysmorphic symptoms are replicated in clinical samples, they suggest that patients' interpretations of their memories of appearance-based teasing may be an important factor to consider in treatments for BDD and body dissatisfaction. Furthermore, the present findings suggest that organizing efforts to decrease bullying, particularly appearance-focused bullying, among youth could potentially lower the risk for both the development of BDD and body dissatisfaction, as well as the trajectory toward the most severe outcomes among those with BDD. Similarly, developing interventions to target appearance-related beliefs in youth who experience such teasing and bullying may also help prevent the trajectory toward BDD or severe body dissatisfaction and associated outcomes.

As noted, although the present study produces novel information about cognitive-behavioral conceptualizations of an understudied disorder, there are several limitations to consider. First, we used self-reported recall of appearance-based teasing, as opposed to observed experiences of appearance-based teasing or children's reports of current teasing. This method limits our ability to draw causal inferences between actual childhood teasing experience and current body dysmorphic symptoms, functional impairment, and depression. It also allows for the possibility that associations were inflated due to biased recall in those with greater body dysmorphic symptoms. Second, we tested our hypotheses within a non-clinical sample. Therefore, it is not possible to know whether these findings will generalize to the clinical BDD population. Future studies would build on the present study by utilizing clinical samples. However, as body dissatisfaction ranges from mild to severe within the general population, the present sample provides a valid and appropriate first step for capturing the relationship between body dissatisfaction, appearance-based teasing, functional impairment and depression. Third, we used survey methods to capture each study variable, rather than utilizing clinician-administered clinical assessments. Thus, although the present study used well-validated measures of BDD and OCD symptoms, these data provide only a first step at looking at the role of appearance-based teasing within individuals with symptoms of these disorders. Last, our sample was primarily female, prohibiting examination of gender effects.

Notwithstanding these limitations, the present study extends the limited literature on risk factors for body dysmorphic symptoms by examining the specificity of results via comparisons to obsessive-compulsive symptoms. In addition, the present study contributes novel information about appearance-based teasing as a potential malleable risk factor for functional impairment and depression, two severe and costly outcomes that are notably elevated among those with body dissatisfaction and BDD symptoms. Last, the present study is the first to demonstrate an interaction effect, in which appearance-based teasing is a risk factor to functional impairment and depression, *in particular* among those with elevated BDD symptoms, as compared to those with low levels of BDD symptoms. As such, the findings lay the foundation for several avenues of future research on this costly disorder.

References

American Psychiatric Association. (2013). *Diagnostic and statistical manual of mental disorders* (5th ed.). Washington, DC: Author.

Antony, M. M., Bieling, P. J., Cox, B. J., Enns, M. W., & Swinson, R. P. (1998). Psychometric properties of the 42-item and 21-item versions of the Depression Anxiety Stress Scales in clinical groups and a community sample. *Psychological Assessment, 10*, 176–181. doi: 10.1037/1040-3590.10.2.176

Beck, A. T., Rush, A. J., Shaw, B. F., & Emery, G. (1979). *Cognitive therapy of depression: A treatment manual.* New York, NY: Guilford Press.

Boyda, D., & Shevlin, M. (2011). Childhood victimisation as a predictor of muscle dysmorphia in adult male bodybuilders. *The Irish Journal of Psychology, 32*, 105–115. doi: 10.1080/03033910.2011.616289

Brown, T. A., Chorpita, B. F., Korotitsch, W., & Barlow, D. H. (1997). Psychometric properties of the Depression Anxiety Stress Scales (DASS) in clinical samples. *Behaviour Research and Therapy, 35*, 79–89. doi: 10.1016/S0005-7967(96)00068-X

Buhlmann, U., Cook, L. M., Fama, J. M., & Wilhelm, S. (2007). Perceived teasing experiences in body dysmorphic disorder. *Body Image, 4*, 381–385. doi: 10.1016/j.bodyim.2007.06.004

Buhlmann, U., Glaesmer, H., Mewes, R., Fama, J. M., Wilhelm, S., Brähler, E., & Rief, W. (2010). Updates on the prevalence of body dysmorphic disorder: A population-based survey. *Psychiatry Research, 178*, 171–175. doi: 10.1016/j.psychres.2009.05.002

Buhlmann, U., Wilhelm, S., Glaesmer, H., Mewes, R., Brähler, E., & Rief, W. (2011). Perceived appearance-related teasing in body dysmorphic disorder: A population-based survey. *International Journal of Cognitive Therapy, 4*, 342–348. doi: 10.1521/ijct.2011.4.4.342

Chosak, A., Marques, L., Greenberg, J. L., Jenike, E., Dougherty, D. D., & Wilhelm, S. (2008). Body dysmorphic disorder and obsessive compulsive disorder: Similarities, differences and the classification debate. *Expert Review of Neurotherapeutics, 8*, 1209–1218. doi: 10.1586/14737175.8.8.1209

Conroy, M., Menard, W., Fleming-Ives, K., Modha, P., Cerullo, H., & Phillips, K. A. (2008). Prevalence and clinical characteristics of body dysmorphic disorder in an adult inpatient setting. *General Hospital Psychiatry, 30*, 67–72. doi: 10.1016/j.genhosppsych.2007.09.004

Cororve, M. B., & Gleaves, D. H. (2001). Body dysmorphic disorder: A review of conceptualizations, assessment, and treatment strategies. *Clinical Psychology Review, 21*, 949–970. doi: 10.1016/S0272-7358(00)00075-1

Didie, E. R., Menard, W., Stern, A. P., & Phillips, K. A. (2008). Occupational functioning and impairment in adults with body dysmorphic disorder. *Comprehensive Psychiatry, 49*, 561–569. doi: 10.1016/j.comppsych.2008.04.003

Feusner, J.D., Neziroglu, F., Wilhelm, S., Mancusi, L., & Bohon, C. (2010). What causes BDD: Research findings and a proposed model. *Psychiatric Annals, 40,* 349−355. doi: 10.3928/00485713-20100701-08

Foa, E. B., Huppert, J.D., Leiberg, S., Langner, R., Kichic, R., Hajcak, G., & Salkovskis, P.M. (2002). The Obsessive-Complusive Inventory: Development and validation of a short version. *Psychological Assessment, 14,* 485−495. doi: 10.1037/1040-3590.14.4.485

Fontenelle, L. F., Telles, L. L., Nazar, B. P., De Menezes, G. B., Do Nascimento, A. L., Mendlowicz, M. V., & Versiani, M. (2006). A sociodemographic, phenomenological, and long-term follow-up study of patients with body dysmorphic disorder in Brazil. *International Journal of Psychiatry in Medicine, 36,* 243−259. doi: 10.2190/B6XM-HLHQ-7x6C-8GC0

Frare, F., Perugi, G., Ruffolo, G., & Toni, C. (2004). Obsessive-compulsive disorder and body dysmorphic disorder: A comparison of clinical features. *European Psychiatry, 19,* 292−298. doi: 10.1016/j.eurpsy.2004.04.014

Henry, J.D., & Crawford, J. R. (2005). The short-form version of the Depression Anxiety Stress Scales (DASS-21): Construct validity and normative data in a large non-clinical sample. *British Journal of Clinical Psychology, 44,* 227−239. doi: 10.1348/014466505x29657

Hollander, E. (1993). *Obsessive-compulsive related disorders.* Washington, DC: American Psychiatric Press.

Koran, L. M., Abujaoude, E., Large, M. D., & Serpe, R. T. (2008). The prevalence of body dysmorphic disorder in the United States adult population. *CNS Spectrums, 13,* 316−322.

Lovibond, P. F., & Lovibond, S. H. (1995). The structure of negative emotional states: Comparison of the Depression Anxiety Stress Scales (DASS) with the Beck Depression and Anxiety Inventories. *Behaviour Research and Therapy, 33,* 335−343. doi: 10.1016/0005-7967(94)00075-U

Marques, L., LeBlanc, N., Weingarden, H., Greenberg, J. L., Traeger, L., & Wilhelm, S. (2011). Body dysmorphic symptoms: Phenomenology and ethnicity. *Body Image: An International Journal of Research, 8,* 163−167. doi: 10.1016/j.bodyim.2010.12.006

Marques, L., Weingarden, H. M., LeBlanc, N. J., & Wilhelm, S. (2011). Treatment utilization and barriers to treatment engagement among people with body dysmorphic symptoms. *Journal of Psychosomatic Research, 70,* 286−293. doi: 10.1016/j.jpsychores.2010.10.002

Peng, C.Y. J., Harwell, M., Liou, S.-M., & Ehman, L. H. (2006). Advances in missing data methods and implcations for educational research. In S. Sawilowsky (Ed.), *Real data analysis* (pp. 31−78). Greenwich, CT: Information Age.

Perugi, G., Akiskal, H. S., Giannotti, D., Frare, F., Di Vaio, S., & Cassano, G. B. (1997). Gender-related differences in body dysmorphic disorder (dysmorphophobia). *Journal of Nervous and Mental Disease, 185,* 578−582. doi: 10.1097/00005053-199709000-00007

Phillips, K. A. (1996). *The broken mirror: Understanding and treating body dysmorphic disorder.* New York, NY: Oxford University Press.

Phillips, K. A., & Diaz, S. F. (1997). Gender Differences in Body Dysmorphic Disorder. *The Journal of Nervous and Mental Disease, 185,* 570−577. doi: 10.1097/00005053-199709000-00006

Phillips, K. A., Didie, E. R., Menard, W., Pagano, M. E., Fay, C., & Weisberg, R. B. (2006). Clinical features of body dysmorphic disorder in adolescents and adults. *Psychiatry Research, 141,* 305−314. doi: 10.1016/j.psychres.2005.09.014

Phillips, K. A., Gunderson, C. G., Mallya, G., McElroy, S. L., & Carter, W. (1998). A comparison study of body dysmorphic disorder and obsessive-compulsive disorder. *Journal of Clinical Psychiatry, 59,* 568−575. doi: 10.4088/JCP.v59n1102

Phillips, K. A., Hollander, E., Rasmussen, S. A., & Aronowitz, B. R. (1997). A severity rating scale for body dysmorphic disorder: Development, reliability, and validity of a modified version of the Yale-Brown Obsessive Compulsive Scale. *Psychopharmacology Bulletin, 33,* 17−22.

Phillips, K. A., McElroy, S. L., Keck, P. E., Pope, H. G., & Hudson, J. I. (1993). Body dysmorphic disorder: 30 cases of imagined ugliness. *The American Journal of Psychiatry, 150,* 302−308.

Phillips, K. A., Menard, W., Fay, C., & Weisberg, R. (2005). Demographic characteristics, phenomenology, comorbidity, and family history in 200 individuals with body dysmorphic disorder. *Psychosomatics: Journal of Consultation Liaison Psychiatry, 46,* 317−325. doi: 10.1176/appi.psy.46.4.317

Rief, W., Buhlmann, U., Wilhelm, S., Borkenhagen, A., & Brahler, E. (2006). The prevalence of body dysmorphic disorder: A population-based survey. *Psychological Medicine, 36*, 877–885. doi: 10.1017/S0033291706007264

Sheehan, D.V., Harnett-Sheehan, K., & Raj, B. A. (1996). The measurement of disability. *International Clinical Psychopharmacology, 11*, 89–95. doi: 10.1097/00004850-199606003-00015

Steiger, J. H.Tests for comparing elements of a correlation matrix. *Psychological Bulletin, 87*, 245–251. doi: 10.1037/0033-2909.87.2.245

Thompson, J. K., Cattarin, J., Fowler, B., & Fisher, E. (1995). The Perception of Teasing Scale (POTS): A revision and extension of the Physical Appearance Related Teasing Scale (PARTS). *Journal of Personality Assessment, 65*, 146–157. doi: 10.1207/s15327752jpa6501_11

Veale, D., Boocock, A., Gournay, K., & Dryden, W. (1996). Body dysmorphic disorder: A survey of fifty cases. *British Journal of Psychiatry, 169*, 196–201. doi: 10.1192/bjp.169.2.196

Wolke, D., & Sapouna, M. (2008). Big men feeling small: Childhood bullying experience, muscle dysmorphia and other mental health problems in bodybuilders. *Psychology of Sport and Exercise, 9*, 595–604. doi: 10.1016/j.psychsport.2007.10.002

Part III

Coherence, Resilience and Recovery

Resilience and Coping as Predictors of Well-Being in Adults

Teresa Mayordomo, Paz Viguer, Alicia Sales, Encarnación Satorres, and Juan C. Meléndez

ABSTRACT

Well-being is one of the keys to successful and optimal development across the lifespan. Based on the idea that development involves changes in individuals' adaptive capacity to meet their needs over time, the changes that occur in the second half of life require effort to adapt to the new reality. This study used a structural model to test the effects of coping strategies and resilience on well-being in a sample of 305 mid-life adults. Several constructs were measured: coping strategies, resilience, and well-being. A final model was obtained with good fit indices; psychological well-being was positively predicted by resilience and negatively by emotional coping. Moreover, positive reappraisal and avoidance form part of both coping strategies (problem-focused and emotion-focused). Considering the characteristics of the model, educational intervention programs could be developed to promote skills that favor good adaptation at this stage in the life cycle and contribute to promoting successful aging.

Well-being is one of the keys to successful and optimal development across the lifespan. Based on the idea that development involves changes in individuals' adaptive capacity to meet their needs over time, the changes that occur in the second half of life require effort to adapt to the new reality, ultimately leading to changes in psychological well-being (Ryff, 1989). Recently, Ryff (2014) reviewed the scientific advances in psychological well-being. The scientific output in the field of development and aging highlights progression through developmental tasks of adult life is linked to greater well-being, even though aging is accompanied by a decline in purpose in life and personal growth. Well-being changes as individuals negotiate challenging events in adult life, with improvements being related to various psychological processes: social comparisons, flexible self-perceptions, and coping strategies. The present study examines the effects of coping strategies and personal resiliency on psychological well-being (as a psychological outcome) in adults, but first we briefly review the literature on psychological well-being, coping strategies and well-being, and personal resiliency and well-being.

Based on the eudaimonic approach, Ryff and Keyes (1995) defined psychological well-being as an effort to grow and fulfill one's potential. Its development is related to having a purpose in life, giving life meaning, facing challenges and making an effort to overcome them, and achieving worthwhile goals through adaptation processes. These authors conceptualized well-being as having six dimensions: self-acceptance (having an accurate perception of one's actions, motivations, and feelings), positive relations with others (mutual trust and empathy), autonomy (ability to maintain independence and individuality in different contexts and resist social pressure), environmental mastery (ability to choose or create environments that allow goals and needs to be met), purpose in life (setting goals and defining objectives to give life direction), and personal growth (dedication to realizing one's potential and to continued growth).

Based on confirmatory factorial analysis, some authors have indicated that the six-dimension model has the best fit (Ryff, 1989; Springer & Hauser, 2006). However, Ryff and Keyes (1995) suggest that a model of second-order factors with four dimensions: self-acceptance, environmental mastery, personal growth, and purpose in life, explains well-being better. However, autonomy and positive relations with others work independently.

According to the existing research, there are other well-known antecedents of well-being, such as emotions, physical health, social class, personality traits, and social support (Ryan & Deci, 2001). One construct that can influence well-being is coping, which emerges as a key factor in adaptation, can influence the appraisal of one's situation, and enables the individual to adequately deal with demands (Boerner, 2004; Boerner & Wang, 2012).

Coping is an important building block in the adult personality and fundamental to adults' social-emotional functioning (Carver & Connor-Smith, 2010). Thus, coping plays a critical role in the way an individual deals with the day-to-day challenges of adult life and in long-term developmental outcomes. Coping strategies tend to be viewed as conscious, intentional, and mostly adaptive (Cramer, 2008).

Following the Lazarus and Folkman (1984) model, coping is defined as constantly changing cognitive and behavioral efforts to manage specific external and/or internal situations thought to exceed or overwhelm the individual's resources, thus helping to achieve well-being. In this model, there are two types of coping, problem- and emotion-focused coping. Problem-focused coping or active coping has the purpose of managing or modifying the problem causing the discomfort, whereas emotion-focused coping or passive coping uses methods that regulate the emotional response to the problem. Each type of coping consists of different adaptive strategies that will be used as required by life situations. One is not better than the other, but just more adaptive at that moment.

Coping has traditionally been conceptualized as something one can do in stressful situations, but recently coping has been seen as having other positive functions. The idea that coping can have a positive use coincides with research highlighting the role of positive beliefs in health promotion (Taylor, Kemeny, Reed, Bower, & Gruenewald, 2000). It has been widely recognized that adapting to change is important in achieving or maintaining well-being. Regarding this idea, authors such as Almássy, Pék, Papp and Greenglass (2014) and Greenglass and Fiksenbaum (2009) have pointed out that coping, and specifically proactive coping, can predict positive outcomes that are important in promoting health and well-being. Because many sources of stress cannot be controlled, effective coping often includes anything that helps the individual to tolerate, minimize, accept, or even ignore the situation.

Another term related to adapting to changes and reaching goals is resilience. Although there is a lack of agreement about its definition, there is consensus in assuming that it means competence or positive and effective coping in response to risk or adversity. Luthar, Crossman and Small (2015) define resilience as a phenomenon characterized by positive outcomes in spite of threats to adaptation or development, where people can emerge even stronger from the situation, improving their coping strategies and improving adaptation and well-being.

Cultivating positive emotions may be particularly useful in building resilience because positive emotions can contribute to resilient individuals' ability to psychologically recover from negative emotional arousal (Tugade & Fredrickson, 2004). Positive emotions can momentarily broaden a person's scope of thinking and facilitate flexible attention, which in turn can improve his or her well-being (Fredrickson, 2001, 2004). For other authors, such as Leipold and Greve (2009), individual stability under significantly adverse conditions stems from coping processes influenced by situational and personal conditions. Through personal resilience, an individual recovers from or avoids negative outcomes of burdensome conditions. A study by Calhoun and Tedeschi (2006), conducted with individuals who faced adverse circumstances, identified changes in variables such as perception of self, philosophy of life, and the scale of values, as well as the strengthening of personal relationships, with these changes being related to well-being.

Thus, following the approaches found in the literature, a relationship between coping, resilience, and psychological well-being can be established. These first two concepts (coping and resilience) help people to adapt to changes or unfavorable situations that occur throughout the life cycle and, therefore, to achieve psychological well-being. People can make use of coping strategies and resilience to perceive their own resources and strengths, thus facilitating the management of contexts where they carry out their day to day lives, establishing new objectives and goals and possible ways to achieve them.

Based on the literature, the aim of this study is to test the effects of coping strategies and personal resiliency on well-being (as an outcome or dependent variable) in a sample of adults, using a structural model with latent variables. The results can provide valuable information about the most adaptive strategies in this period of life. The following study hypotheses are proposed:

Hypothesis 1: Coping strategies are interrelated.

Hypothesis 2: Resilience will be related to the dimensions of psychological well-being and coping strategies.

Hypothesis 3: The dimensions that make up psychological well-being will be related.

Hypothesis 4: The factor structures of the model's components will obtain reliability measured by Cronbach's alpha.

Hypothesis 5: The coping dimensions (problem and emotion coping) will be interrelated.

Hypothesis 6: The coping dimensions predict resilience, positively in the case of problem-focused coping, and negatively in the case of emotion-focused coping.

Hypothesis 7: Resilience positively predicts psychological well-being.

Hypothesis 8: Emotion-focused coping negatively predicts psychological well-being.

Methods

Participants

A convenience sample was used that included 305 Spanish adults between 35 and 64 years old, with an average age of 49.05 (DT = 7.01). Their participation was voluntary and anonymous. They were recruited from civic and social centers that adults attend voluntarily. All the participants were informed about the study protocols and signed informed consent

Table 1. Demographic Data ($N = 305$).

Age	49.05 ($SD = 7.01$)
Gender	
Man	38.7
Women	61.3
Marital status	
Married	84.2
Single	12.1
Widow	3.6
Educational level	
Under primary	2.7
Primary	29.6
Secondary	29.9
University	37.9
Living	
With family members	4.9
In a rented house	10.6
In their own house	84.4
Income	
Less than 600 euros	11.0
601–1000	22.7
1001–1500	34.0
More than 1500	32.3

forms to participate in the study. All the procedures followed the tenets of the Declaration of Helsinki and were approved by the Ethics Committee of the University of Valencia. Table 1 shows the main socio-demographic data for the sample.

Instruments

Participants completed three psychological scales and some socio-demographic indicators. First, we applied the Brief Resilient Coping Scale, created by Sinclair and Wallston (2004) and adapted to Spanish through Confirmatory Factor Analysis (Tomás, Meléndez, Sancho, & Mayordomo, 2012). The results show that the scale has a good factor structure and shows satisfactory reliability and acceptable criterion-related validity. This measure, designed to assess the tendency to cope with stress in a highly adaptive way, has shown adequate levels of reliability and validity. According to Sinclair and Wallston (2004), a single resilient coping factor emerges from the four indicators of the BRCS. The BRCS has 4 items with Likert-type response options ranging from 1 to 5, where 1 means the statement does not describe you at all and 5 means it describes you very well.

The Coping Strategies Questionnaire (*Cuestionario de Afrontamiento al Estrés*) is a self-report measure of general coping made up of 42 items with graduated, Likert-type response options ranging from never (0) to almost always (4). It is designed to assess seven basic coping styles: (1) problem-solving coping, (2) negative self-focused coping, (3) positive reappraisal, (4) overt emotional expression, (5) avoidance coping, (6) seeking social support, and (7) religious coping. The questionnaire was developed and validated in Spain by Sandín and Chorot (2003). Tomás, Sancho, and Meléndez (2013) estimated a confirmatory factor analysis for these seven coping dimensions to test a two-factor solution of problem- and emotion-focused coping. Problem-focused coping included problem-solving coping, positive reappraisal, and seeking social support. Emotion-focused coping included negative self-focused coping, overt emotional expression, avoidance coping, religious coping, and social support seeking. In addition, the homogeneity of the items was adequate, and the alphas of the dimensions obtained values between 0.98 (religion) and 0.65 (positive reappraisal).

Last, Ryff's psychological well-being scales were applied. These scales conceptualize and measure well-being with six dimensions: self-acceptance, positive relations with others, autonomy, environmental mastery, purpose in life, and personal growth; all of the items were scored from 1 (totally disagree) to 6 (totally agree). There are several versions available, depending on the number of items. All the versions have been extensively validated in their original English versions (for example, Ryff, 1989; Ryff & Keyes, 1995). Also the scale has been adapted and validated in Spain (for example, Tomás, Meléndez & Navarro, 2008; Tomas, Meléndez, Oliver, Navarro & Zaragoza, 2010). Meléndez, Tomás, Oliver, and Navarro (2009) obtain the following alphas: autonomy ($\alpha = 0.78$); environmental mastery ($\alpha = 0.78$); personal growth ($\alpha = 0.76$); positive relations with others ($\alpha = 0.83$); self-acceptance ($\alpha = 0.78$); and purpose in life ($\alpha = 0.75$). In the present study, the 29-item version was used (Díaz et al., 2006).

Analysis

The statistical analyses included a structural equation model (SEMs) to test the effects among the constructs, estimated in the EQS 6.0. The plausibility of any CFA and SEM model is assessed by using several fit criteria (Hu & Bentler, 1999). Given that the sample size greatly influences the decision to accept or reject a model based on statistical grounds, a number of fit criteria have emerged to assess the structural model. The following criteria were used: (a) the chi-square statistic; (b) a comparative fit index (CFI) above 0.90 (and, ideally, greater than 0.95); (c) a root mean squared error of approximation (RMSEA) of 0.08 or less; (d) the GFI and AGFI as measures of proportion of variance or covariance explained by the model, with values above 0.90 indicating adequate fit; and (e) standardized root mean squared residuals (SRMRs) of 0.08 or less.

Results

Before explaining the results obtained in the structural model, correlations between the components of the model and their alphas will be presented (see Table 2).

As Table 2 shows, the results obtained respond to the first four hypotheses. Hypothesis 1 is not supported because some of the coping strategies are not related to the others; namely, PR and SSS are not related to NSF, and PSF is not related to any of the emotion-focused strategies, except NSF. Hypothesis 2 is not fully supported because resilience is significantly related to all the dimensions of well-being, but not to all the coping strategies. Hypotheses 3 and 4 are fully supported; all the dimensions of well-being are interrelated, and all the alphas obtained are above .600.

Hypotheses 4, 5, 6, 7, and 8 were analyzed through structural equation modelling. The model was estimated using techniques for latent variables to test the relationships between factors without measurement errors.

Initially, a theoretical measurement model with four latent constructs is proposed: problem-focused coping (problem-solving coping, positive reappraisal, and seeking social support); emotion-focused coping (negative self-focused coping, excessive emotional expression, avoidance coping, religious coping, and social support seeking); resilience; and

Table 2. Correlations Between the Components of the Model and Its Alphas (N = 305).

	SA	PRO	AUT	EM	PG	PL	PSF	PR	SSS	NSF	OEE	AVD	RLG	BRCS
SA	.788													
PRO	.271(**)	.757												
AUT	.347(**)	.266(**)	.796											
EM	.483(**)	.397(**)	.464(**)	.647										
PG	.476(**)	.274(**)	.303(**)	.423(**)	.621									
PL	.668(**)	.258(**)	.272(**)	.526(**)	.515(**)	.755								
PSF	.340(**)	.135(*)	.195(**)	.302(**)	.301(**)	.467(**)	.754							
PR	.229(**)	.125(*)	.062	.245(*)	.312(*)	.322(*)	.360(**)	.692						
SSS	.025	.137(*)	-.077	.001	.015	.096	.245(**)	.265(**)	.879					
NSF	-.318(**)	-.260(**)	-.220(**)	-.329(**)	-.270(**)	-.239(**)	-.290(**)	.022	.067	.666				
OEE	-.241(**)	-.122(*)	-.160(**)	-.113(*)	-.085	-.115(*)	-.076	.183(**)	.212(**)	.410(**)	.739			
AVD	.001	-.056	-.132(*)	-.025	.003	.079	-.065	.185(**)	.297(**)	.278(**)	.318(**)	.778		
RLG	-.051	-.046	-.236(**)	-.044	-.099	.025	.029	.202(**)	.193(**)	.231(**)	.153(**)	.244(**)	.923	
BRCS	.503(**)	.156(*)	.218(**)	.330(**)	.422(**)	.517(*)	.470(**)	.076	.397(**)	-.266(*)	-.129(*)	.123(*)	.071	.708

Note. SA = self-acceptance; PRO = positive relations with others; AUT = autonomy; EM = environmental mastery; PG = personal growth; PL = purpose in life. PSF = problem-solving focus; PR = positive reappraisal; SSS = social support seeking; NSF = negative self-focus; OEE = overt emotional expression; AVD = avoidance; RLG = religion; BRCS = Brief Resilient Coping Scale. Values along the diagonal are alpha coefficients.

*Correlation is significant at the 0.05 level.

**Correlation is significant at the 0.01 level.

psychological well-being (self-acceptance, positive relations with others, autonomy, environmental mastery, personal growth, and purpose in life). An examination of the measurement model would determine whether the observed variables actually measured their respective latent constructs. Obtaining appropriate indexes in this initial and preliminary estimation of the structural model would justify the conceptual relationship between the dimensions.

Thus, the measurement model is computed assuming that each observed variable significantly contributed to its respective latent variable and assuming the existence of significant covariance between each pair of latent constructs. Initially, the indices obtained did not show adequate fit $(c^2(g.l. = 70) = 218.93, p > .001$; CFI $= .845$, RMSEA $= .084$ (90% $=$ CI $= .071, .096$)). The analysis of the results suggests making modifications to the psychological well-being scale, that is, the removal of two dimensions, relationships with others and autonomy; it also suggests including avoidance in problem-focused coping. As indicated in the introduction, these modifications are consistent with the literature, as other authors (Ryff & Keyes, 1995; Springer & Hauser, 2006) found a second-order factor underlying the four dimensions, along with two other independent factors, autonomy and positive relations with others. Avoidance loads on both types of coping, which may be due to the fact that certain sources of stress cannot be controlled and are best ignored.

The proposed modifications were made, and indexes were obtained with optimal fit c^2 (g.l. $= 46$) $= 118.06, p > .001$; in addition, Comparative Fit Indices for this model showed scores within the accepted parameters (CFI $= .910$, RMSEA $= .070$ (90% $=$ CI $= .054$, .086). Each of the observed variables contributes significantly to its respective latent construct with values for $t > 2.56$.

Also, the composite index of each latent variable's reliability was calculated; this statistic is analogous to Cronbach's alpha and estimates the internal consistency of responses. The coefficients, problem-focused coping (0.72), emotion-focused coping (0.70), and psychological well-being (0.82), were within accepted parameters, equal to or above .70. In other words, clusters of observed variables under their respective latent constructs appear to be related. This result supports the delimitation of the constructs as hypothesized.

Given the existence of common dimensions for the latent constructs, the discriminant validity of these constructs was examined to determine whether the dimensions measure different phenomena. First, the chi-square differences test was applied; in this test, the statistical value must exceed the critical value of the chi-square for that level of degrees of freedom. The results obtained when comparing the two models $(Dc^2(Dgl = 1) = 64.12)$ show that the difference is greater than the critical value for any level of significance, confirming the discriminant validity of the two latent constructs. Also, confidence interval tests were performed to evaluate discriminant validity. This involves the calculation of confidence intervals for the covariance of $\pm$ two standard errors around the estimate resulting from the CFA; when the confidence intervals do not include the value 1.0, discriminant validity can be confirmed. This condition was observed for problem-focused coping vs. Emotion-focused coping (0.004 $\pm 0.041 = -0.080 - 0.086$).

As shown, the goodness of fit indices and discriminant validity supported the feasibility of measuring the structural model. The resulting model, consistent with the initial hypotheses (6 and 7), showed suitable fit indices with correct parameters $(c^2(g.l. = 46) = 119.93, p > .001$; CFI $= .910$, RMSEA $= .063$ (90% $=$ CI $= .047, .079$)).

Figure 1 shows the two dimensions of coping, problem-focused and emotion-focused. Regarding the composition of these two dimensions, the analysis indicated that SSS and

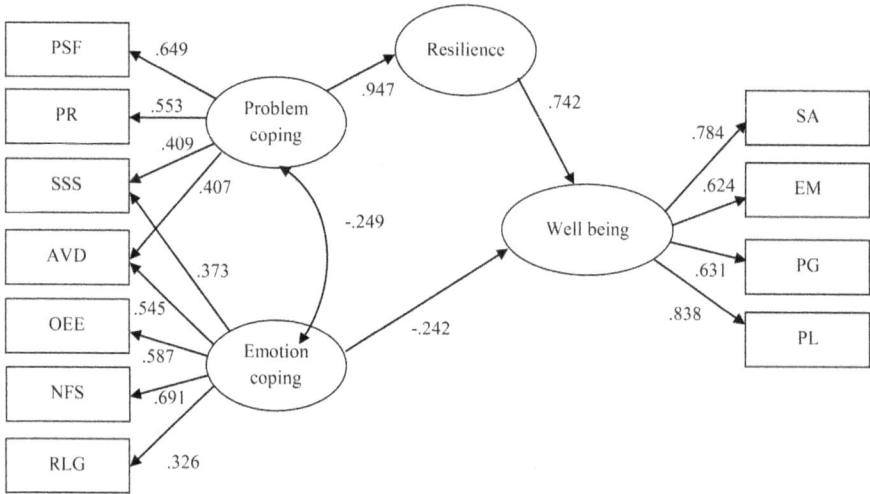

Figure 1. Final Structural Equation Model Predicting Well-being in adults (*N* = 305). *Note.* PSF = problem-solving focus; PR = positive reappraisal; SSS = seeking social support; AVD = avoidance; OEE = overt emotional expression; NSF = negative self-focus; RLG = religion. SA = self-acceptance; EM = environmental mastery; PG = personal growth; PL = purpose in life.

AVD should form part of both dimensions. In addition, these two types of strategies are interrelated negatively, confirming Hypothesis 5.

The next part of the model shows that problem-focused coping positively predicts resilience, whereas the predictive power of emotion-focused coping is not as significant as indicated in the initial model. These results keep us from completely confirming Hypothesis 6. Last, resilience positively predicts psychological well-being, which in turn is negatively predicted by emotion-focused coping, confirming Hypotheses 7 and 8.

Discussion

Adaptation is fundamental throughout the lifespan, and coping strategies and resilience are known to play an important role in attaining this adaptation and, hence, in achieving psychological well-being. This study examined a structural equation model of the relationships among coping strategies, resilience, and well-being in adults. The results provide evidence for the prediction of psychological well-being through a confirmatory model, showing the impact of coping and resilience on psychological well-being. The findings show that problem-focused coping positively predicts resilience, and resilience positively predicts psychological well-being to a large extent, whereas emotion-focused coping negatively predicts it. These results are similar to those from other studies in the Spanish population (Tomás, Sancho, Meléndez, & Mayordomo, 2012; Mayordomo, Meléndez, Viguer, & Sales, 2015). Moreover, the results show that Hypotheses 1, 2, and 6 are not supported, whereas the other hypotheses are.

The final model shows two coping dimensions: problem-focused coping and emotion-focused coping, as proposed by Lazarus and Folkman (1984), which are negatively and moderately correlated. With regard to emotion-focused coping, which uses methods that regulate the emotional response to the problem, these strategies are launched when the problem cannot be solved and the subject is trying to alleviate or mitigate emotional pain. Some of these strategies have a negative nature, which has led to them being considered maladaptive at times. All the coping strategies loaded on the hypothesized second-order factors; however, there were exceptions because seeking social support and avoidance loaded on both coping factors, and this structure was the best one, as the data analysis indicated.

Regarding seeking social support, considering that we define this strategy as support from others to change the stressful situation or feel comfort, this strategy loads on both coping factors, which is quite logical because it can be used to solve a problem (seek advice from someone) or to find emotion relief from a situation with which one does not know how to cope, and these results have been found in several studies (Lazarus & Folkman, 1984).

Avoidance loads on both types of coping, possibly because certain sources of stress cannot be controlled and are best ignored. In this regard, some authors suggest that, through development, people acquire greater skill with emotion-focused strategies (Carver & Connor-Smith, 2010). With age there may be a tendency to react to a stressful situation by stepping back and avoiding rushing into making a decision, focusing more on the problem than on themselves. Thus, using an avoidance strategy can be beneficial because, while avoiding a situation, older people think more and know their own emotions better than in youth, and they produce better and more appropriate strategies to effectively respond to conflictive situations. The use of this strategy for a short time is adaptive, but continuing it for a long time could produce rumination, which impairs the adaptive process (Michl, McLaughlin, Shepherd, and Nolen-Hoeksema, 2013).

With regard to the prediction of resilience, as noted in the final model, this construct is explained largely by the problem-focused strategies, as Hypothesis 6 proposed. Sinclair and Wallston (2004) pointed out that this measure describes an effective, active, problem-solving coping pattern that reflects resilient coping patterns. As noted, emotion-focused coping did not predict this resilience measure. In this regard, it should be noted that the emotions that enhance resilience are positive emotions, not negative as would be those that make up the emotion-focused coping (negative self-focused coping, for example). According to some authors (Fredrickson, Tugade, Waugh, & Larkin, 2003; Ong, Bergeman, Bisconti, & Wallace, 2006), a lot of positive emotions can enhance high levels of resilience, leading indirectly to the preparation of the individual to cope successfully difficulties and future adversities (Fredrickson, 2001). Also, in the dispositional resilience pattern proposed by Polk (1997) it is mentioned that some factors related to the ego positively and the sense of mastery and positive self-esteem (Wagnild & Young, 1993) encourage this pattern of resilience, while negative emotions or no emotional control can result in maladaptive to a stressful or adverse situation.

Last, in the case of psychological well-being, it is positively predicted by resilience, which in turn is predicted by problem-focused coping, as indicated by Hypothesis 7. With regard to resilience, it should be noted that in a study conducted in a young population (17–27 years), results indicated that people with greater resilience had greater life satisfaction (Limonero, Tomás-Sábado, Fernández-Castro, Gómez-Romero, & Ardilla-Herrero, 2012). Moreover, some research shows that active problem-focused coping is strongly linked to well-being outcomes (Carver & Connor-Smith, 2010). Furthermore, maintaining or returning to a balanced mood state is adaptive, contributing to positive outcomes in terms of physical health and well-being. This result is consistent with the recent study by Smith, Saklofske, Keefer, and Tremblay (2015). In addition, as proposed in hypothesis 8, well-being is negatively predicted by emotion-focused coping, which makes us think that the use of emotion-focused strategies plays a slightly beneficial role in the psychological well-being of adults, being these results similar to those obtained by Mayordomo et al. (2015) who in a sample of young obtained a negative prediction of emotion-focused coping to psychological well-being. With regard to the wellness dimensions, a good fit is obtained when considering the four dimensions of well-being (self-acceptance, environmental mastery, personal growth, and purpose in life), and these results are consistent with other studies that indicate the importance of this dimension (Springer & Hauser, 2006).

This study has shown what kind of strategies encourages the improvement or maintenance of psychological well-being and, therefore, life satisfaction. In addition, it also noted that the use of emotional strategies has a negative effect on the mental health of adults because these strategies can lead to the development of emotional disorders such as anxiety or depression. Other studies (Tugade, Fredrickson, & Feldman Barrett, 2004; Tugade & Fredrickson, 2004) have shown that positive emotions contribute to psychological and physical well-being, not negative emotions. Specifically, Tugade and Fredrickson (2004) indicate that the experience of positive emotions contributes, in part, to the ability of participants to achieve the regulation of emotions finding positive meaning in negative circumstances, which leads us to believe that these results should be noted when developing intervention programs to improve psychological well-being in adults.

To conclude, we would mention some shortcomings of this study, as well as directions for future research. The main limitation is that the model was tested in a convenience sample of adults and may not be generalizable to other populations. Moreover, the design is cross-sectional, which always limits our ability to draw causal conclusions from the data.

A future direction for research would be to join two literatures: the literature on coping, resilience, and well-being and the literature on personality development and well-being. Based on major adult developmental theories and empirical evidence showing a relationship among coping, resilience and well-being, we included both personality and adaptation variables in our examination of the paths to adults' well-being in middle adulthood. Given that theories of adult development suggest that personality development is a source of well-being, our aim would be to provide empirical support for the influence of Erikson's developmental tasks, such as generativity and integrity, on well-being.

Another possible line of research would be to study the effects of positive emotions in stressful events that participants have faced in the past year. Also it would be interesting to distinguish between types of events and how they affect mental health and psychological well-being.

Last, given the importance of adaptation at any stage in the life cycle, and specifically in adulthood, it is crucial to develop traits that encourage good adjustment to change and to adverse situations. Moreover, in order to prepare for the potential of the second half of life, it appears useful to shift to optimizing coping and resilience traits. Thus, we can contribute to promoting successful aging by encouraging people to invest in their future by focusing on personal growth and taking advantage of life in middle adulthood. The development of socio-educational programs for adults seems promising. Therefore, we propose the development of a brief intervention program that provides training in coping and resilience strategies.

Programs of this type should aim to promote the use of problem-focused coping strategies, as they play an important role in the development of resilience and well-being. Also they must make known, through psychoeducational sessions, what the emotional strategies are, and that their prolonged use can have a negative effect on quality of life, but their controlled use can help to develop psychological well-being and life satisfaction. Also programs should take into account the development of the perception of the resources that people already have to deal with their daily lives, while teaching them new resources with benefits in terms of adaptation and well-being.

References

Almássy, Z., Pék, G., Papp, G., & Greenglass, E. R. (2014). The psychometric properties of the Hungarian version of the Proactive Coping Inventory: Reliability, construct validity and factor structure. *International Journal of Psychology and Psychological Therapy, 14*, 115–124.

Boerner, K. (2004). Adaptation to disability among middle-aged and older adults: The role of assimilative and accommodative coping. *The Journals of Gerontology Series B: Psychological Sciences and Social Sciences, 59*, 35–42. doi:10.1093/geronb/59.1.P35

Boerner, K., & Wang, S. (2012). Targets for rehabilitation: An evidence base for adaptive coping with visual disability. *Rehabilitation Psychology, 57*, 320–327. doi:10.1037/a0030787

Calhoun, L. G., & Tedeschi, R. G. (2006). *The handbook of posttraumatic growth: Research and practice.* New York, NY: Lawrence Erlbaum.

Carver, C. S., & Connor-Smith, J. (2010). Personality and coping. *Annual Review of Psychology, 61*, 679–704. doi:10.1146/annurev.psych.093008.100352

Cramer, P. (2008). Seven pillars of defense mechanism theory. *Social and Personality Psychology Compass, 2*, 1963–1981. doi:10.1111/j.1751-9004.2008.00135.

Díaz, D., Rodriguez-Carvajal, R., Blanco, A., Moreno-Jimenez, B., Gallardo, I., Valle, C., & van Dierendonck, D. (2006). Spanish adaptation of the Psychological Well-Being Scales (PWBS). *Psicothema, 18*, 572–577.

Fredrickson, B. L. (2001). The role of positive emotions in positive psychology: The broaden-and-build theory of positive emotions. *The American Psychologist, 56*, 218–226.

Fredrickson, B. L. (2004). The broaden-and-build theory of positive emotions. *Philosophical Transactions of the Royal Society B: Biological Sciences, 359*, 1367–1378. doi:10.1098/rstb.2004.1512

Fredrickson, B. L., Tugade, M. M., Waugh, C. E., & Larkin, G. R. (2003). What good are positive emotions in crisis? A prospective study of resilience and emotions following the terrorist attacks on the United States on September 11th, 2001. *Journal of Personality and Social Psychology, 84*, 365–376.

Greenglass, E. R., & Fiksenbaum, L. (2009). Proactive coping, positive affect, and well-being. *European Psychologist, 14*, 29–39. doi:10.1027/1016-9040.14.1.29

Hu, L. T., & Bentler, P. (1999). Cutoff criteria for fit indexes in covariance structure analysis: Conventional criteria versus new alternatives. *Structural Equation Modeling: A Multidisciplinary Journal, 6*(1), 1–55.

Lazarus, R. S., & Folkman, S. (1984). *Stress appraisal and coping.* New York, NY: Springer.

Leipold, B., & Greve, W. (2009). Resilience: A conceptual bridge between coping and development, *European Psychologist, 14*(1), 40–50.

Limonero, J. T., Tomás-Sábado, J., Fernández-Castro, J., Gómez-Romero, M. J. Y., & Ardilla-Herrero, A. (2012). Coping strategies and emotional resilience regulation: Predictors of life satisfaction. *Behavioral Psychology/Psicología Conductual, 20*, 183–196.

Luthar, S. S., Crossman, E. J., & Small, P. J. (2015). Resilience and adversity. In R. Lerner (Ed), *Handbook of child psychology and developmental science.* (Vol. 3, pp. 247–386). New York, NY: Wiley.

Mayordomo, T., Meléndez, J. C., Viguer, P., & Sales, A. (2015). Coping strategies as predictors of well-being in youth adult. *Social Indicators Research, 122*, 479–489. doi:10.1007/s11205-014-0689-4

Meléndez, J. C., Tomás, J. M., Oliver, A., & Navarro, E. (2009). Psychological and physical dimensions explaining life satisfaction among the elderly: A structural model examination. *Archives of Gerontology & Geriatrics, 48*, 291–295. doi:10.1016/j.archger.2008.02.008

Michl, L. C., McLaughlin, K. A., Shepherd, K., & Nolen-Hoeksema, S. (2013). Rumination as a mechanism linking stressful life events to symptoms of depression and anxiety: Longitudinal evidence in early adolescents and adults. *Journal of Abnormal Psychology, 122*, 339–352. doi:10.1037/a0031994

Ong, A. D., Bergeman, C. S., Bisconti, T. L., & Wallace, K. A. (2006). Psychological resilience, positive emotions, and successful adaptation to stress in later life. *Journal of Personal and Social Psychology, 91*, 730–749. doi:10.1037/0022-3514.91.4.730

Polk, L. V. (1997). Toward a middle-range theory of resilience. *Advances in Nursing Science, 19*, 1–13.

Ryan, R. M., & Deci, E. L. (2001). On happiness and human potentials: A review of research on hedonic and eudaimonic well-being. *Annual Review of Psychology, 52*, 141–166. doi:10.1146/annurev.psych.52.1.141

Ryff, C. D. (1989). Happiness is everything, or is it? Explorations on the meaning of psychological well-being. *Journal of Personality and Social Psychology, 57*, 1069–1081. doi:10.1037/0022-3514.69.4.719

Ryff, C. D. (2014). Psychological well-being revisited: Advances in science and practice. *Psychotherapy and Psychosomatics, 83*, 10–28. doi:10.1159/000353263

Ryff, C. D., & Keyes, C. L. M. (1995). The structure of psychological well-being revisited. *Journal of Personality and Social Psychology, 69*, 719–727. doi:10.1037/0022-3514.69.4.719

Sandín, B., & Chorot, P. (2003). Cuestionario de Afrontamiento del Estrés (CAE): Desarrollo y validación preliminar. [The Coping Strategies Questionnaire: Development and preliminary valdation]. *Revista de Psicopatología y Psicología Clínica, 8*, 39–54. doi:10.5944/rppc.vol.8.num.1.2003.3941

Sinclair, V. G., & Wallston, K. A. (2004). The development and psychometric evaluation of the Brief Resilient Coping Scale. *Assessment, 11*, 94–101. doi:10.1177/1073191103258144

Smith, M. M., Saklofske, D. H., Keefer, K. V., & Tremblay, P. F. (2015). Coping strategies and psychological outcomes: The moderating effects of personal resiliency, *The Journal of Psychology: Interdisciplinary and Applied, 150*, 318–332. doi:10.1080/00223980.2015.1036828

Springer, K. W., & Hauser, R. M. (2006). An assessment of the construct validity of Ryff's scales of psychological wellbeing: Method, mode and measurement effects. *Social Science Research, 35*, 1080–1102. doi:10.1016/j.ssresearch.2005.07.004

Taylor, S. E., Kemeny, M. E., Reed, G. M., Bower, J. E., & Gruenewald, T. L. (2000). Psychological resources, positive illusions, and health. *American Psychologist, 55*, 99–109. doi:10.1037/0003-066X.55.1.99

Tomás, J. M., Meléndez, J. C., & Navarro, E. (2008). Modelos factoriales confirmatorios de las escalas de Ryff en una muestra de personas mayores. [Factorial confirmatory models of Ryff's scales in a sample of elderly people]. *Psicothema, 20*, 298–304.

Tomás, J. M., Meléndez, J. C., Oliver, A., Navarro, E., & Zaragoza, G. (2010). Method effects in Ryff's scales: A study in an elderly population. *Psicológica, 31*, 383–400.

Tomás, J. M., Meléndez, J. C., Sancho, P., & Mayordomo, T. (2012). Adaptation and initial validation of the BRCS in an Elderly Spanish sample. *European Journal of Psychological Assessment, 28*, 283–289. doi:10.1027/1015-5759/a000108

Tomás, J. M., Sancho, P., & Meléndez, J. C. (2013). Validación del cuestionario de afrontamiento del estres (CAE) para su uso en población mayor española. *Psicología Conductual, 21*, 103–122.

Tomás, J. M., Sancho, P., Meléndez, J. C., & Mayordomo, T. (2012). Resilience and coping as predictors of general well-being in the elderly: A structural equation modeling approach. *Aging & Mental Health, 16*, 317–326. doi:10.1080/13607863.2011.615737

Tugade, M. M., & Fredrickson, B. L. (2004). Resilient individuals use positive emotions to bounce back from negative emotional experiences. *Journal of Personality & Social Psychology, 86*, 320–333. doi:10.1037/0022-3514.86.2.320

Tugade, M. M., Fredrickson, B. L., & Feldman Barrett, L. (2004). Psychological resilience and positive emotional granularity: Examining the benefits of positive emotions on coping and health. *Journal of Personality, 72*, 1161–1190. doi:10.1111/j.1467-6494.2004.00294.x

Wagnild, G. M., & Young, H. M. (1993). Development and psychometric evaluation of the resilience scale. *Journal of Nursing Measurement, 1*, 165–178.

Loneliness and Suicidal Risk in Young Adults: Does Believing in a Changeable Future Help Minimize Suicidal Risk Among the Lonely?

Edward C. Chang, Liangqiu Wan, Pengzi Li, Yuncheng Guo, Jiaying He, Yu Gu, Yingjie Wang, Xiaoqing Li, Zhan Zhang, Yingrui Sun, Casey N.-H. Batterbee, Olivia D. Chang, Abigael G. Lucas, and Jameson K. Hirsch

ABSTRACT
This study examined loneliness and future orientation as predictors of suicidal risk, namely, depressive symptoms and suicide ideation, in a sample of 228 college students (54 males and 174 females). Results of regression analyses indicated that loneliness was a significant predictor of both indices of suicidal risk. The inclusion of future orientation was found to significantly augment the prediction model of both depressive symptoms and suicide ideation, even after accounting for loneliness. Noteworthy, beyond loneliness and future orientation, the Loneliness × Future Orientation interaction term was found to further augment both prediction models of suicidal risk. Consistent with the notion that future orientation is an important buffer of suicidal risk, among lonely students, those with high future orientation, compared to low future orientation, were found to report significantly lower levels of depressive symptoms and suicide ideation. Some implications of the present findings for studying both risk and protective factors associated with suicidal risk in young adults are discussed.

Mental health concerns are a serious and growing problem in adult populations around the world (World Health Organization [WHO], 2013), including in young adult populations (e.g., college students; Zivin, Eisenberg, Gollust, & Golberstein, 2009). Among young adults, suicide has been found to be the second leading cause of death behind unintentional injury (e.g., fatal traffic accidents, accidental poisoning; Centers for Disease Control & Prevention, 2014). According to the model proposed by Bonner and Rich (1987), both distal (viz., depressive symptoms) and proximal (viz., suicidal behaviors) variables are believed to increase the risk of committing suicide in young adult college students. Indeed, consistent with their framework, findings from numerous studies over the past several decades have consistently implicated depression and suicidal behaviors (e.g., suicide ideation) as important risk factors associated with suicide in college students (e.g., Furr, Westefeld, McConnell, & Jenkins, 2001; Smith et al., 2015; Westefeld & Furr, 1987). Thus, it is not surprising that researchers have been eager to identify variables that predict suicidal risk in young adult populations, including in college student populations.

Loneliness as an Important Predictor of Suicidal Risk in College Students

One variable that has been strongly linked to suicidal risk in college students is loneliness. *Loneliness* is defined by feelings and thoughts of being isolated and disconnected from others (Russell, Peplau, & Cutrona, 1980). According to Baumeister and Leary (1995), all humans have a fundamental need to achieve a sense of belongingness or social connectedness with others. Thus, it is not surprising that findings from studies on loneliness over the past three decades have indicated that it is a robust correlate and predictor of a wide range of negative outcomes (e.g., anxiety, stress, mortality; Blai, 1989; Hawkley & Cacioppo, 2010; Heinrich & Gullone, 2006). Indeed, according to Joiner's (2005) interpersonal theory of suicide, social disconnectedness represents a critical factor involved in the development of suicidal risk. Consistent with this view, findings from studies on loneliness have also implicated it as a reliable predictor of suicidal risk in college student populations (e.g., Chang et al., 2015; Hirsch, Chang, & Jeglic, 2012; Lamis, Ballard, & Patel, 2014; Muyan & Chang, 2015; Weber, Metha, & Nelsen, 1997). For example, in a recent study, Chang, Muyan, and Hirsch (2015) found that loneliness was significantly associated with greater depressive symptoms and suicidal behaviors in college students. Indeed, Westefeld and Furr (1987) found that in 47% of the college students who indicated a history of suicide ideation, loneliness was the most frequently cited cause of suicide ideation. However, what is less clear is the extent to which other variables might add to, or even moderate, the hypothesized negative impact of loneliness on suicidal risk in college students.

Future Orientation as a Protective Factor?: Does Belief in a Changeable Future Make a Difference?

According to Wingate et al. (2006), positive future cognitions represent an important category of protective variables for understanding suicidal risk in adults. Among positive future cognitions, *future orientation*, that is, the belief that one's future can and will change for the better (Hirsch et al., 2006), may be a particularly important variable to examine. First, future orientation is predicated on thoughts about realizing specific outcomes that are associated with positive adjustment within the individual (e.g., feeling good, reaching desired goals, being able to engage in effective action; Hirsch et al., 2006). In that regard, future orientation is conceptually different from more general positive future cognitions that tend to focus more on a general disposition toward a positive expectation for future outcomes (Scheier & Carver, 1985) or a positive expectation of reaching a desired goal in the future (Snyder, 2002). Accordingly, believing that one will soon feel better should serve to broaden an individual's range of perceived options for dealing with painful or stressful situations in their life, and in turn reduce the development of suicidal risk. Second, findings examining future orientation as a predictor of suicidal risk in adults have shown that it significantly augments the prediction model, above and beyond more general positive future cognition variables. For example, Chang et al. (2013) found that the inclusion of future orientation added significant incremental validity in accounting for depressive symptoms and suicidal behaviors in a sample of adult primary care patients. Third, findings from a recent study of emotional victimization point to future orientation as both an important predictor and buffer of suicidal risk in early adolescents aged 12–13 years (Hamilton et al., 2015). Nonetheless, the extent to which future orientation might augment a prediction model involving loneliness as a predictor of suicidal risk in young adults has yet to be clarified. Moreover, beyond an additive role, it would be useful to examine if future orientation might also moderate, or buffer, the extent to which loneliness is associated with suicidal risk in young adults (e.g., Hamilton et al., 2015).

Purpose of the Present Study

Given these concerns and possibilities, we conducted the present study to: (a) determine if future orientation adds to the prediction of suicidal risk, namely, depressive symptoms and suicide ideation in college students; and (b) determine if the Loneliness × Future Orientation interaction would add further incremental validity to these predictions beyond the main effects of loneliness and future orientation.

Consistent with past research findings (e.g., Hirsch et al., 2012; Muyan & Chang, 2015), we expect loneliness to be an important predictor of both depressive symptoms and suicide ideation in college students. However, consistent with the notion that positive future cognitions represent important variables for understanding suicidal risk (Wingate et al., 2006), and past research findings specifically pointing to the value of future orientation in understanding suicidal risk in adults (Chang et al., 2013), we hypothesize that future orientation would significantly augment the prediction model of both indices of suicidal risk, even after accounting for the variance associated with loneliness. Finally, consistent with recent findings indicating that the association between loneliness and suicidal risk in adults partly depends on other factors (e.g., positive life experiences, sexual assault history; Chang et al., 2015; Chang et al., 2015), we tested a moderation model in which future orientation was hypothesized to weaken, or buffer (e.g., Hamilton et al., 2015), the relationship between loneliness and suicidal risk. That is, we expect to find evidence for a significant Loneliness × Future Orientation interaction effect in predicting suicidal risk. Thus, we hypothesize that among lonely individuals, those who do believe that their future will change for the better should report lower levels of suicidal risk compared to those who do not believe that their future will change for the better.

Method

Participants

This study consisted of 228 college students (54 males and 174 females) from a large public university in the Midwest. The sample was predominantly white (68%). Ages ranged from 18 to 28 years, with a mean age of 19.69 years ($SD = 1.38$).

Measures

Loneliness

Loneliness was assessed by the revised UCLA Loneliness Scale (R-UCLA; Russell et al., 1980). The scale consists of 20 items, half of which describe non-lonely thoughts (e.g., "There are people I feel close to"), while the other half describes feelings of loneliness (e.g., "I feel isolated from others"). Respondents are asked to rate the statements on the frequency with which they experience these feelings using a 4-point Likert-type scale, ranging from 1 (*never*) to 4 (*often*). In support of construct validity, scores on the R-UCLA have been found to be positively associated with other measures of social disconnectedness (Russell et al., 1980). Higher scores on the R-UCLA indicate greater levels of loneliness.

Future Orientation

Future orientation was assessed by the Future Orientation Scale (FOS; Hirsch et al., 2006). The FOS is a 6-item self-report measure that was developed to assess for an individual's belief and appreciation that the future will be changed even when experiencing stressful circumstances or negative events (e.g., "No matter how badly I feel, I know it will not last"). Respondents are asked to indicate "how important each reason is to you for dealing with stressors" using a 6-point Likert-type scale, ranging from 1 (*extremely unimportant*) to 5 (*extremely important*). In support of construct validity, scores on the FOS have been found to be positively associated with other measures of positive future cognitions (Yu & Chang, 2016). In general, higher scores on the FOS indicate a greater belief that one's future can be changed for the better.

Suicidal Risk

Suicidal risk was assessed by the Beck Depression Inventory (BDI; Beck, Ward, Mendelson, Mock, & Erbaugh, 1961) and the Frequency of Suicidal Ideation Inventory (FSII; Chang & Chang, 2016). The BDI is a commonly used 21-item self-report measure of depressive symptomatology. Respondents are asked to rate the extent to which they have experienced specific depressive symptoms in the past week, across a 4-point Likert-type scale (e.g., "0 = *I do not feel sad*" to "3 = *I am so sad or unhappy that I can't stand it*"). In support of construct validity, scores on the BDI have been found to be positively associated with other measures of depressive symptoms (Beck et al., 1961). Higher scores on the BDI indicate greater depressive symptoms.

The FSII is a 5-item scale that assesses for the frequency of suicide ideation (e.g., "Over the past 12 months, how often have you thought about killing yourself?"). Respondents are asked to indicate how frequently they have entertained suicidal thoughts over the past twelve months using a 5-point Likert-type scale, ranging from 1 (*never*) to 5 (*almost every day*). In support of construct validity, scores on the FSII have been found to be positively associated with other measures of suicide risk and negatively associated with measures of suicide protection (Chang & Chang, 2016). In general, higher scores on the FSII are indicative of greater suicide ideation.

Procedure

Approval for the study was obtained from the Institutional Review Board at the university where the study was conducted. All participants were enrolled in a psychology course and completed the present survey in partial fulfillment of course requirements. Participants were not made aware of the purpose of the study until after they had completed all measures.

Table 1. Correlations between Measures of Loneliness, Future Orientation, Depressive Symptoms, and Suicide Ideation.

Measures	1	2	3	4
1. Loneliness	—			
2. Future orientation	−.52***	—		
3. Depressive symptoms	.69***	−.49***	—	
4. Suicide ideation	.52***	−.39***	.61***	—
M	34.78	29.82	7.73	7.35
SD	11.68	5.989	8.25	3.96
Score range	20–73	6–36	0–40	5–24
α	.89	.88	.92	.95

Note. $N = 228$.
***$p < .001$.

Results

Correlations, means, standard deviations, and reliability estimates for all study measures are presented in Table 1. Consistent with past findings, both loneliness and future orientation were found to be correlated in the expected manner with the two indices of suicidal risk examined in the present study.

Loneliness and Future Orientation as Predictors of Suicidal Risk in College Students

To examine for loneliness and future orientation as predictors of suicidal risk in college students, we conducted a set of hierarchical regression analyses. Given our primary focus, namely, determining if future orientation augments the prediction model of suicidal risk, above and beyond loneliness, we entered loneliness in Step 1. Future orientation was entered in Step 2. Finally, to determine if there was any evidence for an interaction effect, we entered the multiplicative Loneliness × Future Orientation term in Step 3. To determine whether any of the predictors accounted for a small, medium, or large amount of the variance in suicidal risk, we used Cohen's (1977) convention for small ($f^2 = .02$), medium ($f^2 = .15$), and large effects ($f^2 = .35$) as a general guide.

Results for predicting depressive symptoms and suicide ideation are presented in Table 2. As the table shows, loneliness was found to account for a large ($f^2 = .89$) 47.0% of the variance in depressive symptoms. When future orientation was entered, it was found to account

Table 2. Results of Hierarchical Regression Analyses Showing Amount of Variance in Depressive Symptoms and Suicide Ideation Accounted for by Loneliness and Future Orientation.

Outcome	β	R^2	ΔR^2	F	p
Depressive symptoms					
Step 1: Loneliness	.69***	.47	—	200.42	<.001
Step 2: Future orientation	−.19***	.50	.03	11.92	≤.001
Step 3: Loneliness × Future orientation	−.59**	.52	.02	9.62	<.01
Suicide ideation					
Step 1: Loneliness	.52***	.27	—	83.26	<.001
Step 2: Future orientation	−.16*	.29	.02	5.99	<.05
Step 3: Loneliness × Future orientation	−.99***	.35	.06	19.94	<.001

Note. $N = 228$.
*$p < .05$. **$p < .01$. ***$p \leq .001$.

for a small ($f^2 = .03$), but significant ($p \leq .001$) 2.7% of additional unique variance in depressive symptoms. Noteworthy, after including future orientation (moderator variable), the strength of the effect of loneliness on depressive symptoms decreased ($\Delta\beta = .10$). Finally, when the Loneliness × Future Orientation term was entered, it was found to account for a small ($f^2 = .02$), but significant 2.1% of additional unique variance in depressive symptoms. Thus, evidence for a significant, albeit partial moderation effect was found (Aiken & West, 1991). The total model was found to account for a large ($f^2 = 1.07$) 51.7% of the variance in depressive symptoms, $F(3, 224) = 80.05, p < .001$.

To visually inspect the manner in which loneliness and future orientation interacted with each other in predicting depressive symptoms, we plotted the regression of depressive symptoms on loneliness at low and high levels ($\pm\frac{1}{2}$ SD below and above the mean [26.87 and 32.77], respectively) of low versus high future orientation ($\pm\frac{1}{2}$ SD below and above the mean [28.93 and 40.62], respectively), based on our initial regression results (see Figure 1). As this interaction shows, among lonely students, those with high future orientation, compared to low future orientation, reported significantly lower levels of depressive symptoms, $Ms = 9.30$ vs. 20.41, respectively, $t(42) = 3.31, p < .01$.

In predicting suicide ideation, loneliness was found to account for a large ($f^2 = .37$) 26.9% of the variance in suicide ideation. When future orientation was entered, it was found to account for a small ($f^2 = .02$), but significant ($p < .05$) 1.9% of additional unique variance in suicide ideation. Noteworthy, after including future orientation (moderator variable), the strength of the effect of loneliness on suicide ideation decreased ($\Delta\beta = .08$). Finally, when the Loneliness × Future Orientation term was entered, it was found to account for a small-medium ($f^2 = .06$) 5.8% of additional unique variance in suicide ideation. Again, evidence for a significant, albeit partial moderation effect was found. The total model was found to account for a large ($f^2 = .53$) 34.6% of the variance in suicide ideation, $F(3, 224) = 39.56$, $p < .001$.

Again, to visually inspect the manner in which loneliness and future orientation interacted with each other in predicting suicide ideation, we plotted the regression of suicide ideation on loneliness at low and high levels ($\pm\frac{1}{2}$ SD below and above the mean, respectively) of negative and positive future orientation ($\pm\frac{1}{2}$ SD below and above the mean, respectively)

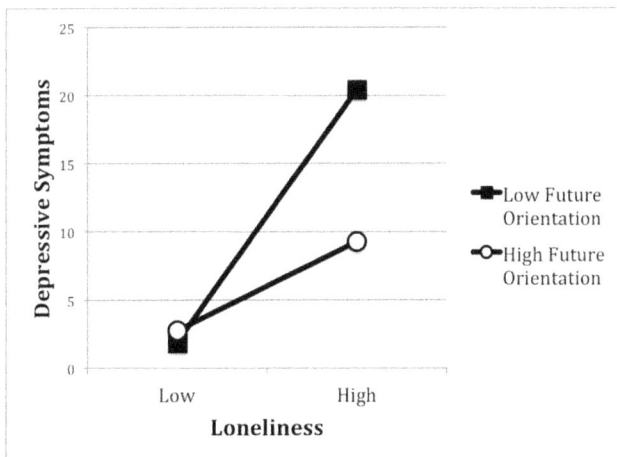

Figure 1. Depressive symptoms at low vs. high future orientation for lonely and non-lonely students.

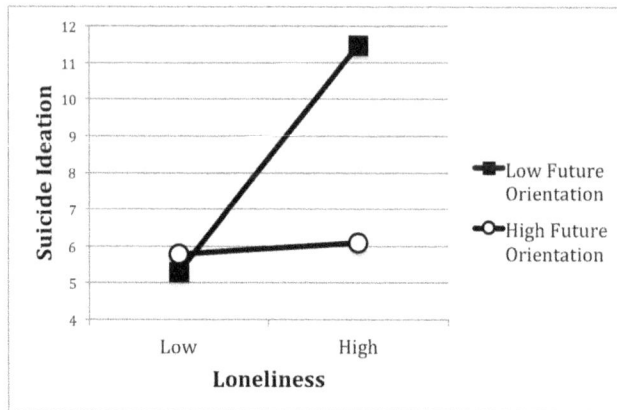

Figure 2. Suicide ideation at low vs. high future orientation for lonely and non-lonely students.

based on our initial regression results (Figure 2). As this interaction also shows, among lonely students, those with high future orientation, compared to low future orientation, reported significantly lower levels of suicide ideation, $Ms = 6.10$ vs. 11.47, respectively, $t(42) = 2.90$, $p < .01$. Interestingly, among students with a positive future orientation, there was no significant difference in levels of suicide ideation between lonely and non-lonely students, $Ms = 6.10$ vs. 5.78, respectively, $t(53) = .49$, $n.s.$

Discussion

Consistent with past research findings pointing to the importance of loneliness as an important predictor of suicidal risk in young adults (e.g., Hirsch et al., 2012; Muyan & Chang, 2015), we found that loneliness was a positive predictor of depressive symptoms and suicide ideation in college students. Indeed, loneliness was found to account for a large amount of variance in both of the indices of suicidal risk examined in the present study. In keeping with various theories that have often posited that interpersonal disconnectedness from others is a critical component of adult suicide (e.g., Baumeister & Leary, 1995; Joiner, 2005; Van Orden et al., 2010), young emerging adults who feel alone and socially disconnected from others during a critical, if not stressful (Dunkel-Schetter & Lobel, 1990), period in their development into adulthood may come to believe that their existence is of little concern to others, thus heightening their general risk for suicide. Overall, the present findings for loneliness join those from other studies to highlight the central role that it plays in predicting suicidal risk in young adults.

Additionally, we found evidence supporting the contention that positive future cognitions, specifically, future orientation (Hirsch et al., 2006; Yu & Chang, 2016), might also represent important predictors of suicidal risk in young adults (Wingate et al., 2006). Indeed, we found believing that one's future can and will change for the better, added significant incremental validity, above and beyond loneliness, to the prediction of both depressive symptoms and suicide ideation in college students. Thus, although feeling socially isolated or disconnected from others might play a strong role in elevating suicidal risk in young adults, our findings clearly indicate that protective factors, such as future orientation, also need to be considered in order to develop comprehensive models of suicide in adults. This view is consistent with the emerging notion that efforts associated with the study and prevention of suicide need to balance an appreciation of processes associated with both risk and protection (WHO, 2014). Given that some studies have pointed to cultural differences in future orientation (Gao, 2016), it would be useful to determine if the present findings might be generalizable to other young adult populations (e.g., East Asians).

Importantly, beyond the main effects of loneliness and future orientation, we also found evidence for a significant Loneliness × Future Orientation interaction effect in predicting both depressive symptoms and suicide ideation. For both indices of suicidal risk, the pattern obtained indicated that among lonely students, those who believed, compared to those who did not believe, that their future would change for the better reported significantly less risk for suicide. Indeed, we found that for those with high future orientation, levels of suicide ideation were not negatively affected by the presence of loneliness. Thus, these findings are important. They not only add to growing evidence for contextualizing our understanding of the potential negative effects of loneliness on suicidal risk (e.g., Chang et al., 2015), but they also highlight how the presence of protective factors, or positive conditions (e.g., positive life events; Chang et al., 2015), might help minimize (e.g., depressive symptoms), and even help resolve (e.g., suicide ideation), the deleterious effects of loneliness on suicidal risk in young adults. Furthermore, our findings build on Hamilton et al.'s (2015) study to indicate that the positive role of future orientation as an important predictor and buffer of suicidal risk is not limited to early adolescents, but remains an important protective factor into young adulthood. Thus, our findings indicate that believing one's future will change for the better makes a positive difference when it comes to determining suicidal risk.

Taken together, the present findings point to at least two practical implications for potentially reducing or lowering suicidal risk in young adults. First, it would be important to identify those who may lack important suicide protective factors. Thus, for example, within a comprehensive suicide prevention program, mental health professionals should routinely not only assess for the presence of suicidal risk and vulnerability factors (e.g., loneliness), but also assess for the absence of specific protective factors like future orientation. Second, and relatedly, it would be important for mental health professionals to consider applying interventions that help decrease experiences of loneliness (e.g., treatments targeting maladaptive social cognitions; Cacioppo, Grippo, London, Goossens, & Cacioppo, 2015), on the one hand, but help increase the belief that one's future will get better (Hirsch et al., 2006), on the other hand, for those at heightened risk for suicide. For example, within cognitive-behavioral models, mental health professionals may consider applying techniques such as cognitive restructuring (Leahy & Rego, 2012) to help promote greater future orientation in adults at risk for suicide (e.g., identifying maladaptive or distorting thoughts about the future, challenging the accuracy of such thoughts, and evaluating the evidence for or against such thoughts).

Despite the importance of the present findings, it is worth noting a few limitations. First, unlike the numerous studies that have examined the construct of loneliness, fewer studies have examined for the construct of future orientation. Thus, it would be important in future research to continue conducting studies that examine the form and function of future orientation in adults. Second, and relatedly, insofar as future orientation represents a positive future cognition, it would be important to determine if similar buffering effects would emerge when examining constructs like optimism and hope as moderators. Third, given that the present sample was predominantly White, it would be important to examine the generalizability of the present findings when studying different cultural or ethnoracial groups. Lastly, although we tested a model examining loneliness and future orientation as predictors of suicide risk, our cross-sectional design precludes drawing any causal inferences. Thus, it would be useful in future studies to apply a prospective design that examines for loneliness and future orientation as predictors of changes in suicide risk across time.

Concluding Thoughts

In summary, we examined and found support for a prediction model involving loneliness and future orientation as predictors of depressive symptoms and suicide ideation in young adults. Importantly, we also found support for a significant Loneliness × Future Orientation interaction effect. Specifically, findings from this study showed that believing that the future will change for the better was associated with lower suicidal risk among lonely adults. Overall, the present findings are important for highlighting the potential power of positive future cognitions like future orientation in minimizing, and possibly resolving, the negative effects of loneliness on suicidal risk in young adults.

Acknowledgments

The first author would like to acknowledge Tae Myung-Sook and Chang Suk-Choon for their encouragement and support throughout this project. The second to ninth coauthors all contributed equally to the present work and, therefore, their authorship order was determined randomly.

References

Aiken, L. S., & West, S. G. (1991). *Multiple regression: Testing and interpreting interactions*. Newbury Park, CA: Sage.

Baumeister, R. F., & Leary, M. R. (1995). The need to belong: Desire for interpersonal attachments as a fundamental human motive. *Psychological Bulletin, 117*, 497–529.

Beck, A. T., Ward, C. H., Mendelson, M., Mock, J., & Erbaugh, J. (1961). An inventory for measuring depression. *Archives of General Psychiatry, 4*, 561–571.

Blai, B., Jr. (1989). Health consequences of loneliness: Review of the literature. *Journal of American College Health, 27*, 162–167.

Bonner, R. L., & Rich, A. R. (1987). Toward a predictive model of suicidal ideation and behavior: Some preliminary data in college students. *Suicide and Life-Threatening Behavior, 17*, 50–63.

Cacioppo, S., Grippo, A. J., London, S., Goossens, L., & Cacioppo, J. T. (2015). Loneliness: Clinical import and interventions. *Perspectives on Psychological Science, 10*, 238–249.

Centers for Disease Control and Prevention [CDC]. (2014). [Graphic representation of 10 leading causes of death in the United States in 2014, for both sexes]. Leading causes of death reports, National and regional, 1999–2014. Retrieved from http://webappa.cdc.gov/sasweb/ncipc/leadcaus10_us.html

Chang, E. C., & Chang, O. D. (2016). Development of the frequency of suicidal ideation inventory: Evidence for validity and reliability of a brief measure of suicidal ideation frequency in a college student population. *Cognitive Therapy and Research, 40*, 549–556.

Chang, E. C., Lian, X., Yu, T., Qu, J., Zhang, B., Jia, W., Hu, Q., Li, J., Wu, J., & Hirsch, J. K. (2015). Loneliness under assault: Understanding the impact of sexual assault on the relation between loneliness and suicidal risk in college students. *Personality and Individual Differences, 72*, 155–159.

Chang, E. C., Muyan, M., & Hirsch, J. K. (2015). Loneliness, positive life events, and psychological maladjustment: When good things happen, even lonely people feel better! *Personality and Individual Differences, 86*, 150–155.

Chang, E. C., Yu, E. A., Lee, J. Y., Hirsch, J. K., Kupfermann, Y., & Kahle, E. R. (2013). An examination of optimism/pessimism and suicide risk in primary care patients: Does belief in a changeable future make a difference? *Cognitive Therapy and Research, 37*, 796–804.

Cohen, J. (1977). *Statistical power analysis for the behavioral sciences* (Rev. ed.). New York: Academic Press.

Dunkel-Schetter, C., & Lobel, M. (1990). Stress among students. *New Directions for Student Services, 49*, 17–34.

Furr, S. R., Westefeld, J. S., McConnell, G. N., & Jenkins, J. M. (2001). Suicide and depression among college students: A decade later. *Professional Psychology: Research and Practice, 32*, 97–100.

Gao, X. (2016). Cultural differences between East Asian and North American in temporal orientation. *Review of General Psychology, 20*, 118–127.

Hamilton, J. L., Connolly, S. L., Liu, R. T., Stange, J. P., Abramson, L. Y., & Alloy, L. B. (2015). It gets better: Future orientation buffers the development of hopelessness and depressive symptoms following emotional victimization during early adolescence. *Journal of Abnormal Child Psychology, 43*, 465–474.

Hawkley, L. C., & Cacioppo, J. T. (2010). Loneliness matters: A theoretical and empirical review of the consequences and mechanisms. *Annals of Behavioral Medicine, 40*, 218–227.

Heinrich, L. M., & Gullone, E. (2006). The clinical significance of loneliness: A literature review. *Clinical Psychology Review, 26*, 695–718.

Hirsch, J. K., Chang, E. C., & Jeglic, E. L. (2012). Social problem solving and suicide ideation and attempts: Ethnic differences in moderating effects of loneliness and life stress. *Archives of Suicide Research, 16*, 303–315.

Hirsch, J. K., Duberstein, P. R., Conner, K. R., Heisel, M. J., Beckman, A., Franus, N., & Conwell, Y. (2006). Future orientation and suicide ideation and attempts in depressed adults ages 50 and over. *The American Journal of Geriatric Psychiatry, 14*, 752–757.

Joiner, T. E., Jr. (2005). *Why people die by suicide*. Cambridge, MA: Harvard University Press.

Lamis, D. A., Ballard, E. D., & Patel, A. B. (2014). Loneliness and suicidal ideation in drug-using college students. *Suicide and Life-Threatening Behavior, 44*, 629–640.

Leahy, R. L., & Rego, S. A. (2012). Cognitive restructuring. In W. T. O'Donohue & J. E. Fisher (Eds.), *Cognitive behavior therapy: Core principles for practice* (pp. 133–158). Hoboken, NJ: John Wiley & Sons Inc.

Muyan, M., & Chang, E. C. (2015). Perfectionism as a predictor of suicidal risk in Turkish college students: Does loneliness contribute to further risk? *Cognitive Therapy and Research, 39*, 776–784

Russell, D., Peplau, L. A., & Cutrona, C. E. (1980). The revised UCLA Loneliness Scale: Concurrent and discriminant validity evidence. *Journal of Personality and Social Psychology, 39*, 472–480.

Scheier, M. F., & Carver, C. S. (1985). Optimism, coping, and health: Assessment and implications of generalized outcome expectancies. *Health Psychology, 4*, 219–247.

Smith, S. S., Carter, J. S., Karczewski, S., Pivarunas, B., Suffoletto, S., & Munin, A. (2015). Mediating effects of stress, weight-related issues, and depression on suicidality in college students. *Journal of American College Health, 63*, 1–12.

Snyder, C. R. (2002). Hope theory: Rainbows in the mind. *Psychological Inquiry, 13*, 249–275.

Van Orden, K. A., Witte, T. K., Cukrowicz, K. C., Braithwaite, S. R., Selby, E. A., & Joiner, T. E., Jr. (2010). The interpersonal theory of suicide. *Psychological Review, 117*, 575–600.

Weber, B., Metha, A., & Nelsen, E. (1997). Relationships among multiple suicide ideation risk factors in college students. *Journal of College Student Psychotherapy, 11*, 49–64.

Westefeld, J. S., & Furr, S. R. (1987). Suicide and depression among college students. *Professional Psychology: Research and Practice, 18*, 119–123.

Wingate, L. R., Burns, A. B., Gordon, K. H., Perez, M., Walker, R. L., Williams, F. M., & Joiner, T. (2006). Suicide and positive cognitions: Positive psychology applied to the understanding and treatment of suicidal behavior. In T. E. Ellis (Ed.), *Cognition and suicide: Theory, research, and therapy* (pp. 261–283). Washington, DC: American Psychological Association.

World Health Organization [WHO]. (2013). *Mental health action plan 2013–2020*. Geneva, Switzerland: Author.

World Health Organization [WHO]. (2014). *Preventing suicide: A global imperative*. Geneva, Switzerland: Author.

Yu, E. A., & Chang, E. C. (2016). Optimism/pessimism and future orientation as predictors of suicidal ideation: Are there ethnic differences? *Cultural Diversity and Ethnic Minority Psychology, 22*, 572–579.

Zivin, K., Eisenberg, D., Gollust, S. E., & Golberstein, E. (2009). Persistence of mental health problems and needs in a college student population. *Journal of Affective Disorders, 117*, 180–185.

Loneliness and Negative Affective Conditions in Adults: Is There Any Room for Hope in Predicting Anxiety and Depressive Symptoms?

Mine Muyan, Edward C. Chang, Zunaira Jilani, Tina Yu, Jiachen Lin, and Jameson K. Hirsch

ABSTRACT
This study examined the role of hope in understanding the link between loneliness and negative affective conditions (viz., anxiety and depressive symptoms) in a sample of 318 adults. As expected, loneliness was found to be a significant predictor of both anxiety and depressive symptoms. Noteworthy, hope was found to significantly augment the prediction of depressive symptoms, even after accounting for loneliness. Furthermore, we found evidence for a significant Loneliness × Hope interaction effect in predicting anxiety. A plot of the interaction confirmed that the association between loneliness and anxiety was weaker among high, compared to low, hope adults. Some implications of the present findings are discussed.

Philosophers have long contended that being with others represents a fundamental way of existing among human beings (Heidegger, 1927/1962). Indeed, modern psychologists have recently expanded on this view by arguing that being connected to others is not only a basic human disposition, but it is also associated with greater positive psychological functioning (Baumeister & Leary, 1995; Townsend & McWhirter, 2005). For example, Lambert et al. (2013) found that a sense of belonging was positively associated with meaning in life in adults. Similarly, Sánchez, Colón, and Esparza (2005) found that students' sense of belonging positively predicted academic effort, expectancy for success, and educational aspirations/expectations. Alternatively, the inability to develop a sense of belonging is associated with loneliness, and is linked to poor psychological functioning (Van Orden et al., 2010).

According to Russell, Peplau, and Cutrona (1980), *loneliness* is defined by feelings and thoughts of being isolated and disconnected from others. Studies on loneliness in adults have found it to be associated with greater negative psychological outcomes (Hawkley & Cacioppo, 2010; Heinrich & Gullone, 2006). In particular, loneliness has consistently been linked to greater negative affective conditions in adults (viz., anxiety & depressive symptoms; Chang, Sanna, Chang, & Bodem, 2008; Russell et al., 1980; Wilbert & Rupert, 1986). For example, in a recent study of ethnically diverse adults (viz., European and Asian Americans), Chang (2013) found that loneliness was not only associated with greater anxiety and depressive symptoms, but it was also a robust predictor of these two negative affective conditions even after controlling for other key variables (e.g., race/ethnicity, perfectionism). Thus, loneliness appears to be a common correlate of negative affective conditions in adults. Yet, little is known about the contexts or conditions under which these associations may be impacted. For example, the presence of psychological strengths might function to mitigate or weaken the association between loneliness and negative affective conditions in adults.

One psychological strength that might be worth considering is hope (Snyder, 2000, 2004). According to Snyder et al. (1991), *hope* represents a cognitive process that is predicated on the belief that one can achieve personal goals and identify effective strategies to attain these goals. Based on Snyder's (1994, 2002) hope theory, high hope is believed to be associated with greater positive outcomes, whereas low hope is believed to be associated with greater negative outcomes. Indeed, findings from studies on hope conducted over the past two decades have generally supported these contentions (Cheavens & Ritschel, 2014). For example, findings from studies of adults indicate that high hope individuals are less anxious and less depressed than low hope individuals (Carretta, Ridner, & Dietrich, 2014; Chang, Yu, & Hirsch, 2013; Geiger & Kwon, 2010; Visser, Loess, Jeglic, & Hirsch, 2013). Thus, as a psychological strength, the presence of hope may weaken the reliable positive association often found between loneliness and negative affective conditions in adults. Put another way, even among lonely individuals, the presence of a strong belief that one might still be able to achieve important personal goals may help thwart the development of negative affective conditions in this group.

To date, no study has examined the potential role of hope as a buffer of the link between loneliness and negative affective conditions in adults. For example, hope might represent an important buffer of the loneliness–anxiety link, the loneliness–depressive symptoms link, or both. Furthermore, in examining for the role of hope as a buffer, it would be useful to also determine if hope adds to the prediction of negative affective conditions beyond loneliness.

Purpose of the Present Study

Given these possibilities, we had three main objectives in conducting the present study. First, we aimed to examine the extent to which loneliness predicts negative affective conditions. Second, beyond examining the prediction of loneliness in negative affective conditions, we aimed to determine the extent to which the inclusion of hope adds to the prediction of negative affective conditions beyond loneliness. Lastly, we aimed to determine if there is a significant Loneliness × Hope interaction effect that accounts for additional variance in negative affective conditions beyond the main effects of both loneliness and hope.

Consistent with past findings (e.g., Hawkley & Cacioppo, 2010; Russell et al., 1980), we expected loneliness to account for a significant amount of the variance in both anxiety and depressive symptoms. Nonetheless, given the presumed robust explanatory power of hope in adjustment (e.g., Snyder, 2000, 2004), we expected hope to account for a significant amount of additional variance in negative affective conditions beyond loneliness. Finally, consistent with the notion that hope might help mitigate or weaken the association between loneliness and negative affective conditions in adults, we expected to find evidence for a significant Loneliness × Hope interaction effect that accounts for additional variance in predicting negative affective conditions beyond loneliness and hope. Specifically, we expected to find the positive association between loneliness and negative affective conditions to be weaker for those high in hope, compared to those low in hope.

Method

Participants

Participants for the present study were 318 college students from a university in the Southeast United States. Two hundred and fifteen were female (67.6%), 101 were male (31.8%), and 2 indicated as transgender (0.6%). Ages ranged from 18 to 58 with a mean of 21.69 years ($SD = 5.05$). The majority of the participants were European American (89.9%), followed by African American (5.3%), Asian American (2.8%), and Latino American (1.9%).

Measures

Loneliness

Loneliness was measured by the revised UCLA Loneliness Scale (R-UCLA; Russell et al., 1980). The scale consists of 20 items, with 10 items (reverse scored) describing non-lonely thoughts (e.g., "There are people I feel close to"), and 10 items characterizing feelings of loneliness (e.g., "I feel isolated from others"). Respondents are asked to rate the statements on the frequency in which they experienced these feelings using a 4-point scale, ranging from 1 (*never*) to 4 (*often*). Research has shown the R-UCLA scale to have good test-retest reliability over a 12-month period (.73) and to have construct validity with other measures of loneliness (Russell, 1996). In the present study, internal reliability for the R-UCLA was .93. Higher scores on the R-UCLA indicate greater levels of loneliness.

Hope

Hope was measured by the Hope Scale (HS; Snyder et al., 1991). The HS is a 12-item measure of hope with 8 items that measure hopeful thinking (e.g., "I can think of many ways to get out of a jam") and 4 filler items. Respondents are asked to indicate how accurately each item described them using an 8-point scale, ranging from 1 (*definitely false*) to 8 (*definitely true*). Evidence for the construct validity of the HS has been reported in Snyder et al. (1991). In the present study, internal reliability for the HS was .91. Higher scores on the HS indicate greater dispositional hope.

Negative Affect

Negative affective conditions were measured using the Beck Anxiety Inventory (BAI; Beck, Epstein, Brown, & Steer, 1988) and the Beck Depression Inventory (BDI; Beck, Ward, Mendelson, Mock, & Erbaugh, 1961). The BAI is a 21-item self-report measure consisting of common symptoms of anxiety (e.g., "Fear of the worst happening"). Respondents are asked to rate the extent to which they had experienced each symptom over the past week using a 4-point scale ranging from 0 (*not at all*) to 3 (*severely*). Research has shown the BAI to have good test-retest reliability over a 1-week period (.75) and to have construct validity with other measures of anxiety (Beck et al., 1988).

In the present study, internal reliability for the BAI was .94. The BDI is a commonly used 21-item self-report measure of depressive symptomatology. Respondents are asked to rate the extent to which they had experienced specific depressive symptoms in the past week across a 4-point scale (for example, "0 = *I do not feel sad*" to "3 = *I am so sad or unhappy that I can't stand it*"). Research has shown the BDI to have good test-retest reliability over a 4-month period (.62) and to have construct validity with other measures of depressive symptoms (Beck, Steer, & Carbin, 1988). In the present study, internal reliability for the BDI was .95. Higher scores on the BAI and BDI are indicative of greater anxiety and depressive symptoms, respectively.

Procedure

Approval for the study was obtained from the Institutional Review Board prior to data collection. By using the convenience sampling procedure, participants taking a general psychology course, such as Introduction to Psychology, were recruited from a regional university in the Southeast United States and received either course-required credit or extra credit upon completion of the survey. All participants were provided with written informed consent, which indicated that all data would be kept strictly confidential. After signing the statement of informed consent, participants were provided with the survey. Upon completion, all participants were debriefed and provided with contact information for local mental health services.

Data Analysis

Data was analyzed using IBM's Statistical Package for the Social Sciences (SPSS) 22. Pearson correlations were computed to examine relations between all study variables. Next, to address our key question of whether hope accounts for additional unique variance in predicting negative affective conditions above and beyond loneliness, a series of hierarchical regression analyses predicting anxiety and depressive symptoms was conducted. For each regression model, loneliness was entered in the First Step, followed by hope in the Second Step. Moreover, the multiplicative term of Loneliness × Hope was included in the Third Step to determine whether hope may potentially interact with loneliness in predicting negative affective conditions. Additionally, to determine whether any of the predictors accounted for a small, medium, or large amount of the variance in negative affective conditions, we used Cohen's (1977) convention for small ($f^2 = .02$), medium ($f^2 = .15$), and large effects ($f^2 = .35$), as a general guide.

Results

Results of the correlations, means, and standard deviations for all study measures are presented in Table 1. Consistent with past research, greater loneliness was significantly associated with greater anxiety ($r = .47$) and depressive symptoms ($r = .58$). Moreover, as expected, hope was found to have a significant negative association with loneliness ($r = -.58$). Additionally, hope was found to have a significant negative association with anxiety ($r = -.34$) and depressive symptoms ($r = -.48$).

Table 1. Correlations between measures of loneliness, hope, anxiety, and depressive symptoms in adults.

Measures	1	2	3	4
1. Loneliness	—			
2. Hope	$-.58^{***}$	—		
3. Anxiety	$.47^{***}$	$-.34^{***}$	—	
4. Depressive symptoms	$.58^{***}$	$-.48^{***}$	$.64^{***}$	—
Range	20–72	10–64	0–55	0–52
M	39.54	48.47	13.60	10.61
SD	11.98	09.82	11.55	11.31

Note. $N = 318$. $^{***}p < .001$.

Examining a Model of Loneliness and Hope as Predictors of Negative Affective Conditions in Adults

The findings of hierarchical regression analyses are presented in Table 2. As the table shows, in predicting anxiety among adults, loneliness was found to be a significant predictor, accounting for a medium ($f^2 = .28$) 22% variance in anxiety, $F(1, 316) = 90.07$, $p < .001$. However, when hope was entered in the Second Step, it did not account for any significant variance in anxiety, beyond loneliness, $F(1, 315) = 2.32$, *n.s.* When the interaction of loneliness and hope was entered in the Third Step, the Loneliness × Hope term was found to account for a small ($f^2 = .02$), but significant 2% of additional variance in anxiety, $F(1, 314) = 8.39$, $p < .01$. The full prediction model including loneliness, hope, and the interaction term was found to account for a medium ($f^2 = .33$) 25% of variance in anxiety, $F(3, 314) = 34.45$, $p < .001$.

In predicting depressive symptoms, loneliness was found to account for a large ($f^2 = .52$) 34% of variance in depressive symptoms, $F(1, 316) = 162.16$, $p < .001$. Additionally, after controlling for loneliness, when hope was entered in the Second Step, it was found to account for a small ($f^2 = .03$), but significant 3% of additional variance in depressive symptoms, $F(1, 315) = 15.68$, $p < .001$. However, when the interaction term involving loneliness and hope was entered in the Third Step, it was not found to account for any additional variance in depressive symptoms, $F(1, 314) = 1.51$, *n.s.* The full prediction model including loneliness, hope, and the interaction term was found to account for a large ($f^2 = .59$) 37% of variance in depressive symptoms, $F(3, 314) = 62.39$, $p < .001$.

To visually inspect the manner in which loneliness and hope interacted in predicting anxiety, we plotted the regression of anxiety on loneliness (shown at low and high levels, using a

Table 2. Results of hierarchical regression analyses showing amount of variance in anxiety and depressive symptoms accounted for by loneliness and hope in adults.

Outcome and Measure	β	R^2	ΔR^2	F
Anxiety				
Step 1: Loneliness	$.47^{***}$	.22	—	90.07^{***}
Step 2: Hope	$-.09$	.23	.01	2.32
Step 3: Loneliness × Hope	$-.66^{**}$	.25	.02	8.39^{**}
Depressive symptoms				
Step 1: Loneliness	$.58^{***}$	.34	—	162.16^{***}
Step 2: Hope	$-.22^{***}$	.37	.03	15.68^{***}
Step 3: Loneliness × Hope	$-.25$	.37	.00	1.51

Note. $N = 318$. $^{**}p < .01$. $^{***}p < .001$.

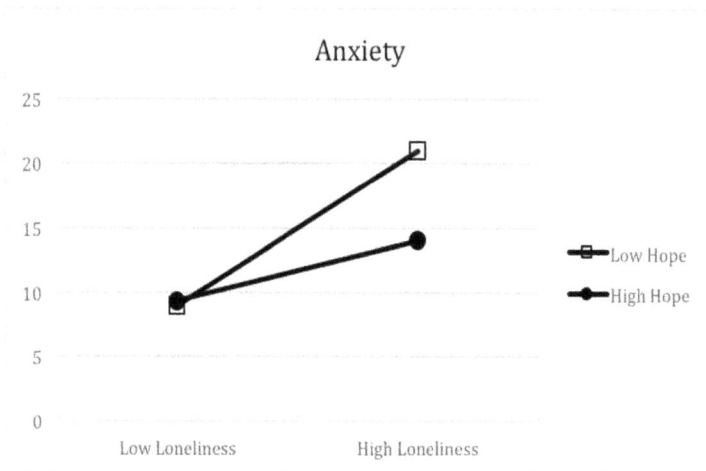

Figure 1. Loneliness and anxiety among low versus high hope adults.

mean split) between low versus high hope individuals (based on using a mean split) based on our initial regression results (Figure 1). As the figure shows, results of plotting this interaction offer support for the role of hope as a buffer of the link between loneliness and anxiety. Overall, the positive association between loneliness and anxiety was weaker for high hope students, compared to low hope students. Indeed, among those highest in experiences of loneliness, those with high hope reported less anxiety than those with low hope.

Discussion

A key objective of the present study was to determine if hope, as a psychological strength (Snyder, 2000, 2004), might be important in understanding the link between loneliness and negative affective conditions in adults. Consistent with past research findings (Heinrich & Gullone, 2006), results of both correlational and regression analyses from the present study affirmed a consistent positive association between loneliness and negative affective conditions, namely, anxiety and depressive symptoms. Noteworthy, findings from the present study indicated two specific ways in which hope played an important role in understanding the link between loneliness and negative affective conditions in adults.

First, beyond loneliness, we found hope to predict additional variance in depressive symptoms, but not in anxiety. This finding suggests that although loneliness may represent a robust predictor of depressive symptoms in adults (Cacioppo, Hawkley, & Thisted, 2010; Cacioppo, Hughes, Waite, Hawkley, & Thisted, 2006), it is useful to consider prediction models of depression that include for other key psychological variables, especially psychological strengths such as hope. In addition, our findings might be taken to suggest the potential value of developing eclectic interventions when working with depressed adults that not only target the reduction of loneliness (Masi, Chen, Hawkley, & Cacioppo, 2011), but also focus on cultivating hope (Cheavens, Feldman, Gum, Michael, & Snyder, 2006). For example, Feldman and Dreher (2012) found that a single-session hope-based intervention that trained individuals to visualize the attainment of important personal goals resulted in both higher hope and better psychological adjustment across a four-week period.

Second, although we did not find hope to directly augment the prediction of additional variance in anxiety, beyond loneliness, we did find that hope moderated the association between loneliness and anxiety in the present study. Consistent with the notion that hope represents a cardinal character strength or protective factor (Ong, Edwards, & Bergeman, 2006), we found that the link between loneliness and anxiety was weaker for adults with high hope, compared to adults with low hope. This pattern is consistent with recent findings supporting the role of hope as an important psychological buffer in predicting other important outcomes. For example, in a study of sexual victimization in adults, Chang et al. (2015) found that regardless of victimization history, levels of suicide behaviors were lowest for adults with high hope, with the highest level of suicide behaviors indicated among victimized adults with low hope. Thus, these findings point to how the general cultivation of hope in adults might help thwart the potential impact of adverse experiences (e.g., loneliness, sexual victimization) that are often associated with negative psychological outcomes (e.g., anxiety, suicidal behaviors).

Some Limitations of the Present Study

Despite the important findings of the present study, some limitations are worth noting. First, as our sample was predominantly European American, it would be important to evaluate the generalizability of the present findings to more diverse racial/ethnic groups. Second, as the participants in the present study were recruited by the convenience sampling procedure, the generalizability of our findings is limited to similar groups. However, to increase the generalizability of the results, further studies may use random sampling procedures. Third, considering the other factors that have been found to be related to loneliness, such as self-esteem (Lasgaard, 2007), we suggest further studies collect data for possible confounding variables to have the power to statistically control those variables in their studies. Fourth, given that hope was found to be an important buffer of the link between loneliness and anxiety, it would be useful to determine if hope represents a general buffer of the link between loneliness and other anxiety-related conditions and outcomes (e.g., worry, obsessive-compulsive problems, Post-Traumatic Stress Disorder). Fifth, and relatedly, it would be important in future research to determine if the buffering effect found in the present study is unique to hope, relative to other positive future cognitions (e.g., optimism, future orientation). Sixth, although we focused on negative affective conditions, it would be interesting to determine if hope operates in different ways in predicting positive affective conditions (e.g., happiness, joy, attention). Finally, given the cross-sectional nature of the present study, it would be useful to build on the present findings to examine how loneliness and hope may interact to predict changes in negative affective conditions in adults across time.

Concluding Thoughts

In the present study, we examined the role of hope in understanding the link between loneliness and negative affective conditions in adults. Findings from our study indicated two ways in which hope plays an important role. First, we found hope to augment the prediction of depressive symptoms, beyond loneliness. Second, we found hope to buffer the link between loneliness and anxiety. Overall, our findings not only underscore the value of hope as an important psychological strength, but they go further to indicate how hope operates in specific ways to account for different negative affective conditions in adults.

References

Baumeister, R. F., & Leary, M. R. (1995). The need to belong: Desire for interpersonal attachments as a fundamental human motivation. *Psychological Bulletin, 117,* 497–529.

Beck, A. T., Epstein, N., Brown, G., & Steer, R. A. (1988). An inventory for measuring clinical anxiety: Psychometric properties. *Journal of Consulting and Clinical Psychology, 56,* 893–897.

Beck, A. T., Steer, R. A., & Carbin, M. G. (1988). Psychometric properties of the Beck Depression Inventory: Twenty-five years of evaluation. *Clinical Psychology Review, 8,* 77–100.

Beck, A. T., Ward, C. H., Mendelson, M., Mock, J., & Erbaugh, J. K. (1961). An inventory for measuring depression. *Archives of General Psychiatry, 4,* 561–571.

Cacioppo, J. T., Hawkley, L. C., & Thisted, R. A. (2010). Perceived social isolation makes me sad: 5-year cross-lagged analyses of loneliness and depressive symptomatology in the Chicago Health, Aging, and Social Relations Study. *Psychology and Aging, 25,* 453–463.

Cacioppo, J. T., Hughes, M. E., Waite, L. J., Hawkley, L. C., & Thisted, R. A. (2006). Loneliness as a specific risk factor for depressive symptoms: Cross-sectional and longitudinal analyses. *Psychology and Aging, 21,* 140–151.

Carretta, C., Ridner, S. H., & Dietrich, M. S. (2014). Hope, hopelessness, and anxiety: A pilot instrument comparison study. *Archives of Psychiatric Nursing, 28,* 230–234.

Chang, E. C. (2013). Perfectionism and loneliness as predictors of depressive and anxious symptoms in Asian and European Americans: Do self-construal schemas also matter? *Cognitive Therapy and Research, 37,* 1179–1188.

Chang, E. C., Sanna, L. J., Chang, R., & Bodem, M. R. (2008). A preliminary look at loneliness as a moderator of the link between perfectionism and depressive and anxious symptoms in college students: Does being lonely make perfectionistic strivings more distressing? *Behaviour Research and Therapy, 46,* 877–886.

Chang, E. C., Yu, E. A., & Hirsch, J. K. (2013). On the confluence of optimism and hope on depressive symptoms in primary care patients: Does doubling up on *bonum futurum* proffer any added benefits? *The Journal of Positive Psychology, 8*, 404–411.

Chang, E. C., Yu, T., Jilani, Z., Fowler, E. E., Yu, E. A., Lin, J., & Hirsch, J. K. (2015). Hope under assault: Understanding the impact of sexual assault on the relation between hope and suicidal risk in college students. *Journal of Social and Clinical Psychology, 34*, 221–238.

Cheavens, J. S., Feldman, D. B., Gum, A., Michael, S. T., & Snyder, C. R. (2006). Hope therapy in a community sample: A pilot investigation. *Social Indicators Research, 77*, 61–78.

Cheavens, J. S., & Ritschel, L. A. (2014). Hope theory. In M. M. Tugade, M. N. Shiota, & L. D. Kirby (Eds.), *Handbook of positive emotions* (pp. 396–410). New York, NY: Guilford Press.

Cohen, J. (1977). *Statistical power analysis for the behavioral sciences* (rev. ed.). New York, NY: Academic Press.

Feldman, D. B., & Dreher, D. E. (2012). Can hope be changed in 90 minutes? Testing the efficacy of a single-session goal-pursuit intervention for college students. *Journal of Happiness Studies, 13*, 745–759.

Geiger, K. A., & Kwon, P. (2010). Rumination and depressive symptoms: Evidence for the moderating role of hope. *Personality and Individual Differences, 49*, 391–395.

Hawkley, L. C., & Cacioppo, J. T. (2010). Loneliness matters: A theoretical and empirical review of consequences and mechanisms. *Annals of Behavioral Medicine, 40*, 218–227.

Heidegger, M. (1962). *Being and time.* Trans. by J. Macquarrie and E. Robinson. New York, NY: Harper & Row. (Original work published 1927).

Heinrich, L. M., & Gullone, E. (2006). The clinical significance of loneliness: A literature review. *Clinical Psychology Review, 26*, 695–718.

Lambert, N. M., Stillman, T. F., Hicks, J. A., Kamble, S., Baumeister, R. F., & Fincham, F. D. (2013). To belong is to matter sense of belonging enhances meaning in life. *Personality and Social Psychology Bulletin, 39*, 1418–1427.

Lasgaard, M. (2007). Reliability and validity of the Danish version of the UCLA Loneliness Scale. *Personality and Individual Differences, 42*, 1359–1366.

Masi, C. M., Chen, H. Y., Hawkley, L. C., & Cacioppo, J. T. (2011). A meta-analysis of interventions to reduce loneliness. *Personality and Social Psychology Review, 15*, 219–266.

Ong, A. D., Edwards, L. M., & Bergeman, C. S. (2006). Hope as a source of resilience in later adulthood. *Personality and Individual Differences, 41*, 1263–1273.

Russell, D., Peplau, L. A., & Cutrona, C. E. (1980). The revised UCLA Loneliness Scale: Concurrent and discriminant validity evidence. *Journal of Personality and Social Psychology, 39*, 471–480.

Russell, D. W. (1996). UCLA Loneliness Scale (Version 3): Reliability, validity, and factor structure. *Journal of Personality Assessment, 66*, 20–40.

Sánchez, B., Colón, Y., & Esparza, P. (2005). The role of sense of school belonging and gender in the academic adjustment of Latino adolescents. *Journal of Youth and Adolescence, 34*, 619–628.

Snyder, C. R. (1994). *The psychology of hope: You can get there from here.* New York, NY: Free Press.

Snyder, C. R. (2000). The past and possible future of hope. *Journal of Social and Clinical Psychology, 19*, 11–28.

Snyder, C. R. (2002). Hope theory: Rainbows in the mind. *Psychological Inquiry, 13*, 249–275.

Snyder, C. R. (2004). Hope and other strengths. Lesson from Animal Farm. *Journal of Social and Clinical Psychology, 23*, 624–627.

Snyder, C. R., Harris, C., Anderson, J. R., Holleran, S. A., Irving, L. M., Sigmon,…Harney, P. (1991). The will and the ways: Development and validation of an individual-differences measure of hope. *Journal of Personality and Social Psychology, 60*, 570–585.

Townsend, K. C., & McWhirter, B. T. (2005). Connectedness: A review of the literature with implications for counseling, assessment, and research. *Journal of Counseling & Development, 83*, 191–201.

Van Orden, K. A., Witte, T. K., Cukrowicz, K. C., Braithwaite, S. R., Selby, E. A., & Joiner Jr., T. E. (2010). The interpersonal theory of suicide. *Psychological Review, 117*, 575–600.

Visser, P. L., Loess, P., Jeglic, E. L., & Hirsch, J. K. (2013). Hope as a moderator of negative life events and depressive symptoms in a diverse sample. *Stress and Health, 29*, 82–88.

Wilbert, J. R., & Rupert, P. A. (1986). Dysfunctional attitudes, loneliness, and depression in college students. *Cognitive Therapy and Research, 10*, 71–77.

Related Changes in Personal Recovery, Benefit Finding, and Sense of Coherence among People with Chronic Mental Illness: A Two-Wave Study

Rie Chiba, Yoshihiko Yamazaki, Yuki Miyamoto, and Akiko Funakoshi

ABSTRACT

Personal recovery is a process of developing new meaning and purpose in life beyond the catastrophic effects of mental illness. Benefit finding (BF) is conceptualized as finding positive changes or benefits through experiences in adversity. Sense of coherence (SOC) focuses on how people can stay healthy and maintain well-being, even in adversity. This study aimed to examine the relationships among the initial levels and longitudinal changes in personal recovery, BF, and SOC among people with chronic mental illness in Japan. In this longitudinal study, a two-wave self-report questionnaire survey was conducted for service users aged 20 or older with mental illness using convenience sampling method in 2014 and 2015. We applied the Latent Change Score approach. Model fit was evaluated according to the CFI and RMSEA. Among 373 eligible participants at baseline, valid responses in both T1 and T2 from 195 respondents were included in the study (valid response rate = 52.3%). Among them, 65.6% were male, with average age of 45.6. The model of the three constructs at the two time points had good to reasonable fit to the data. The initial levels and changes in personal recovery, BF, and SOC were significantly and positively related to each other.

Introduction

Patient-reported outcome measurements (PROMs) have been widely used in mental health research (Gelkopf et al., 2020), as healthcare has come to respect one's subjective assessment and experiences. PROMs, which focus on person's psychological well-being, reflect a shift from the treatment evaluation in terms of symptom management to resilience in the face of illness. One of the most important aspects of PROMs in mental health is personal recovery, which has become a prominent concept in mental health care worldwide (Ellison et al., 2018; van Weeghel et al., 2019; Wood & Alsawy, 2018). While it is a complicated and multidimensional concept (Ellison et al., 2018; van Weeghel et al., 2019), personal recovery is conceptualized as a complex and subjective process of developing new meaning and purpose in life as people grow beyond the catastrophic effects of mental illness (Anthony, 1993). It includes components such as connectedness, hope and optimism, meaning in life, and empowerment. (Ellison et al.,

2018; Leamy et al., 2011; van Weeghel et al., 2019; Wood & Alsawy, 2018). Recovery-oriented interventions are also varied and are implemented within complex systems (Chester et al., 2016; Le Boutillier et al., 2015; van Weeghel et al., 2019; Winsper et al., 2020).

Given that recovery processes include positive changes, to address them from a positive psychology approach is one way to deepen interpretation and broaden further research on personal recovery (Moran et al., 2014; Moran & Russo-Netzer, 2016). Positive psychology is a branch of scientific psychology that focuses on well-being and positive changes, both within and outside the clinical spectrum of mental illness, rather than dysfunction or symptoms (Snyder et al., 2020; Moran & Russo-Netzer, 2016). Among many concepts contained in positive psychology, "benefit finding" (BF) and "sense of coherence" (SOC) have received considerable attention in research focused on people with chronic illness (Andrykowski et al., 2017; Länsimies et al., 2017; Lechner, 2020; Mittelmark et al., 2016; Stansfeld et al., 2017).

BF is conceptualized as finding positive changes or benefits through negative experiences in adversity, such as chronic illness (Tennen & Affleck, 2002: Lechner, 2020). It has been described as a positive reappraisal coping strategy including a construction of positive meaning-making, which facilitates positive emotions and behaviors among people going through life-changing experiences (Gallagher et al., 2020; Liu et al., 2018). An earlier qualitative study revealed that people with mental illness can realize various types of benefits through their experience of illness (Chiba *et al.* 2010).

SOC originated from the salutogenic (as opposed to pathogenic) approach, which focuses on how people can stay healthy and maintain well-being even in adversity, and has three domains: comprehensibility, manageability, and meaningfulness (Antonovsky, 1987; 1993; Mittelmark et al., 2016). Among several types of coping strategies, SOC has been interpreted as "meaning-based" coping, which can help conceptualize how people cope with and adjust to illness (Harrop et al., 2017; Kvåle & Synnes, 2013). Meaning-based coping has been proposed within the context of increasing evidence that positive psychological states are achievable and important for people with illness (Harrop et al., 2017).

Though these three concepts have parallel perspectives and similarity each other (Barley & Lawson, 2016; Chiba et al., 2011; 2014; Griffiths *et al.* 2009), each has different theoretical background. While all of these concepts comprise "meaning," personal recovery signifies finding meaning in their lives themselves, whereas BF and SOC encompass finding meaning in their experiences of adversity. Besides, personal recovery represents their own process of the long way of lives, while BF and SOC are interpreted as coping to deal with difficulties. BF has also been conceptually distinguished from SOC, which places more emphasis on how people resist adversity (Aspinwall & Tedeschi, 2010).

If one can find meaning in the experience of illness as BF or SOC, it may lead to finding meaning for comprehensive life as personal recovery. However, to date, there are no studies that longitudinally and empirically examine the reciprocal correlations of these concepts. While cross-sectional studies revealed a positive relationship between personal recovery and BF (Chiba et al., 2011; 2014), the causal relationship between these concepts has not been examined yet. Besides, while earlier studies theoretically mentioned that SOC is conductive to personal recovery (Izydorczyk et al., 2019; Witkowska-Łuć, 2018), the relevance of these concepts has not yet been empirically clarified. Similarly, though both BF and SOC are regarded as coping, the factual relationship of these concepts is still unknown.

If the correlations among personal recovery processes, BF, and SOC would be revealed, it could contribute to the further facilitation of personal recovery among people with chronic mental illness, since studies on the mechanism and related factors of BF and SOC have been increasing in recent years (Lechner, 2020; Mittelmark *et al.* 2017). Therefore, this study aimed to examine the relationships among the initial levels and longitudinal changes in personal recovery, BF, and SOC among people with chronic mental illness in Japan. Our main hypothesis in this study was that the initial levels and longitudinal changes in personal recovery, BF, and SOC would be positively correlated with each other.

Methods

Participants

A two-wave self-report questionnaire longitudinal survey was conducted for people with chronic mental illness. The settings were six psychiatric day treatment centers in six hospitals, and sixteen facilities operated by six incorporated nonprofit organizations in the Kanto region of Japan. In this study, we adopted convenience sampling method. The inclusion criteria were as follows: (1) diagnosed with a mental illness by a psychiatrist, (2) 20 years of age and older, (3) living in the community, and (4) a service-user of a facility for people with mental illness. People who diagnosed with developmental disabilities or dementia, as well as who had difficulty in answering the questionnaire in Japanese were excluded.

The baseline survey (T1) was conducted from August to September 2014. Of the 373 eligible people whom the first author contacted, 295 agreed to participate in the study and returned the questionnaire. Among them, 30 responses were excluded due to the missing value on Recovery Assessment Scale (RAS), Benefit Finding Questionnaire (BFQ), or Sense of Coherence Scale (SOC-13) as described later, or having developmental disabilities or dementia turned out later. After all, 265 participants provided valid responses in T1. In the follow-up survey (T2) conducted from August to September 2015, 195 participants out of 265 provided valid responses. 70 participants were excluded, due to the dropout or missing value. The conclusive valid response rate was 52.3% for the initial accessible population (Figure 1).

Measures

Recovery Assessment Scale (RAS)

The RAS is a scale developed in US to assess personal recovery in people with mental illness (Corrigan et al., 1999; 2004). Twenty-four items, such as "I have goals in life that I want to reach" and "I have people I can count on" are rated on a 5-point Likert scale. Higher total scores indicate further progress in personal recovery. Japanese RAS, developed by researchers based on the guideline for the translation and adaptation of

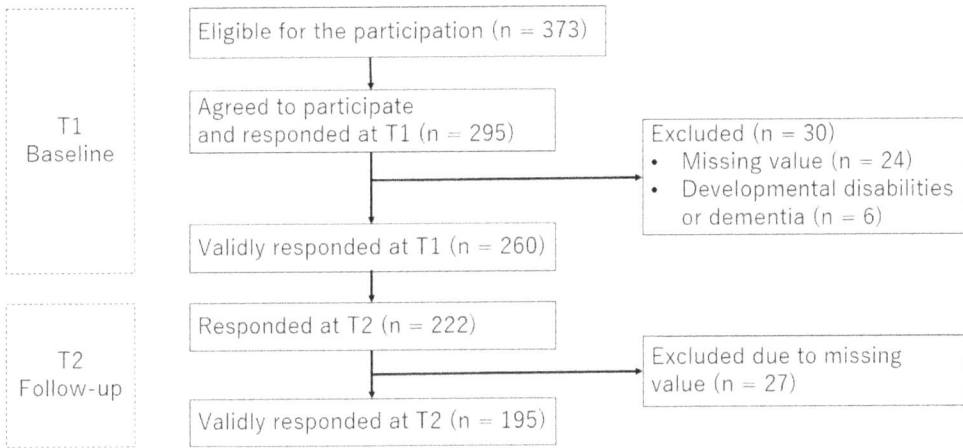

Figure 1. The flowchart of participants selection in this study ($N = 195$).

psychometric scales, showed high overall internal consistency reliability (Cronbach's alpha $= .89$). It also indicated good factorial validity and concurrent validity. Factor analyses of Japanese RAS revealed five factors: goal/success orientation and hope, reliance on others, personal confidence, no domination by symptoms, and willingness to ask for help (CFI $= 0.90$; RMSEA $= 0.06$). (Chiba et al., 2010b). Cronbach's alpha for each factor in the sample in this study ($N = 195$) were .65 to .91.

Benefit Finding Questionnaire (BFQ)

The BFQ is a scale developed by Japanese researchers through adequate process including literature review and focus group interview, to assess BF among people with chronic mental illness (Chiba *et al.* 2020). It comprises 21 items, such as "Trustworthy friends or peers you would not have met if you did not have mental illness have been gained" and "New something to live for or enjoyment in life has been gained," that are rated on a 5-point Likert scale ranging from such as "None" to "A lot." Higher total scores mean greater experiences of BF. It has demonstrated good factorial validity with two factors: changes in sense of values and way of thinking, and changes in relationships with others (CFI $= 0.94$; RMSEA $= 0.055$). Concurrent and divergent validity was also good. Each factor showed reasonable internal consistency reliability (Cronbach's alpha $= .93$ and .81, respectively) (Chiba *et al.* 2020). Cronbach's alphas for each factor in the sample in this study ($N = 195$) were .93 and .81, respectively.

Sense of Coherence Scale (SOC-13)

The SOC-13 is a scale developed in the US to assess SOC (Antonovsky, 1987; 1993). It comprises 13 items, such as "Do you have the feeling that you're being treated unfairly?" and "Do you have the feeling that you are in an unfamiliar situation and don't know what to do?," that are rated on a 5-point Likert scale ranging from such as "1 = Very often" to "7 = Very seldom or never" (Antonovsky, 1987; 1993). This study used the Japanese version of the SOC-13 whose reliability and validity has been confirmed (Cronbach's alpha = .76 to .79; CFI = 0.94; RMSEA = 0.036) (Togari et al., 2008). Cronbach's alpha for total items in the sample in this study ($N = 195$) were .79.

Sociodemographic and clinical data, including age, sex, illness duration, and diagnosis were also obtained in the baseline study.

Statistical Analysis

The analysis began by comparing sociodemographic and clinical characteristics between T1 respondents and T2 respondents, excluding dropouts, using t-tests and Chi-squared tests. Then, we calculated intercorrelations among personal recovery, BF, and SOC at T1 and T2. Subsequently, each score for personal recovery, BF, and SOC was standardized. Next, the study sample was divided into three subgroups: increase, no change, or decrease, by tertile of the degree of changes (T2-T1) in BF and SOC scores. Average RAS scores at T1 and T2 were compared by three subgroups in BF and SOC changes, to better demonstrate how changes in personal recovery were related to changes in BF and SOC.

Next, to examine the relationships among changes in personal recovery, BF and SOC, we applied the Latent Change Score (LCS) approach, using a structural equation model. This method can straightforwardly examine changes as the difference between latent scores from two measurement points. It has been suggested as an explicit method to examine mean changes in scores and predict change over time (Bakic & Ajdukovic, 2019; Henk & Castro-Schilo, 2016; Iimura & Taku, 2018; Takahashi et al. 2013). In this model, the level of a latent construct and the change of it over time are extrapolated, and all latent initial and change factors are allowed to covary (Takahashi et al. 2012). When multiple variables are modeled concurrently, LCS models can function as structural regression models in which the initial level and change in one variable predict the initial level and change in another variable (Schwartz et al., 2020; Takahashi et al. 2012). Figure 2 shows an illustration of the model examined in this study. Latent constructs were identified by the same observed indicators at each time point using parcels as suggested by earlier studies (Bakic & Ajdukovic, 2019; Little et al., 2013; Shimizu & Miho, 2011). Personal recovery was parceled into five RAS factors, and SOC was parceled into its three factors. Since at least three parcels per scale were recommended (Little et al., 2013), BF with two factors was further parceled from each of the two factors into a total of four factors, using methods described in previous studies (Bakic & Ajdukovic, 2019; Shimizu & Miho, 2011). Latent constructs were estimated by constraining the indicator loadings to an average of 1.0 and the indicator intercepts sum to zero for each construct (effects coding) (Bakic & Ajdukovic, 2019). LCSs are generated by setting the regression path between baseline and follow-up equal to 1, entailing that some portion of the follow-up score is equal to the baseline score, and the residual variable is regarded as a change score (McArdle & Nesselroade, 2014). Model fit was evaluated using the comparative fit index (CFI) and root mean square error of approximation (RMSEA). CFI values above 0.90 was considered to be adequate (Hu & Bentler, 1999). RMSEA values below 0.08 indicated an acceptable model fit (Hooper et al., 2008). For structural equation modeling, we used IBM SPSS Amos ver.26. Other statistical analyses, including descriptive analyses, were conducted using IBM

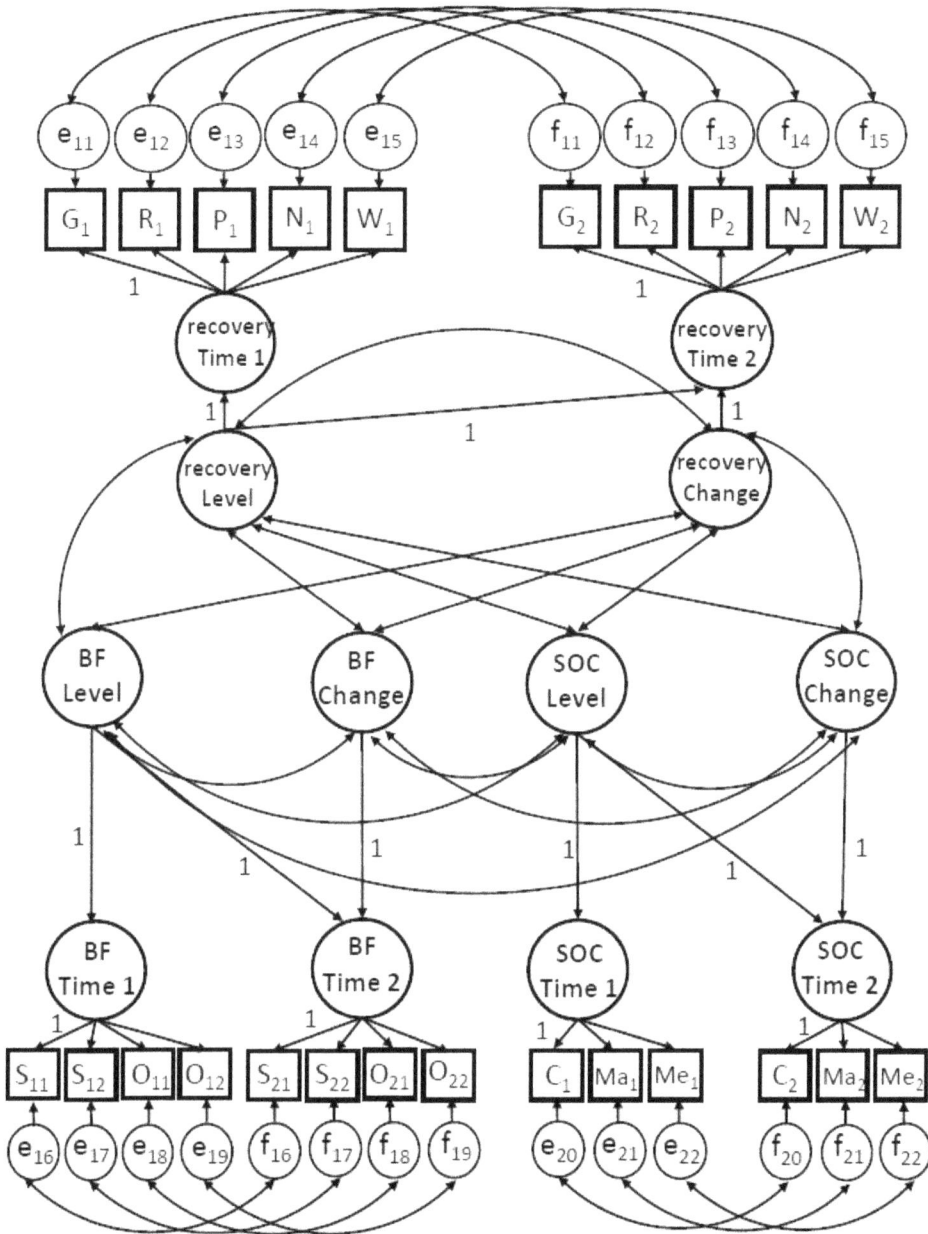

Figure 2. Multiple latent change score model as estimated in this study.

Note

Indicators of each latent variable were measured at two time points (Times 1 and 2). Regression coefficients shown in the figure were fixed at 1, defining the latent variable of VLevel as equal to V at Time 1 and VChange as the difference between V at Time 1 and Time 2. Factor loadings for the indicators of V were restricted to be equal over time.

BF: benefit finding; SOC: sense of coherence

G: Goal/success orientation and hope; R: Reliance on others; P: Personal confidence;

N: No domination by symptoms; W: Willingness to ask for help

S: Changes in one's sense of values and way of thinking; O: Changes in relationships with others

C: Comprehensibility; Ma: Manageability; Me: Meaningfulness

SPSS ver.26. *P* values of less than 0.05 were considered statistically significant (two-tailed tests).

While there are several suggestions about sample size in LCS approach (Zhang & Liu, 2018), there is not solid way to estimate it for a trivariate LCS approach. Thus, based on earlier studies which used LCS model with sample sizes with around 200 to 300 (Shimizu & Miho, 2011; Shimizu et al., 2011), we estimated the required number of samples to be around 200.

Ethical Consideration

This study was approved by the ethical committee of Jichi Medical University (No. EKI 14-27). All participants received oral explanations with written documentation relevant to the purpose and methods. Providing an answer represented their agreement to participate in the study. The survey was conducted anonymously, and ID number was assigned to each questionnaire to link the same respondent in T1 and T2.

Results

Characteristics of Respondents

Descriptive statistics of sociodemographic and clinical variables in this study are presented in the "Time 2" column in Table 1. No significant differences were found between the variables at T1. Although 70 participants dropped out after T1, no evidence was found for systematic dropout. In this study ($N = 195$), 65.6% of respondents were

Table 1. Sample Descriptive Information and Drop-out Analysis.

	Time 1 ($N = 265$)			Time 2 ($N = 195$)			
	M/n	SD	%	M/n	SD	%	t/χ^2 (*p*)
Age (years)	45.3	12.9		45.6	12.5		0.25 (0.80)
Sex (male)	173		65.3	128		65.6	0.01 (0.94)
Duration of the illness (years)	16.1	11.9		16.6	12.1		0.44 (0.66)
Diagnosis							1.36 (0.72)
Schizophrenia	187		70.6	145		74.4	
Depression	24		9.1	17		8.7	
Bipolar disorder	16		6.0	12		6.2	
Others, Unknown	38		14.3	21		10.7	
Coexisting physical illness (yes)	102		38.5	72		36.9	0.12 (0.73)
Experience of hospitalization for psychiatric wards (yes)	201		75.8	159		81.5	2.14 (0.14)
Recipient of Mental disability certificate (yes)	169		36.2	126		64.6	0.03 (0.85)
Recipient of Disability pension (yes)	162		61.1	119		61.0	0.00 (0.98)
Recipient of Livelihood protection (yes)	71		26.8	52		26.7	0.00 (0.94)
Place of living							0.57 (0.45)
Home of one's own or apartment	206		77.7	148		75.9	
Group-home	56		21.1	47		24.1	
Unknown	3		1.1				
Cohabitation (multiple answers allowed)							1.95 (0.74)
With parents	122		46.0	90		46.2	
With siblings	51		19.2	35		17.9	
With a partner	10		3.8	3		1.5	
With children	10		3.8	7		3.6	
Single living	96		36.2	70		35.9	

Table 2. Zero-order Correlation Coefficients of Variables in the Model ($N = 195$).

	1	2	3	4	5	6
1. personal recovery (T1)	1					
2. personal recovery (T2)	.69***	1				
	[.61– 76]					
3. benefit finding (T1)	.83***	.61***	1			
	[.78–.87]	[.51–.69]				
4. benefit finding (T2)	.55***	.84***	.63***	1		
	[.44–.64]	[.79–.88]	[.54–.71]			
5. sense of coherence (T1)	.59***	.38***	.52***	.35***	1	
	[.54–.82]	[.25–.49]	[.41–.62]	[.22–.47]		
6. sense of coherence (T2)	.46***	.49***	.41***	.49***	.64***	1
	[.34–.56]	[.38–.59]	[.29–.52]	[.38–.59]	[.55–.72]	

Note.
T1: baseline (Time 1); T2: follow up (Time 2).
***: $p < 0.001$.
95% confidence intervals are reported in brackets.

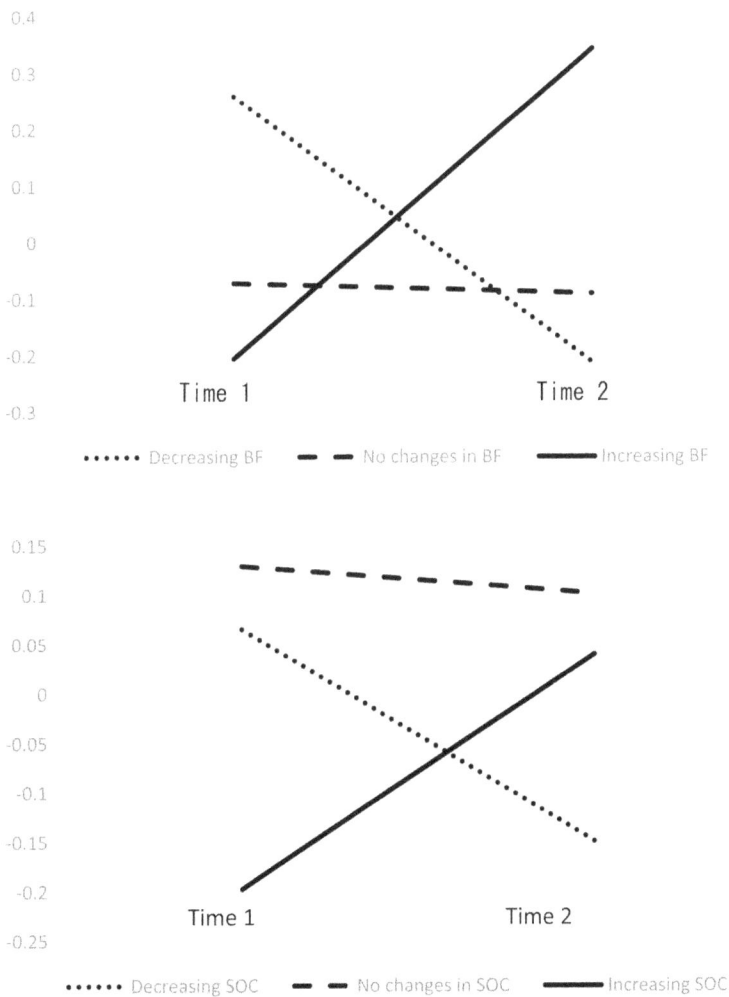

Figure 3. Changes in z scores of latent means of personal recovery ($N = 195$).
Note.
T1: baseline (Time 1); T2: follow up (Time 2)

Table 3. Estimated Correlations and Covariates Between Each Latent Level and Change in Multiple Latent Change Score Model (N = 195).

| | | Levels | | | | | | Changes | | | |
| | | Recovery | | BF | | SOC | | Recovery | | BF | |
		Correlation	covariate	correlation	covariate	correlation	covariate	correlation	covariate	correlation	covariate
Levels	BF	.92*** [.90–.94]	.76***								
	SOC	.61*** [.52–.69]	.39***	.52*** [.41–.62]	.35***						
Changes	Recovery	-.37*** [-.49– -.24]	-.23***	-.32*** [-.44– -.19]	-.20***	-.29*** [-.41– -.16]	-.14**				
	BF	-.38*** [-.49– -.25]	-.27***	-.44*** [-.55– -.32]	-.33***	-.22** [-.35– -.08]	-.13*	.85*** [.81–.89]	.47***		
	SOC	-.14 [-.28– -.00]	-.07	-.09 [-.23–.05]	-.05	-.33*** [-.45– -.20]	-.13*	.45*** [.33–.55]	.16***	.44*** [.32–.55]	.19***

Note.
BF: benefit finding; SOC: sense of coherence.
***: $p < 0.001$;
**: $p < 0.01$;
*: $p < 0.05$.
95% confidence intervals are reported in brackets.

male. Respondents were between the ages of 23 and 76 years ($M = 45.6$, $SD = 12.5$), with an average illness duration 16.6 years ($SD = 12.1$). Additionally, 81.5% of respondents had been previously hospitalized in a psychiatric ward.

Correlations among Personal Recovery, BF, and SOC

Bivariate correlations among personal recovery, BF, and SOC at both T1 and T2 are provided in Table 2. All variables showed significant and positive relationships with all other variables ($p < 0.001$). Figure 3 showed that average RAS score at T1 and T2 changed or continued to be almost flat along with changes in BF and SOC scores.

Relationships among Latent Levels and Changes in Personal Recovery, BF, and SOC in the Multiple LCS Model

The model of the three constructs at the two time points in Figure 2 showed good to reasonabe fit to the data: $\chi^2 = 574.46$, $df = 243$, $p < .001$, CFI $= 0.92$, RMSEA $= 0.08$.

In accordance with the results shown in Table 2, latent levels in personal recovery, BF, and SOC were significantly and positively associated each other (from .52 to .92). Regarding the relationships among levels and changes in personal recovery, BF, and SOC, all correlations were negative (from $-.44$ to $-.09$). This suggested that lower levels of personal recovery, BF, and SOC at T1 were associated with further positive changes in personal recovery, BF, and SOC, while the associations between level of personal recovery and change in SOC, as well as between level of BF and change in SOC were not significant. Regarding the relationships among changes in personal recovery, BF, and SOC, all correlations were significant and positive; change in personal recovery was related to change in BF (.85, $p < .001$), change in personal recovery was associated with change in SOC (.45, $p < .001$); and change in BF was also correlated with change in SOC (.44, $p < .001$) (Table 3).

Discussion

In this study, we examined the relationships among initial levels and changes in personal recovery, BF, and SOC in people with chronic mental illness, using two-wave longitudinal data. The model of the three constructs at the two time points showed good to reasonable fit to the data. The initial levels and changes in personal recovery, BF, and SOC were significantly and positively related to each other, whereas each level of the three constructs showed negative relationships with each change in the three constructs.

Several studies have described that the sense of a meaningful life is one component of personal recovery (Leamy et al., 2011; Weinberg, 2013; van Weeghel et al., 2019). Though the sense of a meaning in the whole life is not the same as meaning-making in adversity, significant relationships between initial levels of personal recovery and BF are consistent with earlier qualitative findings. One could argue that finding meaning in experiences of adversity, such as chronic mental illness, would eventually lead to a perception of more comprehensive meaning in one's own life. Additionally, meaning-making and meaning in life are theoretically connected to SOC, which includes the meaningfulness domain (Kvåle & Synnes, 2013; Winger et al., 2016). Thus, empirically positive relationships among personal recovery, BF, and SOC at baseline in this study are reasonable as hypothesized.

The current study indicated the reciprocal relationships among changes in personal recovery, BF, and SOC. It was also consistent with our hypothesis, while the longitudinal relationships may be more complicated and rounded. For example, personal recovery is sometimes regarded as non-liner process with going forward and backward (Anthony, 1993). It means that, for example, interventions to facilitate BF or SOC may contribute to further progress in personal recovery. Additionally, advances in personal recovery may also facilitate BF or SOC as well. Recently, many interventional studies on BF using such methods as writing, self-disclosure, or stress management techniques have been implemented for people with chronic physical illness and their caregivers (Crawford et al., 2019; Rosenberg et al., 2019; Zhang et al., 2019). Future studies on BF for people with mental illness could be helpful for personal recovery. Similarly, personal recovery may be facilitated through seeking to strengthen SOC and using a salutogenic approach (Bengtsson-Tops & Hansson, 2001; Griffiths, 2009). Recent studies have suggested that SOC can be enhanced through appropriate interventions or as one ages (Arvidsdotter et al., 2015; Heggdal & Lovaas, 2018; Slootjes et al., 2017). It has also been posited that the sense of meaningfulness in SOC among people with mental illness can be facilitated through offering activities with a sufficient level of challenge and by providing a variety of social activities. (Bengtsson-Tops & Hansson, 2001; Griffiths, 2009). Thus, such research for people with mental illness may provide clues to facilitating personal recovery. Furthermore, as an earlier study noted (Chiba et al., 2016), interventions to facilitate personal recovery could also contribute to enhancing BF. Therefore, the findings in this study suggest there can be many approaches to improve personal recovery, BF, and SOC sequentially. Future studies could also focus on more precise mechanisms underlying these changes, including relationships with other associated concepts, such as mental health, quality of life, and resilience (Lansimies *et al.* 2018; Song, 2017).

Notably, each T1 score of personal recovery, BF, and SOC showed negative relationships with each change in these three constructs. As contrasted to it, Rassart et al. (2017) mentioned that trajectories of BF among adolescents with type 1 diabetes in US were differed by baseline level of BF, i.e. low and decreasing, moderate and decreasing, and high and stable. Therefore, the relationship between T1 state and the level of change of these concepts may be influenced by factors such as their types of the illness, the process of the illness, and culture.

The result in this study indicates that people at a lower stage of personal recovery, BF, or SOC may make progress, even without any special interventions. For service providers, to believe the strengths in people with mental illness is important to support their process of personal recovery, even if they seem to be in a stressful and closed world due to the psychiatric symptoms. On the other hand, those who at middle or higher stage of personal recovery, BF, or SOC tend to show unchanged or decreased levels for these constructs. This indicates that maintaining higher levels of personal recovery, BF, and SOC is not necessarily easy. To support such people with mental illness for further personal recovery, coping-focused interventions to meet their aims may be effective, while appropriate involvement may vary depending on the initial level of personal recovery, BF, or SOC.

We need to mention the cultural applicability of the current findings. The mutual relationships among personal recovery, BF, and SOC can be applied to not only Japan, but also to other countries including Western countries, since these concepts are theoretically relevant globally. However, the components of each concept and the actual situations among people are different. For example, hope as the key component of personal recovery are emphasized more in the context of self-cultivation in the Eastern culture, whereas it is expressed more in the context of mastery over events in Western culture (Fukui et al., 2012). Besides, spirituality is not a significant component of BF in Japan, while it is one of the constructs in Western countries (Chiba et al., 2010a). Such differences may affect the process of the development of personal recovery and BF. Moons *et al.* (2020) showed that SOC in Japanese sample was the lowest among fifteen countries including Western countries. Such original characteristics of SOC may impact on the progress of SOC, and reciprocal relationship with personal recovery and BF. Therefore, cultural differences on the relationship of these concepts may be a focus of future research.

Limitations

Some limitations in the present study should be addressed. First, the LCS model we used was restricted to only two measurement points. This means that the model naturally postulates linear changes between these two time points, and that it cannot verify nonlinear changes. Future longitudinal studies with three or more waves would provide further findings on the form and structure of the change process in personal recovery, BF, and SOC, and would enable more detailed consideration. Second, most of the participants in this study were male people with schizophrenia, and community residents who used mental health services. Thus, we cannot infer whether the results in this study can be applied to people with other mental illnesses, hospitalized people or those who do not use mental health services. Besides, the sample size in this study was rather small. Additionally, non-response bias might have occurred, since valid response rate was not high in this study. Therefore, future large-scale study among more participants with various mental illnesses may reveal more elaborate findings. However, despite these limitations, the current study is significant and unique, in that it is the first to reveal the positive relationships among changes in personal recovery, BF, and SOC over time.

Conclusion

In this study, the initial levels and changes in personal recovery, BF, and SOC in people with chronic mental illness were found to be significantly and positively related to each other, whereas each level of the three constructs showed negative relationships with each change. The relationships among changes in these tripartite constructs implies that they can be sequentially facilitated by many approaches.

Acknowledgements

The authors acknowledge the work of Prof. Yuko Nagai (Jichi Medical University) in contributing to data collection for this study.

Disclosure Statement

The authors declare no conflict of interest.

Funding

This study was supported by The Research Grant of Clinical Epidemiology, St Luke's Life Science Institute, as well as Research grant from Faculty of Nursing, Jichi Medical University. And it was also supported by JSPS KAKENHI under Grant Numbers 25862241, 17K17513, 16K12269, 19K11216, and 19K10923.

References

Andrykowski, M. A., Steffens, R. F., Bush, H. M., & Tucker, T. C. (2017). Posttraumatic growth and benefit-finding in lung cancer survivors: The benefit of rural residence? *Journal of Health Psychology*, *22*(7), 896–905. https://doi.org/10.1177/1359105315617820

Anthony, W. A. (1993). Recovery from mental illness: The guiding vision of the mental health service system in the 1990s. *Psychosocial Rehabilitation Journal*, *16*(4), 11–23. https://doi.org/10.1037/h0095655

Antonovsky, A. (1987). *Unravelling the mystery of health: how people manage stress and stay well.* Jossey-Bass.

Antonovsky, A. (1993). The structure and properties of the sense of coherence scale. *Social Science & Medicine (Medicine)*, *36*(6), 725–733. https://doi.org/10.1016/0277-9536(93)90033-z https://doi.org/10.1016/0277-9536(93)90033-Z

Arvidsdotter, T., Marklund, B., Taft, C., & Kylén, S. (2015). Quality of life, sense of coherence and experiences with three different treatments in patients with psychological distress in primary care: A mixed-methods study. *BMC Complementary and Alternative Medicine*, *15*(1), 132https://doi.org/https://doi.org/10.1186/s12906-015-0654-z

Aspinwall, L. G., & Tedeschi, R. G. (2010). The Value of Positive Psychology for Health Psychology: Progress and Pitfalls in Examining the Relation of Positive Phenomena to Health. *Ann Behav Med*, *39*(1), 4–15. https://doi.org/10.1007/s12160-009-9153-0

Bakic, H., & Ajdukovic, D. (2019). Stability and change post-disaster: Dynamic relations between individual, interpersonal and community resources and psychosocial functioning. *European Journal of Psychotraumatology, 10*(1), 1614821 https://doi.org/10.1080/20008198.2019.1614821

Barley, E., & Lawson, V. (2016). Using health psychology to help patients: Promoting wellbeing. *Br J Nurs), 25*(15), 852–855. https://doi.org/10.12968/bjon.2016.25.15.852

Bengtsson-Tops, A., & Hansson, L. (2001). The validity of Antonovsky's Sense of Coherence measure in a sample of schizophrenic patients living in the community. *Journal of Advanced Nursing, 33*(4), 432–438. https://doi.org/10.1046/j.1365-2648.2001.01692.x

Chester, P., Ehrlich, C., Warburton, L., Baker, D., Kendall, E., & Crompton, D. (2016). "What is the work of Recovery Oriented Practice? A systematic literature review". *International Journal of Mental Health Nursing, 25*(4), 270–285. https://doi.org/10.1111/inm.12241

Chiba, R., Funakoshi, A., Yamazaki, Y., & Miyamoto, Y. (2020). The Benefit Finding Questionnaire (BFQ): Scale Development, Validation, and Its Psychometric Properties Among People with Mental Illness. *Healthcare, 8*(3), 303. https://doi.org/10.3390/healthcare8030303

Chiba, R., Kawakami, N., & Miyamoto, Y. (2011). Quantitative relationship between recovery and benefit-finding among persons with chronic mental illness in Japan. *Nursing & Health Sciences, 13*(2), 126–132. https://doi.org/10.1111/j.1442-2018.2011.00589.x

Chiba, R., Miyamoto, Y., & Funakoshi, A. (2010a). Characteristics of Benefit-finding in People with Mental Illness. *Journal of Japan Academy of Nursing Science, 30*(3), 32–40. (in Japanese) https://doi.org/10.5630/jans.30.3_32

Chiba, R., Miyamoto, Y., & Harada, N. (2016). Psychological transformation by an intervention to facilitate benefit finding among people with chronic mental illness in Japan. *Perspectives in Psychiatric Care, 52*(2), 139–144. https://doi.org/10.1111/ppc.12110

Chiba, R., Miyamoto, Y., & Kawakami, N. (2010b). Reliability and validity of the Japanese version of the Recovery Assessment Scale (RAS) for people with chronic mental illness: Scale development. *International Journal of Nursing Studies, 47*(3), 314–322. https://doi.org/10.1016/j.ijnurstu.2009.07.006

Corrigan, P. W., Giffort, D., Rashid, F., Leary, M., & Okeke, I. (1999). Recovery as a psychological construct. *Community Mental Health Journal, 35*(3), 231–239. https://doi.org/10.1023/a:1018741302682

Corrigan, P. W., Salzer, M., Ralph, R. O., Sangster, Y., & Keck, L. (2004). Examining the Factor Structure of the Recovery Assessment Scale. *Schizophrenia Bulletin, 30*(4), 1035–1041. https://doi.org/10.1093/oxfordjournals.schbul.a007118

Crawford, J., Wilhelm, K., & Proudfoot, J. (2019). Web-Based Benefit-Finding Writing for Adults with Type 1 or Type 2 Diabetes: Preliminary Randomized Controlled Trial. *JMIR Diabetes, 4*(2), e13857 https://doi.org/10.2196/13857

Ellison, M. L., Belanger, L. K., Niles, B. L., Evans, L. C., & Bauer, M. S. (2018). Explication and Definition of Mental Health Recovery: A Systematic Review. *Adm Policy Ment Health, 45*(1), 91–102. https://doi.org/10.1007/s10488-016-0767-9

Fukui, S., Shimizu, Y., & Rapp, C. A. (2012). A Cross-cultural Study of Recovery for People with Psychiatric Disabilities Between U.S. and Japan. *Community Mental Health Journal, 48*(6), 804–812. https://doi.org/10.1007/s10597-012-9513-2

Gallagher, S., O'Sullivan, L., Hughes, Z., & O'Connell, B. H. (2020). Building Resources in Caregivers: Feasibility of a Brief Writing Intervention to Increase Benefit Finding in Caregivers. *Applied Psychology. Health and Well-Being, 12*(2), 513–531. https://doi.org/10.1111/aphw.12195

Gelkopf, M., Mazor, Y., & Roe, D. (2020). A systematic review of patient-reported outcome measurement (PROM) and provider assessment in mental health: Goals, implementation, setting, measurement characteristics and barriers. *International Journal for Quality in Health Care.* https://doi.org/10.1093/intqhc/mzz133

Griffiths, C. A. (2009). Sense of coherence and mental health rehabilitation. *Clinical Rehabilitation, 23*(1), 72–78. https://doi.org/10.1177/0269215508095360

Harrop, E., Noble, S., Edwards, M., Sivell, S., Moore, B., & Nelson, A. (2017). Managing, making sense of and finding meaning in advanced illness: A qualitative exploration of the coping and wellbeing experiences of patients with lung cancer. *Sociology of Health & Illness*, *39*(8), 1448–1464. https://doi.org/10.1111/1467-9566.12601

Heggdal, K., & Lovaas, B. J. (2018). Health promotion in specialist and community care: How a broadly applicable health promotion intervention influences patient's sense of coherence. *Scandinavian Journal of Caring Sciences*, *32*(2), 690–697. https://doi.org/10.1111/scs.12498

Henk, C. M., & Castro-Schilo, L. (2016). Preliminary Detection of Relations Among Dynamic Processes With Two-Occasion Data. *Structural Equation Modeling: A Multidisciplinary Journal*, *23*(2), 180–193. https://doi.org/10.1080/10705511.2015.1030022

Hooper, D., Coughlah, J., & Mullen, M. (2008). Structural Equation Modelling: Guidelines for Determining Model Fit. *Electronic Journal of Business Research Methods*, *6*(1), 53–60.

Hu, L., & Bentler, P. M. (1999). Cutoff criteria for fit indexes in covariance structure analysis: Conventional criteria versus new alternatives. *Structural Equation Modeling: A Multidisciplinary Journal*, *6*(1), 1–55. https://doi.org/10.1080/10705519909540118

Iimura, S., & Taku, K. (2018). Positive Developmental Changes after Transition to High School: Is Retrospective Growth Correlated with Measured Changes in Current Status of Personal Growth? *Journal of Youth and Adolescence*, *47*(6), 1192–1207. https://doi.org/10.1007/s10964-018-0816-7

Izydorczyk, B., Sitnik-Warchulska, K., Kühn-Dymecka, A., & Lizińczyk, S. (2019). Resilience, Sense of Coherence, and Coping with Stress as Predictors of Psychological Well-Being in the Course of Schizophrenia. The Study Design. *International Journal of Environmental Research and Public Health*, *16*(7), 1266. https://doi.org/10.3390/ijerph16071266

Kvåle, K., & Synnes, O. (2013). Understanding cancer patients' reflections on good nursing care in light of Antonovsky's theory. *European Journal of Oncology Nursing : The Official Journal of European Oncology Nursing Society*, *17*(6), 814–819. https://doi.org/10.1016/j.ejon.2013.07.003

Länsimies, H., Pietilä, A.-M., Hietasola-Husu, S., & Kangasniemi, M. (2017). A systematic review of adolescents' sense of coherence and health. *Scandinavian Journal of Caring Sciences*, *31*(4), 651–661. https://doi.org/10.1111/scs.12402

Le Boutillier, C., Chevalier, A., Lawrence, V., Leamy, M., Bird, V. J., Macpherson, R., Williams, J., & Slade, M. (2015). Staff understanding of recovery-orientated mental health practice: A systematic review and narrative synthesis. *Implementation Science*, *10*(1), 87. https://doi.org/10.1186/s13012-015-0275-4

Leamy, M., Bird, V., Boutillier, C. L., Williams, J., & Slade, M. (2011). Conceptual framework for personal recovery in mental health: Systematic review and narrative synthesis. *The British Journal of Psychiatry : The Journal of Mental Science*, *199*(6), 445–452. https://doi.org/10.1192/bjp.bp.110.083733

Lechner, S. C. (2020). Benefit-Finding. In Snyder, C.R., Lopez, S.J., Edwards, L.M.,. (Eds.): *The Oxford Handbook of Positive Psychology*. (3rd ed.). 907–918. Oxford University Press.

Little, T. D., Rhemtulla, M., Gibson, K., & Schoemann, A. M. (2013). Why the items versus parcels controversy needn't be one. *Psychological Methods*, *18*(3), 285–300. https://doi.org/10.1037/a0033266

Liu, Z., Zhang, L., Cao, Y., Xia, W., & Zhang, L. (2018). The relationship between coping styles and benefit finding of Chinese cancer patients: The mediating role of distress. *European Journal of Oncology Nursing : The Official Journal of European Oncology Nursing Society*, *34*, 15–20. https://doi.org/10.1016/j.ejon.2018.03.001

McArdle, J. J., & Nesselroade, J. R. (2014). *Longitudinal Data Analysis Using Structural Equation Models*. American Psychological Association.

Mittelmark, M. B., Sagy, S., Eriksson, M., Bauer, G. F., Pelikan, J. M., Lindström, B., & Espnes, G. A. (2017). *The Handbook of Salutogenesis*. (1st ed. 2017 ed.). Springer.

Moons, P., Apers, S., Kovacs, A. H., Thomet, C., Budts, W., Enomoto, J., Sluman, M. A., Wang, J.-K., Jackson, J. L., Khairy, P., Cook, S. C., Chidambarathanu, S., Alday, L., Oechslin, E., Eriksen, K., Dellborg, M., Berghammer, M., Johansson, B., Mackie, A. S., … Luyckx, K. (2020). Sense of coherence in adults with congenital heart disease in 15 countries: Patient characteristics, cultural dimensions and quality of life. *European Journal of Cardiovascular Nursing*, 147451512093049. https://doi.org/10.1177/1474515120930496

Moran, G. S., Russinova, Z., Yim, J. Y., & Sprague, C. (2014). Motivations of Persons with Psychiatric Disabilities to Work in Mental Health Peer Services: A Qualitative Study Using Self-Determination Theory. *Journal of Occupational Rehabilitation*, 24(1), 32–41. https://doi.org/10.1007/s10926-013-9440-2

Moran, G., & Russo-Netzer, P. (2016). Understanding universal elements in mental health recovery: A cross-examination of peer providers and a non-clinical sample. *Qualitative Health Research*, 26(2), 273–287. https://doi.org/10.1177/1049732315570124

Rassart, J., Luyckx, K., Berg, C. A., Oris, L., & Wiebe, D. J. (2017). Longitudinal trajectories of benefit finding in adolescents with Type 1 diabetes. *Health Psychology : official Journal of the Division of Health Psychology, American Psychological Association*, 36(10), 977–986. https://doi.org/10.1037/hea0000513

Rosenberg, A. R., Bradford, M. C., Barton, K. S., Etsekson, N., McCauley, E., Curtis, J. R., Wolfe, J., Baker, K. S., & Yi-Frazier, J. P. (2019). Hope and benefit finding: Results from the PRISM randomized controlled trial. *Pediatric Blood & Cancer*, 66(1), e27485 https://doi.org/10.1002/pbc.27485

Schwartz, E., Ayalon, L., & Huxhold, O. (2020). Exploring the Reciprocal Associations of Perceptions of Aging and Social Involvement. *The Journals of Gerontology: Series B*, https://doi.org/10.1093/geronb/gbaa008

Shimizu, K., & Miho, N. (2011). Modeling for change by latent difference score model: Adapting process of the student of freshman at half year intervals. *Bulletin of the Faculty of Sociology, Kansai University*, 42(3), 1–28.

Shimizu, K., Miho, N., Konda, H., Hanai, Y., & Yamamoto, R. (2011). Modeling of psychological change: Latent Difference Score Model for three wave longitudinal data. *Kansai University Psychological Research*, 2, 19–28.

Slootjes, J., Keuzenkamp, S., & Saharso, S. (2017). The mechanisms behind the formation of a strong Sense of Coherence (SOC): The role of migration and integration. *Scand J Psychol*, 58(6), 571–580. https://doi.org/10.1111/sjop.12400

Snyder, C. R., Lopez, S. J., Edwards, L. M., & Marques, S. C. (2020). *The Oxford Handbook of Positive Psychology (OXFORD LIBRARY OF PSYCHOLOGY SERIES)*. (3rd ed.). Oxford University Press.

Song, L. (2017). Predictors of personal recovery for persons with psychiatric disabilities: An examination of the Unity Model of Recovery. *Psychiatry Research*, 250, 185–192. https://doi.org/10.1016/j.psychres.2017.01.088

Stansfeld, J., Stoner, C. R., Wenborn, J., Vernooij-Dassen, M., Moniz-Cook, E., & Orrell, M. (2017). Positive psychology outcome measures for family caregivers of people living with dementia: A systematic review. *International Psychogeriatrics*, 29(8), 1281–1296. https://doi.org/10.1017/S1041610217000655

Takahashi, Y., Edmonds, G. W., Jackson, J. J., & Roberts, B. W. (2013). Longitudinal Correlated Changes in Conscientiousness, Preventative Health-Related Behaviors, and Self-Perceived Physical Health. *Journal of Personality*, 81(4), 417–427. https://doi.org/10.1111/jopy.12007

Tennen, H., & Affleck, G. (2002). Benefit-finding and benefit-reminding. In C. R. Snyder, & S. J. Lopez (Ed.), *Handbook of Positive Psychology*. (pp. 584–597). Oxford University Press.

Togari, T., Yamazaki, Y., Nakayama, K., Yamaki, C., & Takayama, T. (2008). Construct validity of Antonovsky's sense of coherence scale: Stability of factor structure and predictive validity with regard to the well-being of Japanese undergraduate students from two-year follow-up data. *Japanese Journal of Health and Human Ecology*, 74(2), 71–86. https://doi.org/10.3861/jshhe.74.71

van Weeghel, J., van Zelst, C., Boertien, D., & Hasson-Ohayon, I. (2019). Conceptualizations, assessments, and implications of personal recovery in mental illness: A scoping review of systematic reviews and meta-analyses. *Psychiatric Rehabilitation Journal*, 42(2), 169–181. https://doi.org/10.1037/prj0000356

Weinberg, C. M. (2013). Hope, meaning, and purpose: Making recovery possible. *Psychiatric Rehabilitation Journal*, 36(2), 124–125. https://doi.org/10.1037/prj0000011

Winger, J. G., Adams, R. N., & Mosher, C. E. (2016). Relations of meaning in life and sense of coherence to distress in cancer patients: A meta-analysis. *Psycho-Oncology, 25*(1), 2–10. https://doi.org/10.1002/pon.3798

Winsper, C., Crawford-Docherty, A., Weich, S., Fenton, S.-J., & Singh, S. P. (2020). How do recovery-oriented interventions contribute to personal mental health recovery? A systematic review and logic model. *Clinical Psychology Review, 76*, 101815. https://doi.org/10.1016/j.cpr.2020.101815

Witkowska-Łuć, B. Ł. (2018). Schizophrenia and sense of coherence. *Psychiatria Polska, 52*(2), 217–226. https://doi.org/10.12740/PP/OnlineFirst/69697

Wood, L., & Alsawy, S. (2018). Recovery in psychosis from a service user perspective: A systematic review and thematic synthesis of current qualitative evidence. *Community Ment Health J, 54*(6), 793–804. https://doi.org/10.1007/s10597-017-0185-9

Zhang, Z., & Liu, H. (2018). Sample size and measurement occasion planning for Latent Change Score Models through Monte Carlo Simulation 1. In E. Ferrer, M. S. Boker, & J. K. Grimm (Ed.), *Longitudinal Multivariate Psychology (Multivariate Applications Series)*. (1st ed.). Routledge.

Zhang, M. M., Yang, Y. J., Su, D., Zhang, T., Jiang, X. X., & Li, H. P. (2019). A randomized controlled trial of a guided self-disclosure intervention to facilitate benefit finding in Chinese breast cancer patients: Study protocol. *Journal of Advanced Nursing, 75*, 1805–1814. https://doi.org/10.1111/jan.14042

Index

For Product Safety Concerns and Information please contact our EU
representative GPSR@taylorandfrancis.com
Taylor & Francis Verlag GmbH, Kaufingerstraße 24, 80331 München, Germany